The 2003 Year Book Series

Year Book of **Allergy, Asthma, and Clinical Immunology**™: Drs Rosenwasser, Boguniewicz, Milgrom, Routes, and Spahn

Year Book of **Anesthesiology and Pain Management**™: Drs Chestnut, Abram, Black, Lang, Roizen, Trankina, and Wood

Year Book of **Cardiology**®: Drs Gersh, Graham, Kaplan, and Waldo

Year Book of **Critical Care Medicine**®: Drs Dellinger, Parrillo, Balk, Bekes, Roberts, and Dries

Year Book of **Dentistry**®: Drs Zakariasen, Boghosian, Dederich, Hatcher, Horswell, and McIntyre

Year Book of **Dermatology and Dermatologic Surgery**™: Drs Thiers and Lang

Year Book of **Diagnostic Radiology**®: Drs Osborn, Birdwell, Dalinka, Groskin, Maynard, Oestreich, Pentecost, and Ros

Year Book of **Emergency Medicine**®: Drs Burdick, Cone, Cydulka, Hamilton, Kassutto, and Niemann

Year Book of **Endocrinology**®: Drs Mazzaferri, Becker, Kannan, Kennedy, Kreisberg, Meikle, Molitch, Osei, Poehlman, and Rogol

Year Book of **Family Practice**®: Drs Bowman, Apgar, Dexter, Gilchrist, Neill, and Scherger

Year Book of **Gastroenterology**™: Drs Lichtenstein, Dempsey, Ginsberg, Katzka, Kochman, Morris, Nunes, Rosato, and Stein

Year Book of **Hand Surgery**®: Drs Berger and Ladd

Year Book of **Medicine**®: Drs Barkin, Frishman, Klahr, Loehrer, Mazzaferri, Phillips, and Pillinger

Year Book of **Neonatal and Perinatal Medicine**®: Drs Fanaroff, Maisels, and Stevenson

Year Book of **Neurology and Neurosurgery**®: Drs Bradley, Gibbs, and Verma

Year Book of **Nuclear Medicine**®: Drs Gottschalk, Blaufox, Coleman, Strauss, and Zubal

Year Book of **Obstetrics, Gynecology, and Women's Health**®: Drs Mishell, Kirschbaum, and Miller

Year Book of **Oncology**®: Drs Loehrer, Arceci, Glatstein, Gordon, Johnson, Morrow, and Thigpen

Year Book of **Ophthalmology**®: Drs Rapuano, Cohen, Eagle, Grossman, Myers, Nelson, Penne, Regillo, Sergott, Shields, and Tipperman

Year Book of **Orthopedics**®: Drs Morrey, Beauchamp, Peterson, Swiontkowski, Trigg, and Yaszemski

Year Book of **Otolaryngology-Head and Neck Surgery**®: Drs Paparella, Keefe, and Otto

YEAR BO
NUCLEAR MEDI

2003

The Year Book of NUCLEAR MEDICINE®

Editor-in-Chief
Alexander Gottschalk, MD

Associate Editors
M. Donald Blaufox, MD, PhD
R. Edward Coleman, MD
H. William Strauss, MD
I. George Zubal, PhD

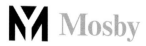 Mosby

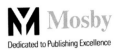
Dedicated to Publishing Excellence

Vice President, Continuity Publishing: Glen P. Campbell
Developmental Editor: Beth Martz
Senior Manager, Continuity Production: Idelle L. Winer
Issue Manager: Donna M. Skelton
Composition Specialist: Betty Dockins
Illustrations and Permissions Coordinator: Kimberly E. Hulett

2003 EDITION

Printed in the United States of America
Composition by Thomas Technology Solutions, Inc.
Printing/binding by Sheridan Books, Inc.

Editorial Office:
Elsevier
The Curtis Center
Suite 300
Independence Square West
Philadelphia, PA 19106-3399

International Standard Serial Number: 0084-3903
International Standard Book Number: 0-323-02072-0

Editorial Board

Table of Contents

Journals Represented

Mosby and its editors survey approximately 500 journals for its abstract and commentary publications. From these journals, the editors select the articles to be abstracted. Journals represented in this YEAR BOOK are listed below.

Acta Neurologica Scandinavica
Acta Paediatrica
Acta Radiologica
American Journal of Cardiology
American Journal of Gastroenterology
American Journal of Medicine
American Journal of Neuroradiology
American Journal of Psychiatry
American Journal of Roentgenology
Annals of Emergency Medicine
Annals of Neurology
Annals of Surgery
Annals of Surgical Oncology
Annals of Thoracic Surgery
Brain
British Journal of Cancer
British Journal of Radiology
British Journal of Surgery
Cancer
Cancer Research
Chest
Circulation
Clinical Cancer Research
Clinical Endocrinology (Oxford)
Clinical Nuclear Medicine
Clinical Radiology
Diabetes Care
Epilepsia
European Heart Journal
European Journal of Nuclear Medicine
European Journal of Surgery
Foot & Ankle International
Gastrointestinal Endoscopy
Gynecologic Oncology
Head and Neck
Heart
Hypertension
Journal of Bone and Joint Surgery (American Volume)
Journal of Clinical Endocrinology and Metabolism
Journal of Clinical Oncology
Journal of Computer Assisted Tomography
Journal of Neurosurgery
Journal of Nuclear Cardiology
Journal of Nuclear Medicine
Journal of Pediatric Orthopaedics
Journal of Rheumatology
Journal of Thoracic and Cardiovascular Surgery

Journal of the American College of Cardiology
Journal of the American Medical Association
Medical Physics
Nephrology, Dialysis, Transplantation
Neurology
Neuroradiology
Neurosurgery
Otolaryngology-Head and Neck Surgery
Radiology
Surgery
Thyroid
Urology
World Journal of Surgery

STANDARD ABBREVIATIONS

The following terms are abbreviated in this edition: acquired immunodeficiency syndrome (AIDS), cardiopulmonary resuscitation (CPR), central nervous system (CNS), cerebrospinal fluid (CSF), computed tomography (CT), deoxyribonucleic acid (DNA), electrocardiography (ECG), [fluorine-18]-fluorodeoxyglucose (FDG), gadolinium-diethylenetriamine-pentaacetic acid (Gd-DTPA), health maintenance organization (HMO), human immunodeficiency virus (HIV), intensive care unit (ICU), intramuscular (IM), intravenous (IV), magnetic resonance (MR) imaging (MRI), nuclear magnetic resonance (NMR), positron emission tomography (PET), ribonucleic acid (RNA), single-photon emission CT (SPECT), ultrasound (US), and ultraviolet (UV).

NOTE

The YEAR BOOK OF NUCLEAR MEDICINE is a literature survey service providing abstracts of articles published in the professional literature. Every effort is made to assure the accuracy of the information presented in these pages. Neither the editors nor the publisher of the YEAR BOOK OF NUCLEAR MEDICINE can be responsible for errors in the original materials. The editors' comments are their own opinions. Mention of specific products within this publication does not constitute endorsement.

To facilitate the use of the YEAR BOOK OF NUCLEAR MEDICINE as a reference tool, all illustrations and tables included in this publication are now identified as they appear in the original article. This change is meant to help the reader recognize that any illustration or table appearing in the YEAR BOOK OF NUCLEAR MEDICINE may be only one of many in the original article. For this reason, figure and table numbers will often appear to be out of sequence within the YEAR BOOK OF NUCLEAR MEDICINE.

Introduction

And Now Good-Bye

Both James L. Quinn and Paul B. Hoffer, my predecessors as Editor-in-Chief of this YEAR BOOK, retired for health reasons. My health is as good as one can expect for a septuagenarian. My main reason for retiring as editor-in-chief was well articulated by Yogi Berra when he said, "It's déjà vu all over again." I believe Yogi's comment was made during the year both Roger Marris and Mickey Mantle were hitting home runs at an alarming rate—more than 110 between them for the season. After one impressive blast from one of these sluggers, Yogi turned to his dugout teammates and articulated this now classic sentence. I have been working on this YEAR BOOK for 23 years and have selected more than 1600 articles for inclusion. That likely means I have reviewed some 4 to 5 times that many. Recently I have had the disturbing reaction articulated by Yogi. In particular it has bothered me most of this past year. I cannot help but feeling every time I write a comment that I have said it somewhere before in one of our earlier volumes. I believe that any YEAR BOOK editor should have constructive biases, but I now believe you know all of mine and when I restate them "it's déjà vu all over again."

Just to cite a few examples, I have consistently reminded you when I select articles that compare one modality to another that it is only fair if state-of-the-art equipment comparisons are made. Similarly, it is only fair when state-of-the-art technique comparisons are made. For example, it is not fair to point out that brain nuclear medicine perfusion studies may find more abnormality than standard MRI studies. I would argue that if you want to compare brain perfusion studies to MRI you should include MRI perfusion studies as well. There is an article in this YEAR BOOK that does just that.

I also get annoyed when I am never given enough "housekeeping" details to figure out how a technique was performed or an image was made. When this happens, I cannot tell whether the data—in which I may find some shortcoming—is a little substandard because the technique was bad or because the concept was bad.

I firmly believe that it is important for professionals in nuclear medicine to be up to date on all of the diseases we can diagnose and techniques that nuclear medicine can perform even if some of these are not clinically relevant for the moment. For example, you may have read my comments on many occasions about our ability to diagnose Parkinson's disease at an early stage ending with a comment like "know about this now because when Parkinson's disease becomes treatable, patients will be lined up around the block to get into your nuclear medicine center."

I have been pushing fusion between tracer slices and other cross sectional techniques for years. I am convinced that if you do not believe this is a good idea, there is likely no hope for you. There is now little doubt that we should get on the PET bandwagon. And finally, I believe it is imperative that we practice quality nuclear medicine. Turf wars are commonplace these days. If your examination is not optimum, or if you are only available for 4 hours a day during the yachting season, there seems to be little chance that nuclear medicine will win in your shop against a dedicated competitor trying to introduce or takeover your modality. If you read this volume, you will recognize that I have written all of the above ideas, and others, in some form or another for some time.

For more than two decades I have been amazed that I have never received any real hate mail. You might think that someone writing comments about articles that were not always couched in glowing terms would get serious missiles back from the authors. Surprisingly, this has not been the case. On rare occasions, an author would tell me I had misinterpreted his or her data, but I can count those instances on the fingers of one hand, and I will admit that in the cases I can remember at this time, I believe the authors were correct. I never tried to be mean, although I often tried to be constructive. I recognize that mean and constructive can get very close together on occasion, but the lack of disgruntled feedback leads me to believe I succeeded in this effort more often than I failed.

Somewhere in my contract with the publishers it says that I am responsible for "riding herd on" my associate editors, and being sure that they do their work on time, in appropriate fashion, and with pizzazz, etc. This has been the easiest part of my job. In fact, it has required no work at all. There is a simple trick to this—get real professionals and just leave them alone to do their thing. It has been a great pleasure in my years as editor-in-chief to have worked with John G. McAffee, Barry L. Zaret, Frans J. T. Wackers, Ronald D. Neumann, H. William Strauss, and R. Edward Coleman. Special thanks go to I. George Zubal and M. Donald Blaufox who have been with me my entire tenure as editor-in-chief. They deserve some type of tenacity award with oak leaf clusters. With this group of consummate pros, it is easy to see why I never had a problem with their contributions. I believe sincerely that the bulk of the success this volume has enjoyed over the years is due to their efforts.

Finally, I usually tried to select articles that provide information the practicing nuclear medicine physician could use. In the past few years, however, I have altered this approach somewhat to try to select more articles at the leading edge of our specialty. I think the new emphasis the Society of Nuclear Medicine puts on molecular imaging is entirely appropriate. I believe we begin an era when proteinomics and genomics (and other "-omics") should provide us with an array of tracers unlike any we have had before. It is probably time for the YEAR BOOK OF NUCLEAR MEDICINE to switch its emphasis from providing articles indicating better ways to do what you know how to do, to providing a framework for you to assimilate leading-edge knowledge to help you better understand this new molecular era.

It has been a good run. I have enjoyed it. I hope that all of you who have looked through the pages of this volume at some time or other in the past 23 years have found it useful.

Alexander Gottschalk, MD

1 Pulmonary

Introduction

This chapter starts with several articles using PET for the diagnosis of pulmonary nodules and related problems. This year, this topic has replaced pulmonary embolism as the major focus of the pulmonary section. Tumor detection with single photon tracers follows. Pulmonary embolism is not omitted, and articles about MAA perfusion scanning have been selected. The section ends with the uses of Xe-133 to diagnose an air leak.

Alexander Gottschalk, MD

Accuracy of F-18 Fluorodeoxyglucose Positron Emission Tomography for the Evaluation of Malignancy in Patients Presenting With New Lung Abnormalities: A Retrospective Review

Lee J, Aronchick JM, Alavi A (Univ of Pennsylvania, Philadelphia)
Chest 120:1791-1797, 2001   1–1

Background.—The role of PET with FDG for patients with lung cancer has not been fully defined. The accuracy of this modality in determining the presence of malignancy in patients with new lung findings was further investigated.

Methods.—One hundred ninety-six patients referred for the evaluation of new lung findings between 1997 and 1999—either as an incidental finding or after definitive treatment of a primary carcinoma—were identified in the PET database at the authors' center. For 71 patients, the diagnosis of a malignant or benign condition was established by histopathology from biopsy or subsequent imaging showing disease progression, resolution, or stability of initial findings.

Findings.—For the 37 patients with new lung findings but no history of carcinoma, PET had a sensitivity of 95% and a specificity of 82%. In this group, the negative predictive value was 93% and the positive predictive value was 86%. The sensitivity and specificity of PET were lower for assessing metastatic or recurrent disease in patients previously treated for carcinoma. In the 13 patients with previously treated primary lung cancer, PET had a sensitivity and specificity of 70% and 67%, respectively. Its negative and positive predictive values were 40% and 88%, respectively, in this subgroup. Among 21 patients with an extrapulmonary primary carcinoma with

1

new lung nodules, PET's sensitivity was 92% and its specificity was 63%. Its positive and negative predictive values in this setting were 80% and 83%, respectively. Overall, PET had an 88% sensitivity, a 75% specificity, an 81% negative predictive value, and an 84% positive predictive value.

Conclusion.—The sensitivity of PET appears to be best for assessing new malignancy in patients without a known primary carcinoma. This modality is less sensitive for evaluating metastatic or recurrent disease.

▶ In an article like this one, I have come to expect the PET data to unfold like a bouquet of roses. This bouquet has some dandelions in it. The authors suggest we could learn to love the dandelions if they were presented with dual time point FDG-PET imaging. I hope they are right—the sooner they tell us, the better.
(Read on please).

A. Gottschalk, MD

Dual Time Point ^{18}F-FDG PET for the Evaluation of Pulmonary Nodules
Matthies A, Hickeson M, Cuchiara A, et al (Univ of Pennsylvania, Philadelphia)
J Nucl Med 43:871-875, 2002   1–2

Objective.—^{18}F-FDG PET is now widely used for diagnostic assessment of pulmonary nodules. Although higher standardized uptake values (SUVs) are generally associated with malignancy, there is still significant overlap between benign and malignant lesions. Dual time point ^{18}F-FDG PET imaging was compared with conventional ^{18}F-FDG PET for distinguishing between benign and malignant pulmonary nodules.

Methods.—Two sequential PET scans were performed in 36 patients with known or suspected malignant pulmonary nodules: an initial whole-body scan followed by a second scan of the chest. The patients were 21 women and 15 men with a mean age of 67 years; a total of 38 pulmonary nodules were evaluated. The first scan was performed 70 minutes after IV injection of ^{18}F-FDG, 2.5 MBq/kg, and the second scan after 123 minutes. A dedicated C-PET scanner was used for all scans; the first and second scans were performed a mean of 56 minutes apart. For each corrected image, regions of interest were overlaid in areas of radiographically detected lung densities. Standardized uptake values for the first and second scans were calculated and compared.

Results.—Pathologic examination and clinical followup showed a total of 20 malignant tumors in 19 patients; the remaining 16 patients had benign nodules. Mean tumor SUV increased from 3.66 on the first scan to 4.43 on the second scan. Twenty percent of the malignant tumors showed initial SUVs of less than 2.5 (Fig 1). The benign lesions had similarly low SUVs on both the first and second scans: 1.14 and 1.11, respectively. Sensitivity increased from 80% with standard PET at an SUV threshold of 2.5 to 100% with dual time point scanning. Specificity values were 94% and 89%, respectively.

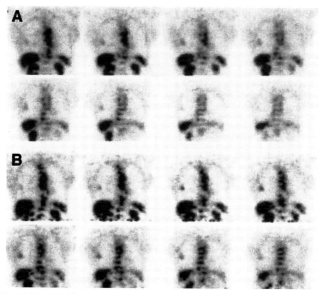

FIGURE 1.—A 72-year-old woman presented with right lower lobe nodule measuring 1.8 × 1.0 cm. SUV increased from 1.45 on scan 1 at 65 minutes after injection (**A**) to 1.72 on scan 2 at 123 minutes after injection (**B**). Biopsy of the lesion revealed moderately differentiated adenocarcinoma. (Reprinted by permission of the Society of Nuclear Medicine from Matthies A, Hickeson M, Cuchiara A, et al: Dual time point ^{18}F-FDG PET for the evaluation of pulmonary nodules. *J Nucl Med* 43:871-875, 2002.

Conclusions.—For patients with pulmonary nodules, dual time point ^{18}F-FDG PET may improve the diagnostic assessment of malignant versus benign lesions, compared with conventional ^{18}F-FDG PET. The dual time point protocol is simple and readily applicable in clinical practice. However, more study in larger samples is needed to confirm the results.

▶ OK. So they did not exactly tell us. They used a different type of patient. But the results clearly seem improved by the dual time point technique. The authors admit that the patient series is small and lacking in both tough true positive histology (bronchoalveolar carcinoma) and the expected false-positives from some granulomas. So be encouraged, but await a bigger series.

A. Gottschalk, MD

Two Incorrect FDG Positron Emission Tomographic Interpretations of a Pulmonary Mass and Mediastinal Lymphadenopathy
Kao C-H, Tsai S-C, Hung G-U (China Med College, Taichung, Taiwan; Show-Chwan Mem Hosp, Chunghua, Taiwan; Taichung Veterans Gen Hosp, Taiwan)
Clin Nucl Med 26:1049-1050, 2001   1–3

Introduction.—FDG PET can be used to assess pulmonary masses. A patient with 2 distinct misleading results on FDG-PET scanning of a pulmonary mass was reported.

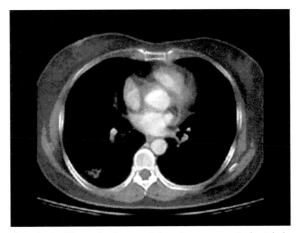

FIGURE 1.—A routine health examination revealed a pulmonary mass in the right lower lobe of a 50-year-old woman. CT of the chest showed a consolidative mass that measured approximately 2.5 cm in the greatest dimension in the posterior aspect of the right lower lobe. In addition, multiple areas of lymphadenopathy involving the para-aortic, subaortic, and subcarinal regions of the mediastinum are shown. (Courtesy of Kao C-H, Tsai S-C, Hung G-U: Two incorrect FDG positron emission tomographic interpretations of a pulmonary mass and mediastinal lymphadenopathy. *Clin Nucl Med* 26(12):1049-1050, 2001.)

Case Report.—Woman, 50, had an incidentally detected pulmonary mass of the right lower lung field associated with mediastinal lymphadenopathy (Fig 1). Whole-body FDG PET showed increased tracer uptake—standardized uptake value greater than 2.5—in the mediastinal lymphadenopathy, suggesting a malignant lesion. However, pathologic examination of a surgical specimen showed only benign anthracosis. In contrast, the right lower lung mass—which had a standardized uptake value of 1.69—proved to be a moderately differentiated adenocarcinoma (Fig 2).

Discussion.—In these scans, an area of elevated tracer uptake represents a benign process, whereas a mass with low uptake proves to be an adenocarcinoma.

▶ We cannot win them all. But common sense often wins out when the numbers fail. If the PET makes you believe the mediastinal nodes are malignant and you have an associated speculated lung lesion with a benign standard uptake value, I doubt if too many of us would stop short of suggesting another test (eg, biopsy) to assess the lung histology.

A. Gottschalk, MD

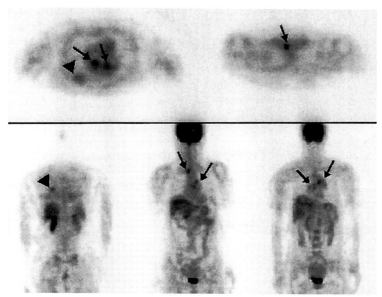

FIGURE 2.—The patient underwent whole-body FDG PET for further evaluation. The mass in the posterior right lower lobe (*arrowhead*) showed mildly increased tracer uptake (standard uptake value, 1.69), which indicated a benign process (eg, nonspecific inflammation). In addition, multiple foci (*arrows*) of intense FDG uptake were visible in the mediastinum and were thought to be associated with a malignant process, in which the standard uptake values were 2.82 when measured in the right paratracheal region and 2.56 when measured in the subcarinal region. Because adenocarcinoma was found on cytologic analysis performed after bronchial brushing, the patient had a right lower radical lobectomy with extended lymph node dissection. Pathologic examination showed that the mass in the posterior right lower lobe was a moderately differentiated adenocarcinoma. However, no malignant cells were found in all of the 10 groups of lymph nodes, with only anthracosis seen in parts of them. (Courtesy of Kao C-H, Tsai S-C, Hung G-U: Two incorrect FDG positron emission tomographic interpretations of a pulmonary mass and mediastinal lymphadenopathy. *Clin Nucl Med* 26(12):1049-1050, 2001.)

FDG-PET as a "Metabolic Biopsy" Tool in Non-Lung Lesions With Indeterminate Biopsy

Beggs AD, Hain SF, Curran KM, et al (Guy's Kings and St Thomas' School of Medicine, London)
Eur J Nucl Med 29:542-546, 2002   1–4

Introduction.—Histologic verification of anatomic abnormalities observed on imaging is usually a prerequisite for optimum management. Yet, there are many circumstances in which this is not always possible. It is often difficult for the clinician to decide how hard to pursue a histologic diagnosis. FDG-PET scanning has demonstrated its usefulness as a "metabolic biopsy" in lung lesions. It is not known whether it can be used as a metabolic biopsy tool in imaging lesions outside the lung. The role of FDG PET in helping identify patients with malignant lesions outside the lung was examined in 50 patients.

Methods.—Fifty patients with a mean age of 52.2 years underwent FDG PET for evaluation of either a single or multiple (27 and 23 patients, respectively) abnormalities suspected to be malignant. Patients had either undergone biopsy with indeterminate findings or had a lesion not amenable to biopsy. The final diagnosis was verified by histologic findings or by clinical follow-up. Absence of malignancy was assumed if no clinical deterioration occurred and the lesions remained stable or demonstrated resolution on subsequent imaging review (minimum follow-up, 1 year). Both visual and quantitative analyses were performed.

Results.—The positive and negative predictive values on visual analysis were 89% and 100%, respectively; for quantitative (standard uptake value >2.5) analysis, these values were 93% and 86%, respectively.

Conclusion.—Negative FDG-PET findings in patients with lesions outside the lung and indeterminate biopsy findings virtually exclude malignancy and permit the patient to be reassured. A positive scan encourages the clinician to pursue further biopsy to verify a diagnosis histologically. Thus, FDG PET can be used to decide which patients need to undergo further evaluation.

▶ I find it hard to recognize that FDG-PET is becoming the "evil messenger"—the test that brings the bad news. A positive PET in a lung cancer patient usually means "school is out—get on the palliative bus." A negative PET invites a "go for broke to cure attitude." I understand that the unnecessary morbidity of surgery and curative chemotherapy and decreased expense is an overall good thing, but I grieve for the patient whose optimistic balloon is about to sail with hope for corrective surgery when it gets deflated by an FDG arrow. We induce months of dismay in these folks, but I guess it is the right thing to do.

A. Gottschalk, MD

3-Deoxy-3-[¹⁸F]Fluorothymidine-Positron Emission Tomography for Noninvasive Assessment of Proliferation in Pulmonary Nodules

Buck AK, Schirrmeister H, Hetzel M, et al (Universit of Ulm, Germany)
Cancer Res 62:3331-3334, 2002   1–5

Background.—3-Deoxy-3-[¹⁸F]fluorothymidine ([¹⁸F]FLT) is a new thymidine analogue developed as a PET tracer for noninvasive assessment of tumor proliferation. The use of [¹⁸F]FLT to evaluate proliferation in solitary pulmonary nodules was evaluated.

Methods.—The prospective study included 30 patients, with a mean age of 62 years, with CT-detected pulmonary nodules. Confirmation was obtained at surgical resection in 19 patients and core biopsy in 11, with proliferation evaluated by a monoclonal antibody MIB-1 specific for nuclear antigen Ki-67 used for immunostaining. The findings were correlated with measures of [¹⁸F]FLT uptake.

Results.—Twenty-two malignant tumors were detected. On Ki-67 evaluation, the mean proliferation fraction was 30.9% in malignant lesions compared with less than 5% in benign pulmonary nodules. The mean standardized uptake value of [¹⁸F]FLT in pulmonary nodules was 2.8, increasing to

3.5 in non–small-cell lung cancers. Benign lesions showed no [¹⁸F]FLT uptake. On linear regression analysis, [¹⁸F]FLT uptake was significantly correlated with the Ki-67 index in malignant lesions.

Conclusions.—In assessment of solitary pulmonary nodules, [¹⁸F]FLT uptake appears to be specifically associated with malignant lesions. This new PET tracer may be of value for differential diagnosis of pulmonary nodules and evaluation of proliferation. Although sensitivity and specificity are high in this series of untreated patients with suspicious lesions, diagnostic performance may differ in previously treated patients.

▶ We need to remember as we all get into a positron mode that FDG is good but is unlikely to be the "be-all and end-all" of the technique. This article points out the potential of other F-18 tracers.

A. Gottschalk, MD

Improved Image Interpretation With Registered Thoracic CT and Positron Emission Tomography Data Sets

Aquino SL, Asmuth JC, Moore RH, et al (Massachusetts Gen Hosp, Boston; Sarnoff Corp, Princeton, NJ)
AJR 178:939-944, 2002   1–6

Introduction.—As the traditional imaging modality for lung cancer staging, CT provides anatomic accuracy but is limited in its ability to detect metastatic spread to mediastinal lymph nodes. With FDG PET, detection of metastatic spread to the mediastinum is improved, but anatomic accuracy is limited. In an attempt to improve the interpretation of cancer imaging studies, a computational algorithm was used to register the CT and PET data sets of patients who were imaged for lung cancer staging or reassessment after therapy.

Methods.—The analysis included data sets of 15 patients, 11 men and 4 women with a mean age of 50.6 years. Scans were obtained for lung cancer in 12 cases and for 1 case each of lymphoma, renal cell carcinoma, and esophageal carcinoma. The CT scans were obtained with HiSpeed or Light-Speed scanners; whole-body and thoracic FDG PET studies were performed with the ECAT-HR+ camera about 45 minutes after approximately 10 mCi of FDG was injected IV as a bolus. Registered PET CT data sets were analyzed for areas of increased uptake and for registration accuracy. All regions were anatomically specified on the basis of CT anatomy.

Results.—In 4 patients, data set evaluation showed excellent registration of regions of increased FDG uptake with correlative CT masses or enlarged lymph nodes in the mediastinum. There was increased FDG in the esophagus in 5 patients and in the left ventricle in 8 patients. Unregistered PET suggested tumor activity in a number of cases, but these areas were often interpreted as normal on registration (Table 1).

Discussion.—Image information from FDG PET is based on glucose uptake rather than on the anatomic and structural characteristics of the tissue.

TABLE 1.—Results of Interpretation of Registered CT and PET Versus Individual PET

Patient	History	Study	Interpretation	Abnormal Uptake in Lymph Nodes	Follow-up
1	Lung cancer restaging	Registered	Uptake in mass; no pleural dz	No	12 mo: tumor progress in mass, no pleural mets
2	Lung cancer restaging	PET alone	Uptake in mass and pleura	No	12 mo: no recurrence
		Registered	Radiation changes, no tumor	No	
3	Lung cancer restaging	PET alone	Uptake in apex c/w tumor	No	4 mo: pericardial mets
		Registered	Tumor in pericardium	No	Deceased
			Rad changes in upper lungs		
		PET alone	Tumor in left lung? location	No	
			Tumor vs rad changes in upper lungs		
4	Renal cancer	Registered	No tumor	No	12 mo: no recurrence
		PET alone	No tumor	No	
5	Lung cancer restaging	Registered	No tumor	No	11 mo: no recurrence
		PET alone	No tumor	No	
6	Lung cancer staging	Registered	No tumor activity	No	Rounded atelectasis
		PET alone	No tumor activity	Hilar uptake? tumor	
7	Esophageal cancer	Registered	Uptake in gastric pull-through	No	14 mo: no recurrence
		PET alone	Tumor in lower mediastinum	No	
8	Lung cancer restaging	Registered	Residual uptake in lung mass	No hilar or mediastinal dz	Surgical resection: no hilar dz
		PET alone	Residual uptake in lung mass	R hilar uptake	
9	Lung cancer restaging	Registered	Physiologic uptake GE jxn	R paratracheal	15 mo: no dz in lower thorax
		PET alone	Tumor activity in lower thorax	R paratracheal	
10	Lung cancer staging	Registered	Uptake in mediastinum	R paratracheal	Thoracotomy, resection
		PET alone	Uptake in mediastinum	R paratracheal	Mediastinal dz present
11	Lung cancer restaging	Registered	No tumor	No	12 mo: new R hilum, supraclav. dz
		PET alone	Mediastinal tumor vs radiation	No	

12	Lymphoma	Registered	Anterior mediastinal mass	Prevascular only	12 mo: no recurrence
		PET alone	Anterior mediastinal mass	Prevascular, L tracheal	
13	Lung cancer restaging	Registered	No tumor activity	No	1 yr: pulmonary, hilar mets
		PET alone	No tumor activity	No	
14	Lung cancer staging	Registered	See next entry	R hilum, tracheal; subcarinal	Preoperative chemo rad
				Diffuse bilateral	
14	Lung cancer restaging	PET alone	See next entry	No	No mediastinal dz at surgery
		Registered	See next entry	No	
		PET alone	See next entry		
15	Lung cancer staging	Registered	Inc uptake in RUL mass	R tracheal; subcarinal	5 mo: tumor progression in lung, mediastinum
		PET alone	Inc uptake in entire upper lobe	R tracheal; R hilum	Deceased

Note: Restaging = staging after chemotherapy and radiation therapy.
Abbreviations: dz, Disease; *mets,* metastases; *clu,* consistent with; *rad,* radiation; *R,* right; *GE jnx,* gastroesophageal junction; *supraclav,* supraclavicular; *L,* left; *chemo rad,* chemotherapy and radiation therapy; *inc,* increase; *RUL,* right upper lobe.

(Courtesy of Aquino SL, Asmuth JC, Moore RH, et al: Improved image interpretation with registered thoracic CT and positron emission tomography data sets. *AJR* 178:939-944, 2002. Reprinted with permission from the American Journal of Roentgenology.)

To make use of this information, an individual anatomic reference CT scan is required. The patient cannot be scanned in an identical position with the 2 methods, and body geometry differs between PET and CT. Registered data sets can have a major impact in cancer treatment by improving the distinction between therapeutic changes and recurrent disease or metastasis. In the cases reported here, registration of thoracic CT and PET data sets accurately downgraded some suspected positive findings on clinical PET interpretation.

► I would have been devastated if these results had not supported fusion. It would have been even more interesting if the authors assessed "side-by-side" CT with PET versus fusion. If the case is complicated, fusion will win this hands down as well. This concept was elegantly illustrated by Dr G. Von Schulthess in his refresher course "PET/CT Imaging" at the Los Angeles Society of Nuclear Medicine meeting in 2002. If you are interested in the topic and he gives this course again, I suggest you attend it.

A. Gottschalk, MD

^{99m}TC-Tetrofosmin Scintigraphy in Lung Carcinoma Staging and Follow-up Evaluations

Buccheri G, Biggi A, Ferrigno D, et al (Ospedale A Carle, Cuneo, Italy; Ospedale S Croce, Cuneo, Italy)
Cancer 94:1796-1807, 2002   1–7

Introduction.—A radiopharmaceutical initially developed for myocardial imaging, ^{99m}TC-tetrofosmin also accumulates in lung carcinoma. This is the first comprehensive investigation of the ability of ^{99m}TC-tetrofosmin scintigraphy to detect primary and metastatic cancer deposits in the lung and to recognize treatment-induced responses.

Methods.—The target sample for the study was 60 new unselected patients evaluated for surgical cure of a highly suspected lung carcinoma. All patients underwent ^{99m}TC-tetrofosmin scan (both planar and SPECT images), ^{99m}TC-methilene diphosphate bone scan, and CT of the thorax, abdomen, and brain. Follow-up clinical reassessments were obtained at 3- to 4-week intervals during chemotherapy and at 3- to 6-month intervals when radical surgery was performed. Twenty-one patients had a complete restaging evaluation 3 months after the initial evaluation.

Results.—Sixty-one patients were registered and assessable. Twenty-one had a final diagnosis of squamous cell carcinoma, 8 had small-cell carcinoma, 18 had adenocarcinoma, 5 had large-cell anaplastic carcinoma, 5 had an undefined cell type of mixed histology lung carcinoma, and 4 had nonmalignant lung lesions. All 57 carcinomas showed accumulation of the radiotracer (100% sensitivity), but so did 3 of the 4 nonmalignant lesions. The radiotracer was highly sensitive (97%) for detection of T0-T2 disease and highly specific (83%) for N0-N1 disease. In 16 pathologically staged mediastina, sensitivity, specificity, and accuracy rates were 73%, 100%, and

81%, respectively. Most skeleton (9 of 10) and brain (5 of 7) metastases were correctly identified with ^{99m}TC-tetrofosmin, and radiotracer findings at response evaluation corresponded to the clinical estimate in almost half of the cases.

Conclusion.—The ^{99m}TC-tetrofosmin scan was judged relatively accurate in the evaluation of lung carcinoma. Surgical maneuvers, however, remain essential for a correct staging classification.

▶ When 57 of 66 patients have lung carcinoma in the series you are evaluating, to worry about patient selection bias seems understated. When the authors conclude that "thoracic CT is the standard test for pretreatment and post treatment evaluation of lung carcinoma," I get tossed backward in time. If you are into this problem, the authors present a large easy-to-use bibliography (see Table 1 in the original article) discussing most of the recent tracers evaluated for lung carcinoma except for new additions like Neotect.

A. Gottschalk, MD

Thymic Lesions in Patients With Myasthenia Gravis: Characterization With Thallium 201 Scintigraphy

Higuchi T, Taki J, Kinuya S, et al (Kanazawa Univ, Ishikawa, Japan)
Radiology 221:201-206, 2001   1–8

Background.—Myasthenia gravis (MG) is associated with impaired neuromuscular transmission. The clinical characteristics of MG include exercise-induced increasing fatigue caused by an antibody-mediated autoimmune response against nicotinic acetylcholine receptors. Most patients with MG have thymic abnormalities, including thymic lymphoid follicular hyperplasia (LFH) and thymoma. The pathogenesis of MG is not well understood, but it is thought that the thymus plays a critical role. The value of thallium 201 SPECT in the evaluation of thymic lesions associated with MG, including LFH and thymoma, was assessed.

Methods.—A group of 46 patients with MG who had undergone thymectomy were evaluated preoperatively with ^{201}Tl SPECT and CT. SPECT studies were performed at 15 minutes (early image) and 180 minutes (delayed image) after ^{201}Tl injection. The results were visually assessed, and ^{201}Tl uptake ratios were measured for quantitative analysis. ^{201}Tl uptake was analyzed among the normal thymus, LFH, and thymoma patient groups.

Results.—Histopathologic studies indicated a normal thymus in 19 patients, LFH in 16 patients, and thymoma in 11 patients. Mean uptake ratios in the normal thymus, LFH, and thymoma were 0.96, 1.14, and 1.87, respectively, for early images and 1.09, 1.65, and 2.03, respectively, for delayed images. Thymoma demonstrated more intense ^{201}Tl accumulation than did the normal thymus and LFH on early images. Both thymoma and LFH demonstrated more intense uptake than did the normal thymus on delayed images.

Conclusions.—The evaluation of patients with MG with use of ^{201}Tl SPECT can allow the differentiation of a normal thymus from LFH and thymoma.

▶ The SPECT observations are probably dependent on good technique and instrumentation. These authors used a triple-headed camera and provided all the necessary "housekeeping" details to tell you how to recreate their images if you want to replicate these data (good for them). As the data suggest, if I had a possible thymic lesion, I would get both a CT and a ^{201}Tl SPECT scan. All in all, these authors have given us a good piece of work.

A. Gottschalk, MD

Recurrent Pulmonary Embolism Despite the Use of a Greenfield Filter
Barreras JR, Agarwal DM, Maximin ST, et al (St Vincent's Med Ctr, Staten Island, NY)
Clin Nucl Med 26:1040-1041, 2001   1–9

Case Report.—Man, 71, had been treated 6 months earlier with a Greenfield inferior vena cava (IVC) filter after experiencing multiple episodes of sudden substernal chest pressure and shortness of breath; he also had a history of pulmonary embolism (PE). At presentation, a ventilation-perfusion scan showed a high probability of PE. Neck and upper extremity venous system thrombi were excluded with Doppler US and venography. A lower extremity venogram revealed a thrombus in the right iliac vein and a small vessel arising caudal to the IVC filter anastomosed with the left renal vein.

Conclusions.—The diagnosis in this patient was recurrent PE resulting from thrombus migration through a circumaortic left renal vein bypassing a normally positioned filter.

▶ This case reminds me of a case I saw with a much simpler explanation for a recurrent embolism after proper IVC filter placement. In my case, new emboli formed around and through the limbs of the filter extending through the cranial aspect of the filter. When these broke off, a new acute PE occurred.

A. Gottschalk, MD

Lung Ventilation/Perfusion SPECT in the Artificially Embolized Pig
Bajc M, Bitzén U, Olsson B, et al (Lund Univ, Sweden)
J Nucl Med 43:640-647, 2002   1–10

Background.—In the diagnosis of lung embolism, although planar lung scintigraphy offers the advantages of being noninvasive, easy to apply, low in cost, low in radiation exposure, and highly sensitive, the incidence of nondiagnostic findings, and thus the lack of specificity, is high. Ventilation/perfusion (V/P) SPECT has been offered to improve the specificity and decrease the number of intermediate probability results, while maintaining the low cost and low radiation dose. Tomographic and planar techniques were compared for their usefulness in diagnosing low-degree embolism in pigs.

Methods.—The 16 pigs were anesthetized, then injected with 0 to 4 thallium-201 labeled latex emboli (35 emboli total), with the first 7 pigs receiving cylindric emboli and the last 9 receiving flat, 3-tailed emboli. Ventilation scintigraphy was performed with the pigs inhaling 30 MBq of [99m]technetium (^{99m}Tc)-diethylenetriaminepentaacetic acid aerosol. A double-head gamma camera was used to perform planar scintigraphy and SPECT. The cylindric emboli findings were interpreted by 2 readers and the 3-tailed flat emboli findings by 3 readers. A normalized V/P quotient image set was calculated after subtracting the ventilation background from the perfusion tomograms.

Results.—With the use of the [201]thallium (^{201}Tl) window, all the injected emboli were found within the lungs. Twenty-four emboli were impacted in the right lung and some lodged close together. Each doublet or triplet of cylindric emboli created a single perfusion defect (Fig 1), so 19 cylindric emboli caused 14 perfusion defects. Ten true-positive perfusion defects were identified, along with 4 false-negative results, of which 2 were agreed on by the 2

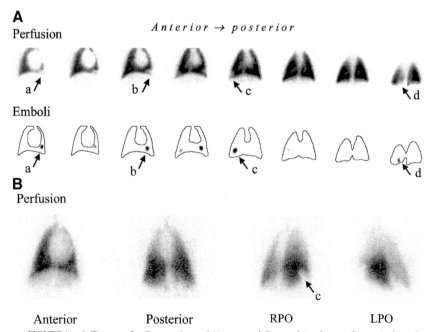

A

Perfusion

A n t e r i o r → *p o s t e r i o r*

Emboli

B

Perfusion

Anterior　　　　Posterior　　　　RPO　　　　LPO

FIGURE 1.—**A**, Tomography. Consecutive perfusion coronal slices and simultaneously acquired matching ^{201}Tl images of emboli. In left lung, 2 emboli (*a* and *b*) cause 1 large perfusion defect. In right lung, 2 emboli caused 2 perfusion defects (*c* and *d*). **B**, Planar images of same pig as in A. Both readers observed only 1 perfusion defect (*c*). *Abbreviations: RPO*, Right posterior oblique; *LPO*, left posterior oblique. (Reprinted with permission of the Society of Nuclear Medicine from Bajc M, Bitzén U, Olsson B, et al: Lung ventilation/perfusion SPECT in the artificially embolized pig. *J Nucl Med* 43:640-647, 2002.)

readers. The average sensitivity and specificity for the 2 readers were 71% and 91%, respectively. The tomographic images revealed 14 true-positive and no false-positive perfusion defects, for a sensitivity and specificity of 100% each. At 15 of the 3-tailed emboli sites, perfusion defects were found. By using the planar modality, the 3 readers averaged 64% in sensitivity and 79% in specificity. By using tomography, the 3 readers averaged 91% in sensitivity and 87% in specificity. The addition of the V/P quotient facilitated interpretation and the joint 3-dimensional cine presentation of ventilation, perfusion, and V/P quotient helped further.

Conclusions.—The sensitivity and accuracy of lung V/P SPECT exceeded those of planar imaging in detecting emboli in the pig model. In addition, specificity did not suffer, so lung V/P SPECT would appear to be a good alternative to planar imaging.

▶ The figure seems to show that 8 SPECT slices are better than ½ of a good perfusion series—especially if you do not count the embolus (b) seen on the LPO view.

Ordinarily, I tend not to select data from animal studies, but no one presents human data with both good SPECT and 8 view planar studies to compare. I knew an excellent nuclear physician who told me SPECT is clearly the way to go. But every time I am involved with a human study with a serious reference standard,[1] I find no compelling reason to abandon the planar technique.

A. Gottschalk, MD

Reference

1. Gottschalk A, Stein PD, Goodman LR, et al: Overview of prospective investigation of pulmonary embolism diagnosis II. *Semin Nucl Med* 32:173-182, 2002.

Quantitative Analysis of Lung Perfusion in Patients With Primary Pulmonary Hypertension

Fukuchi K, Hayashida K, Nakanishi N, et al (Natl Cardiovascular Ctr, Suita, Osaka, Japan)
J Nucl Med 43:757-761, 2002
1–11

Background.—Primary pulmonary hypertension (PPH) is characterized by a progressive increase in pulmonary vascular pressure and resistance, which leads to right ventricular hypertrophy and cor pulmonale. PPH usually takes a prolonged period to diagnose, so the diagnosis most likely depends on making a diagnosis when the pulmonary circulation is responsive to vasodilator therapy. Thus, there is a need for noninvasive methods to assess the severity of pulmonary hypertension and the effects of various therapies for PPH. The ventilation-perfusion scan is used primarily to exclude thromboembolism in patients with PPH; however, lung perfusion scans often show patchy loss of lung perfusion, commonly known as a mottled pattern. The pathogenesis and cause of this phenomenon have not been elucidated. The nonuniform distribution of lung perfusion scans in patients with

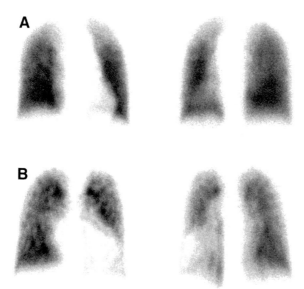

FIGURE 2.—Representative anterior and posterior views of lung perfusion scan derived from patient with mild pulmonary hypertension (**A**) and from patient with severe pulmonary hypertension (**B**). (Reprinted with permission of the Society of Nuclear Medicine from Fukuchi K, Hayashida K, Nakanishi N, et al: Quantitative analysis of lung perfusion in patients with primary pulmonary hypertension. *J Nucl Med* 43:757-761, 2002.)

PPH was evaluated and the association between lung perfusion scan heterogeneity and the severity of PPH was assessed.

Methods.—Lung perfusion scans were obtained in 22 patients with PPH and 12 age-matched control participants (Fig 2). Perfused area rates (PARs) were calculated by dividing the lung area in each 10% threshold width from 10% to 100% of maximal counts by total lung area. The total absolute difference in the PAR between each patients and the mean control value was assumed as the perfusion index of the lung (P index).

Results.—The P index was significantly correlated with the mean pulmonary artery pressure. However, no significant correlation was observed between the P index and the total pulmonary resistance. In patients who underwent vasodilator therapy, the P index was significantly improved after therapy and associated with a reduction in pulmonary arterial pressure.

Conclusions.—These findings suggest that quantitative assessment of lung function irregularity, in addition to providing routine visual representation, may be useful in providing information about the severity of disease and the effects of therapy.

▶ Although I doubt this technique to quantify the perfusion would vary much from a visual stratification scheme used by "experienced eyeballs," it is straight forward. Certainly, "inexperienced eyeballs" can be replaced by this technique.

A. Gottschalk, MD

Diagnosis of an Air Leak by Radionuclide Scan

Unterreiner N, Weiss PE (Rochester Gen Hosp, NY)
Clin Nucl Med 26:1039, 2001   1–12

Background.—The utility of xenon-133 for the demonstration of a bronchopleural fistula on a CT scan is highlighted.

Case Report.—Man, 80, with emphysema was evaluated for spontaneous pneumothorax that was first treated with a chest tube. On CT, a 3-cm spiculated mass was visualized in the right upper lobe. This mass was subsequently proven to be a squamous cell carcinoma. Bilateral lung fibrosis and emphysema with upper lobe bullae and right-sided pneumothorax were also seen. A preoperative ventilation-perfusion scan with quantitation of lung perfusion was performed. Delayed wash-in of xenon was seen peripherally on the right. Washout images demonstrated peripheral air trapping on the right, which was a finding that was compatible with an air leak and pneumothorax. A leaking right upper lobe bulla was found at surgery and was repaired.

Conclusions.—The diagnosis of an air leak with a radionuclide scan is not a new technique. Xenon-133 ventilation CT scanning was used to demonstrate a bronchopleural fistula.

▶ This is an old idea—so old, I thought I would remind you again what bronchopleural fistulas look like with xenon-133. You may wish to look them up; the YEAR BOOK OF NUCLEAR MEDICINE has an example.[1]

The point is that the xenon-133 ventilation scanning is a wonderful technique to show this lesion very easily when there is a problem making or proving the diagnosis.

A. Gottschalk, MD

Reference

1. 1994 YEARBOOK OF NUCLEAR MEDICINE, pp 116-117.

2 Oncology

Introduction

A large number of important articles related to oncologic nuclear medicine were published last year. PET continues to be the hot topic, but articles on thyroid cancer imaging, scintimammography, and lymphoscintigraphy are appearing in large numbers. Articles on PET in lung cancer are still the most frequently encountered, but PET in women's cancers, particularly breast cancer, are being published with increasing frequency. Now that Medicare is reimbursing for staging and restaging as well as therapeutic monitoring of breast cancer, I anticipate an even greater utilization of PET in breast cancer and an increasing number of publications on the topic.

PET/CT is just beginning to hit the literature this year, and its impact is definitely being seen. It is my impression that all of PET will be PET/CT in 3 to 5 years.

Articles on scintimammography continue to demonstrate its value. Even though my colleagues at Duke are working on improved methodology for single photon imaging of breast cancer, we have never been asked to do a single patient with scintimammography.

R. Edward Coleman, MD

Lung Tumors Evaluated With FDG-PET and Dynamic CT: The Relationship Between Vascular Density and Glucose Metabolism

Tateishi U, Nishihara H, Tsukamoto E, et al (Natl Cancer Ctr Hosp, Tokyo; Hokkaido Univ, Sapporo, Japan)
J Comput Assist Tomogr 26:185-190, 2002   2–1

Background.—FDG PET and contrast-enhanced dynamic CT are each useful in the diagnosis of pulmonary tumors. How well the results of FDG PET correlate with those of dynamic CT was examined.

Methods.—The subjects were 40 patients (26 men and 14 women; mean age, 60.4 years) with a pulmonary tumor (mean diameter, 2.6 cm). All patients underwent whole-body FDG PET to determine FDG standardized uptake values (SUVs). They also underwent contrast-enhanced dynamic CT, during which peak attenuation (A_{PA}) and relative flow (RF) of blood to the tumor were measured. Within 2 weeks of the radiologic examinations, all

FIGURE 1

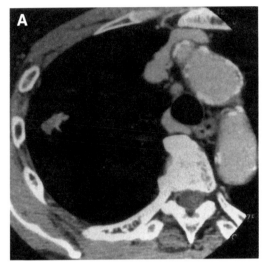

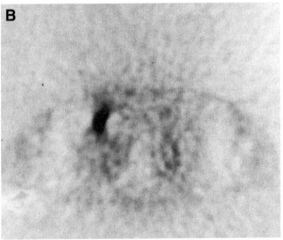

(Continued)

patients underwent surgery. Tumor specimens were submitted for histologic examination, including measurements of microvessel density (MVD).

Results.—The histologic examination revealed 18 adenocarcinomas, 12 squamous cell carcinomas, and 10 benign lesions. Compared with benign tumors, malignant tumors had significantly higher mean A_{PA} (41.6 vs 7.6 Hounsfield units), mean RF (0.019 per second vs 0.005 per second), and mean SUV (4.7 vs 1.1). No significant correlation was found among the mean A_{PA}, RF, SUV, and MVD of the benign lesions. In the malignant lesions, however, both A_{PA} and RF correlated significantly with SUV ($r = 0.665$ and $r = 0.848$, respectively). MVD was also significantly higher in the malignant tumors than in the benign ones (62.4 vs 19.6 microvessels/field). MVD cor-

FIGURE 1 (cont.)

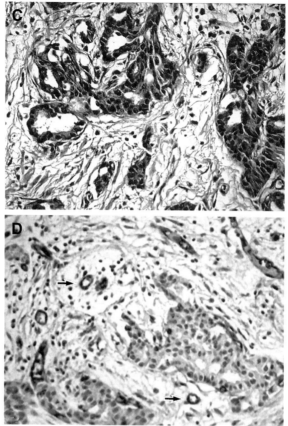

FIGURE 1.—Case of a 64-year-old woman with well-differentiated adenocarcinoma. **A**, Dynamic CT image 140 seconds after administration of contrast agent reveals peak attenuation of 46 HU. **B**, The standardized uptake value of FDG-PET scan is 3.8. **C**, Hematoxylin-eosin–stained specimen demonstrates well-differentiated adenocarcinoma. **D**, Immunohistochemical staining of anti-CD34 antibody is shown. Delineated CD34-positive cells are counted as microvessels (*arrows*). Microvessel density is counted as 87. (Courtesy of Tateishi U, Nishihara H, Tsukamoto E, et al: Lung tumors evaluated with FDG-PET and dynamic CT: The relationship between vascular density and glucose metabolism. *J Comput Assist Tomogr* 26 (2):185-190, 2002.)

related significantly with A_{PA} ($r = 0.801$), RF ($r = 0.723$), and SUV ($r = 0.612$) in the malignant lesions (Fig 1), but not in the benign tumors.

Conclusion.—There are significant and strong positive correlations between FDG PET findings and those of contrast-enhanced dynamic CT in patients with lung cancer. This suggests that blood pooling (as reflected by A_{PA} and RF) may be related to increased glucose metabolism (as reflected by FDG uptake) in malignant tumors.

▶ Much interest is now being shown in the evaluation of tumors by using contrast-enhanced dynamic CT. With the use of antiangiogenic therapies, evalua-

tion of perfusion or a parameter of perfusion may provide important information. Furthermore, the possible relationship between vascular density and
glucose metabolism is of interest. FDG accumulation in tumors is not flow-de-
pendent. This study demonstrates that there is a relationship between the
SUV of lung cancer and the peak attenuation on the contrast-enhanced dynamic CT scan.

R. E. Coleman, MD

**Fluoro-deoxi-glucose Uptake and Angiogenesis Are Independent Bio-
logical Features in Lung Metastases**
Veronesi G, Landoni C, Pelosi G, et al (European Inst of Oncology, Milan, Italy;
Ospedale San Raffaele, Milan, Italy)
Br J Cancer 86:1391-1395, 2002   2–2

Background.—Evidence suggests that the increased glucose uptake of
cancer tumors may be an adaptive response to hypoxia. Hypoxia may also
explain angiogenesis in neoplasms, as the rapidly growing tumor com-
presses existing blood vessels. Thus, the relationship between glucose uptake, as measured by FDG PET, and microvessel density (MVD), as determined from a pathologic examination, in lung cancer was examined.

Methods.—The subjects were 19 patients (10 men and 9 women; mean
age, 61 years) with 43 lung metastases. All patients underwent FDG PET to
identify malignant tumors and to determine the FDG standard uptake value
(SUV) of each nodule. After tumor resection, the surgical specimens were examined to determine MVD.

Results.—The results of FDG PET were positive in 26 of the 43 lesions
(sensitivity, 60%). MVD did not differ significantly between the FDG PET–
positive and the FDG PET–negative tumors (12.9 vs 11.3 microvessels/field,
respectively). MVD was significantly higher in metastatic tumors of sarcoma (n = 8) than in metastatic tumors of colon cancer (n = 16) (16.6 vs
10.2 microvessels/field), but MVD did not correlate with nodule size. Conversely, SUV did correlate with nodule size and was significantly greater in
larger lesions. In addition, SUVs were significantly higher in metastatic tumors of colon cancer than in metastatic tumors of sarcoma (3.04 vs 1.18).
Multivariate analysis confirmed the absence of a significant correlation between SUV and MVD.

Conclusion.—The lack of a significant correlation between glucose metabolism and angiogenesis suggests that these are independent biological
features of metastatic lung tumors.

▶ A wide variety of primary tumor types were included in this study. The absence of correlation between the SUV and the MVD is interesting. In the study
by Tateishi et al (Abstract 2–1) a correlation was found between vascular density and glucose metabolism in the evaluation of patients with suspected primary lung tumors.

R. E. Coleman, MD

Can FDG-PET Reduce the Need for Mediastinoscopy in Potentially Resectable Nonsmall Cell Lung Cancer?

Kernstine KH, McLaughlin KA, Menda Y, et al (Univ of Iowa, Iowa City; Iowa City VA Med Ctr, Iowa)

Ann Thorac Surg 73:394-402, 2002   2–3

Background.—Although mediastinal staging must be accomplished to accurately assess the prognosis and management of patients with non–small-cell lung cancer (NSCLC), the surgical biopsy required involves significant risk and cost factors. Other methods have been tested for their capability to provide the necessary information. Although FDG-PET NSCLC studies have been done, too few patients have been involved to make accurate assessments of FDG PET's capability to stage the mediastinum. Whether PET could eliminate or reduce the need for surgical biopsy in staging the mediastinum in NSCLC was assessed in patients at one surgical clinic.

Methods.—Data were obtained from the FDG-PET assessments performed from 1995 to 2000 and included 265 potential candidates for study; the final study comprised 237 patients (137 men and 100 women; mean age, 65 years). All were operable and had known or suspected NSCLC. Surgical mediastinal nodal sampling was carried out by mediastinoscopy within 31 days of the PET scan, and a definitive diagnosis was made.

Results.—Ninety-nine patients (55 men and 44 women; mean age, 64 years) were known to have NSCLC, and 138 (82 men and 56 women; mean age, 66 years) had suspected NSCLC. PET was performed 0 to 29 days before mediastinoscopy; patients in the known group waited an average of 7 days before mediastinoscopy, and those in the suspect group waited an average of 9 days. In 9 primary lesions, no FDG uptake occurred; 1 was benign, and the other 8 were NSCLC. The known group had higher standardized uptake values (SUVs) than did the suspect group, and more of the known group had mediastinal metastases (26% in the NSCLC group and only 13% in the suspect group). On PET, a higher metastatic cancer rate was noted in both groups; PET found 30% to 50% more than on mediastinoscopy. Among the known group, PET's sensitivity and specificity for N2 were both 0.80, its positive predictive value was 0.57, and its negative predictive value was 0.92. Among the suspect group, PET's sensitivity and specificity were both 0.81, its positive predictive value was 0.36, and its negative predictive value was 0.97. For N3, these values were 0.25 (sensitivity) and 0.96 (specificity) in the known group and 0.00 and 0.99 in the suspect group. For N3 in the known group, the positive predictive value was 0.20, and the negative predictive value was 0.97; these values were 0.00 and 0.96, respectively, for the suspect group. Six patients who had positive findings on PET imaging even though their mediastinal node biopsy results had been negative were found to have positive results on further biopsy. Overall, the sensitivity of PET was 82%, its specificity was 82%, its accuracy was 82%, its negative predictive value was 95%, and its positive predictive value was 51%. In 29 primary lesions, negative histologic results confirmed an SUV of less than

2.5 and negative mediastinal results for PET, which yielded a 100% specificity for PET in these patients.

Conclusions.—PET, although not eliminating the need for mediastinoscopy, was capable of supplying important clinical information on patients who had or were suspected of having operable NSCLC. It can also identify patients who do not require mediastinoscopy and can improve the accuracy of staging based on mediastinal surgical methods.

▶ Farrell et al[1] demonstrated that negative mediastinum results on FDG-PET scanning in patients with stage 1 NSCLC were predictive of negative mediastinum results at mediastinoscopy; thus, mediastinoscopy was not needed. This study performs a different evaluation to conclude that mediastinoscopy is not necessary when the SUV is less than 2.5 and the mediastinum result is PET negative. There are ways to decrease the number of patients needing mediastinoscopy; however, most patients will still undergo mediastinoscopy.

R. E. Coleman, MD

Reference

1. Farrell MA, McAdams HP, Herndon JE, et al: Non-small cell lung cancer: FDG PET for nodal staging in patients with stage I disease. *Radiology* 215:886-890, 2000.

FDG PET for Staging of Advanced Non-Small Cell Lung Cancer Prior to Neoadjuvant Radio-Chemotherapy
Eschmann SM, Friedel G, Paulsen F, et al (Univ Hosp Tübingen, Germany; Schillerhoehe-Hosp for Lung Diseases, Gerlingen, Germany)
Eur J Nucl Med 29:804-808, 2002   2–4

Background.—Preoperative chemotherapy alone or combined with radiotherapy is increasingly being used to reduce tumor size and lymph node metastases in patients with non–small-cell lung cancer (NSCLC), so that subsequent resection may prove more curative. Candidates for neoadjuvant radiochemotherapy are those patients with stage III disease (T2-T4, N2-N3) who are free of distant metastases. The utility of FDG PET in the staging of NSCLC, and thus in the selection of patients eligible for neoadjuvant radiochemotherapy, was investigated.

Methods.—The subjects were 101 patients (75 men and 26 women; mean age, 56.2 years) with histologically or cytologically proven NSCLC. All patients had stage IIIA/B disease and no evidence of lymph node involvement or distant metastasis. All patients had previously undergone mediastinoscopy, CT, bone scintigraphy, and abdominal ultrasonography. For this trial, they also underwent whole-body FDG PET, and these results were compared with those of earlier studies. Any discrepancies were confirmed by biopsy or repeat CT.

Results.—PET revealed hypermetabolic tumors in 99 of the 101 patients; tumors in the other 2 patients were ultimately reassessed to be nonmalignant. Compared with histologic findings, PET allowed the correct identification of 75% of patients without lymph node metastases, 85% of patients with limited (N1-N2) involvement, and 90% of patients with extensive (N3) lymph node metastases. The overall sensitivity, specificity, positive predictive value, and negative predictive value of FDG PET for detecting lymph node metastasis were 96%, 73%, 88%, and 89%, respectively. The overall accuracy of FDG PET was higher than that of CT (84% vs 70%), and FDG PET revealed 6 patients with unsuspected contralateral lymph node metastases that CT missed. FDG PET was incorrect in 14 patients, and the CT results were also false-positive in 5 of these patients. Even though all patients were believed to be free of distant metastasis, FDG PET revealed distant metastatic sites in 25 patients. In total, the results of FDG PET changed clinical management in 29 of 101 patients (29%). Two patients (previously mentioned) did not undergo radiochemotherapy because a malignant tumor was excluded, 1 patient underwent surgery without neoadjuvant therapy after lymph node metastasis was excluded, 1 patient was reclassified as having a seminoma and treated appropriately, and 25 patients with previously unknown distant metastases were excluded from preoperative radiochemotherapy.

Conclusion.—FDG PET was more accurate than CT in staging advanced NSCLC, and it was particularly useful in detecting metastatic disease. FDG PET should be incorporated into the workup of patients with NSCLC who are being considered for neoadjuvant therapy or for other treatments that are dependent on the stage of disease.

▶ This article makes a good argument for the use of PET for selecting patients for neoadjuvant therapy. The PET study resulted in a change in therapy in 29% of patients, primarily by detecting previously unknown distant metastases.

R. E. Coleman, MD

The Impact of PET on the Management of Lung Cancer: The Referring Physician's Perspective

Seltzer MA, Yap CS, Silverman DH, et al (Univ of California, Los Angeles; Northern California PET Imaging Ctr, Sacramento)
J Nucl Med 43:752-756, 2002

2–5

Background.—[18]F-FDG PET has become an important clinical tool for diagnosing, staging, and monitoring cancer therapy. The utility of ^{18}F-FDG PET is based on the observation that many types of malignant tumors have an accelerated rate of glycolysis. Numerous studies have shown that ^{18}F-FDG PET is highly accurate for diagnosing and staging lung cancer, providing diagnostic information beyond that obtained through standard anatomic imaging modalities such as CT or MRI. It has been reported that ^{18}F-FDG PET has a significant effect on the management of lung cancer, but referring physicians' perspectives on the impact of ^{18}F-FDG PET on the staging and management of lung cancer are unknown. Referring physicians' perspectives on the impact of ^{18}F-FDG PET on lung cancer staging and management were studied and determined.

Methods.—A questionnaire was sent to 292 physicians of 744 consecutive patients with known or suspected lung cancer who were evaluated with PET. Questionnaires were returned for 274 patients, for a response rate of 37%. Management changes were categorized as intermodality, which included surgery to medical, surgery to radiation, and medical to no treatment, or intramodality, including altered medical, surgical, or radiotherapy approach.

Results.—The most common reason for PET referral was staging of lung cancer (61% of patients), followed by diagnosis in 20% of patients, and monitoring of therapy or the course of the disease in 6% of patients. According to the physicians who responded to the questionnaire, PET caused them to change their decision on clinical stage in 44% of all patients, with upstaging of the disease in 29% of patients and downstaging in 15% of patients. PET findings resulted in intermodality management changes in 39% of patients, whereas 15% of patients had an intramodality change.

Conclusions.—The findings of this survey indicate that ^{18}F-FDG PET has a significant effect on the staging and management of lung cancer.

▶ This article is 1 of a series of articles from the group at UCLA on determining the impact of PET on management of patients with cancer. The cancer that is most frequently evaluated with PET is lung cancer, and lung cancer patients make up approximately one third of all patients studied with FDG PET. This study documents the major impact that PET has in the management of lung cancer patients.

R. E. Coleman, MD

The Utility of ^{18}F-FDG PET for Suspected Recurrent Non–Small Cell Lung Cancer After Potentially Curative Therapy: Impact on Management and Prognostic Stratification

Hicks RJ, Kalff V, MacManus MP, et al (Pratt Found Statistical Centre, East Melbourne, Victoria, Australia; Peter MacCallum Cancer Inst, East Melbourne, Victoria, Australia)
J Nucl Med 42:1605-1613, 2001   2–6

Introduction.—For patients who have undergone potentially curative therapy of non–small-cell lung cancer (NSCLC), masses or symptoms suggestive of relapse are common, but may be challenging to characterize. Early detection is crucial because salvage therapies are available for localized recurrence. The utility of ^{18}F-FDG PET for such patients was investigated to ascertain a possible association between disease status as assessed by PET and survival rate.

Methods.—The study included 63 consecutive patients referred for clinical assessment of suspected relapse of NSCLC between November 1996 and December 1998 who were prospectively entered into a database. They experienced suspected relapse during 6 months after definitive treatment of NSCLC. The apparent extent of disease on conventional restaging was compared with that on FDG PET. Patients who already had verified systemic metastases were excluded unless aggressive treatment was being considered. Patients underwent serial imaging and pathologic evaluations at a median follow-up of 19 months to validate diagnostic findings. The prognostic significance was determined by the Cox proportional hazards regression model.

Results.—Of 42 patients with confirmed relapse, 41 had positive PET findings (sensitivity, 98%). No disease was identified during a minimum follow-up of 12 months in 14 of 15 patients with clinically suspected relapse (negative predictive value, 93%). A major change was made in patient management as a result of PET findings in 40 (63%) patients, including 6 patients whose treatment was changed from curative to palliative, 3 patients whose treatment was changed from palliative to curative, and 9 patients for whom negative PET findings prevented active management. Both the presence ($P = .012$) and the degree ($P < .0001$) of relapse on PET were highly significant prognostic factors. After adjusting for treatment, a significant prognostic stratification was noted based on the treatment delivered after PET testing ($P = .011$). The PET status continued to be highly predictive of patient survival.

Conclusion.—Compared with conventional staging, PET better evaluates disease status, stratifies prognosis, and affects patient management. It should be incorporated into paradigms for suspected recurrent NSCLC.

▶ This restaging study demonstrates that PET has a high sensitivity for detecting residual disease and a high specificity for excluding recurrent disease. The 63% change in management demonstrates that PET does have a major impact on therapy. Previous studies have documented the prognostic information of PET at the time of diagnosis, and this study demonstrates the prognostic information at the time of restaging.

R. E. Coleman, MD

The Impact of Fluorodeoxyglucose F 18 Positron-Emission Tomography on the Surgical Staging of Non–Small Cell Lung Cancer
Vesselle H, Pugsley JM, Vallières E, et al (Univ of Washington, Seattle)
J Thorac Cardiovasc Surg 124:511-519, 2002   2–7

Background.—Surgical staging of non–small-cell lung cancer (NSCLC) typically involves bronchoscopy, mediastinoscopy, mediastinotomy, thoracoscopy, thoracotomy, and CT. The accuracy and anatomic information provided by FDG PET were compared with those of current methods in the surgical staging of NSCLC.

Methods.—The subjects were 142 patients with potentially resectable NSCLC (stage I or II or T3 N1 M0) as determined by thoracic CT. All patients underwent FDG PET from the neck to the pelvis. PET scans and CT scans were read prospectively. Patients in whom PET revealed no distant metastases were staged with bronchoscopy and mediastinoscopy, with or without mediastinotomy or thoracoscopy, before proceeding to surgery. Patients in whom PET revealed distant metastasis, pleural implants, or N2 or N3 involvement were referred for chemotherapy.

Results.—FDG PET revealed that 24 of the 142 patients (16.9%) had unsuspected distant metastases. PET identified 15 cases of T4 lesions, whereas CT revealed only 8 cases; 6 of the 7 unsuspected cases found exclusively by PET had pleural implants. Nodal status could be determined at surgery in 118 cases. PET correctly staged N status in 83 of the 118 cases (70.3%) and could accurately differentiate N0 or N1 disease from N2 or N3 disease in 101 cases (85.6%). PET did not underestimate any cases of N3 disease, but it did underestimate N2 disease in 8 of these 118 patients (6.8%); in all 8 patients, N2 disease was detected during mediastinoscopy or thoracotomy. In 5 cases, however, PET revealed mediastinal lymph node disease in locations that were not accessible during bronchoscopy or mediastinoscopy. The sensitivity, specificity, positive predictive value, and negative value of FDG PET in the diagnosis of N2 or N3 disease were 80.9%, 96.0%, 91.9%, and 90.1%, respectively. Overall, PET findings influenced management in 35 of 142 cases (24.6%).

Conclusion.—FDG PET is highly accurate in the surgical staging of patients with NSCLC. FDG PET can ensure accurate discrimination between N0 and N1 and N2 and N3 disease in 90% of cases and thus provides localizing information for planning surgical resection. FDG PET is also extremely useful in identifying previously unsuspected distant metastasis, and its results can significantly affect management decisions.

▶ This study is one of many that have demonstrated the accuracy of PET in staging NSCLC. The detection of unsuspected distant metastases in 16.9% of the patients and unsuspected pleural implants in 6 of the 142 patients is slightly greater than the other studies.

R. E. Coleman, MD

An Initial Experience With FDG-PET in the Imaging of Residual Disease After Induction Therapy for Lung Cancer

Akhurst T, Downey RJ, Ginsberg MS, et al (Mem Sloan-Kettering Cancer Ctr, New York; Toronto Gen Hosp)
Ann Thorac Surg 73:259-266, 2002   2–8

Introduction.—For the staging of untreated non–small-cell lung cancer (NSCLC), FDG-PET imaging has an advantage over CT alone. Other than 1 small, 9-patient investigation, no data are available that compare FDG PET with the surgical staging of NSCLC after induction therapy. The accuracy of FDG PET after induction therapy for lung cancer was investigated retrospectively for 56 patients with NSCLC.

Methods.—Systematic queries of PET and thoracic surgical databases were reviewed. A nuclear physician blinded to surgical findings examined the FDG-PET scans and gave a clinical tumor node metastasis (TNM) stage, and a thoracic surgeon assigned a pathologic TNM stage. The clinical and pathologic TNM stages were compared for equivalence.

Results.—The study included 56 patients (30 men, 26 women; mean age, 60 years). Forty patients underwent chemotherapy, 11 had chemoradiation, and 5 had radiation alone, followed by PET and surgery. The positive predictive value of PET for identifying residual viable disease in the primary tumor was 98%. The nodal status was overstaged by PET in 33% of patients, understaged in 15%, and was accurate in 52%. All patients with M1 disease were correctly classified.

Conclusion.—It is not possible to ascertain whether a change observed between PET scans performed before and after induction correlates with pathologic estimates of response or with survival.

▶ FDG PET has demonstrated a high accuracy in the diagnosis of lung cancer and the initial staging of lung cancer. Very little data are available on the use of FDG PET in restaging of lung cancer, and even less data are available on the use of FDG PET in evaluating induction therapy for lung cancer. This study found PET accurate in characterizing the primary lesion and in characterizing distant metastatic disease. However, the nodal status was not accurately characterized, with FDG PET having a sensitivity of 77%, specificity of 57%, positive predictive value of 63% and negative predictive value of 27%. The authors did not have a PET scan before therapy to compare with the PET scan after therapy, and the comparative data might have been helpful.

R. E. Coleman, MD

Intraoperative Sentinel Lymph Node Mapping in Non–Small-Cell Lung Cancer Improves Detection of Micrometastases

Liptay MJ, Grondin SC, Fry WA, et al (Northwestern Univ, Evanston, Ill)
J Clin Oncol 20:1984-1988, 2002   2–9

Background.—The most important prognostic factor in localized non–small-cell lung cancer (NSCLC) is the presence of lymph node metastasis. Whether intraoperative sentinel lymph node (SN) mapping can identify nodal micrometastasis in patients with potentially resectable NSCLC was examined.

Methods.—The subjects were 100 patients (54 men and 46 women; mean age, 70 years) suspected of having potentially resectable NSCLC. At thoracotomy, 0.25 to 2 mCi of ^{99m}Tc was injected into the primary tumor and allowed to migrate throughout the mediastinal lymph nodes for 10 to 15 minutes. Then a hand-held gamma probe was used to obtain intraoperative radiotracer readings from the lymph nodes. An *SN* was defined as any lymph node with a ^{99m}Tc count more than 3 times the background count. Anatomical resection with mediastinal node dissection was performed, and both SNs and non-SNs were submitted for histologic and immunohistochemical examination.

Results.—Of the 100 patients evaluated, 9 did not have NSCLC and were excluded from the analysis. In the remaining 91 patients with NSCLC, the ^{99m}Tc sulfur colloid successfully migrated through the pulmonary lymphatic system in 78 patients (86%). An SN was identified in all 78 patients, including 4 patients who had 2 separate SNs. The identified SNs were classified as true-positive in 69 of these 78 patients (88.5%), in that no metastases were found in other nodes that did not have concurrent SN involvement. Of the 78 patients with SNs, 21 (27%) were determined to have metastatic disease. The SN was the only positive node in 9 of these 21 patients. Histologic or immunohistochemical examination revealed micrometastasis in 7 of these 21 patients (33%), and prompted the upstaging of disease in all 7 cases.

Conclusion.—Intraoperative SN mapping can accurately identify the first site of lymphatic tumor drainage in patients with NSCLC. It may also improve the accuracy of disease staging in these patients and may be particularly useful in patients with small tumors and clinically negative lymph nodes.

▶ This article is the second one from this group on the use of the SN technique in lung cancer. The results are quite encouraging that the procedure will be beneficial. The surgeons at my institution are interested in trying it.

R. E. Coleman, MD

Biologic Correlates of ^{18}Fluorodeoxyglucose Uptake in Human Breast Cancer Measured by Positron Emission Tomography

Bos R, van der Hoeven JJM, van der Wall E, et al (Vrije Universiteit, Amsterdam; Amstelveen Hosp, The Netherlands; Johns Hopkins Univ, Baltimore, Md)
J Clin Oncol 20:379-387, 2002   2–10

Background.—Tumor metabolism can be evaluated in vivo using PET and the glucose analogue ^{18}FDG. However, the mechanisms underlying the uptake of ^{18}FDG in tumors remain uncertain, with different patterns of uptake characteristic of different tumor types. ^{18}FDG uptake varies in breast cancer perhaps more than in many other cancers. Various markers that indicate the rate of glucose metabolism in breast cancer patients (Glut-1; HKs I, II, and III; HIF-1α; and VEGF) were identified and links with ^{18}FDG sought, as well as whether the low ^{18}FDG uptake of lobular breast cancers was explicable.

Methods.—Fifty-five patients were scanned preoperatively, then the tissue samples taken at operation were evaluated using immunohistochemical techniques for the various markers as well as the density of microvessels. Measurements included the mitotic activity index (MAI), amount of necrosis, number of lymphocytes, and tumor cells and volume.

Results.—Intense ^{18}FDG uptake was noted in 24 cancers. Glut-1 and HIF-1α were overexpressed around areas of necrosis as well as heterogenously in some of the tumors. The HKs and VEGF were also expressed heterogeneously in some cases, but most tumors had a homogeneous expression of these markers throughout the tumor. A statistically significant positive correlation with [18]FDG uptake was found with Glut-1 membrane staining, presence of necrosis, tumor cell density, intensity of cytoplasmic HK I, and presence of lymphocytic infiltrate. A significant but weak positive correlation was also found between density of microvessels and PET score. The strongest combination of variables that predicted positive [18]FDG uptake was MAI, Glut-1, HIF-1α, and HK II. The ability to detect PET depended particularly on Glut-1, MAI, tumor cell density, and necrosis.

Conclusion.—The variables that determine the amount of [18]FDG uptake in breast cancer include microvessels that provide glucose, Glut-1 to transport [18]FDG into the cell, HKs to put [18]FDG into glycolysis, number of tumor cells per unit volume, rate of tumor cell proliferation, amount of inflammatory cells in the tumor, and HIF-1α, which is upregulated by hypoxia and induces Glut-1 expression and angiogenesis.

▶ The accumulation of FDG in tumors is a complex process. This study compares the multiple factors associated with FDG accumulation. Many of the parameters that were evaluated were shown to be correlated with the amount of FDG uptake. The multiple parameters involved in the process explain the variability in uptake by the various cell types.

R. E. Coleman, MD

Whole-Body ^{18}F-FDG PET and Conventional Imaging for Predicting Outcome in Previously Treated Breast Cancer Patients
Vranjesevic D, Filmont JE, Meta J, et al (Univ of California, Los Angeles; Northern California PET Imaging Ctr, Sacramento)
J Nucl Med 43:325-329, 2002   2–11

Background.—Breast cancer can be accurately identified, staged, and restaged by using ^{18}F-FDG PET. This modality has also been used successfully in monitoring tumor response to chemotherapy. Whether FDG PET predicts outcome in patients with breast cancer after primary treatment with similar or superior accuracy than that of conventional imaging (CI) is not known. The ability of ^{18}F-FDG PET and CI to predict outcomes in patients with breast cancer who had undergone primary treatment was examined.

Methods.—Sixty-one women with a median age of 54 years (range, 32-91 years) were re-evaluated with ^{18}F-FDG PET and CI at a median interval between last treatment and PET of 0.4 years (range, 0-16 years). Patients underwent PET within 3 months of CI (median interval, 25 days; range, 2-84 days). To ascertain the independent effect of PET on outcome, PET images were reinterpreted in blinded fashion. The availability of clinical information after PET scanning (median, 21 months) was required for study inclusion. End points were clinical evidence of progression of disease or death.

Findings.—At the time of last follow-up, 19 (31.1%) of 61 patients were considered free of disease, 38 (62.3%) had clinical evidence of stable or progressive disease, and 4 (6.6%) had died. The positive predictive value (PPV) of PET was 93%, and the negative predictive value (NPV) was 84%. The PPV and NPV of CI were 85% and 59%, respectively. The prognostic accuracy of a single whole-body PET image was better than that of multiple procedures with CI (90% vs. 75%; $P < .05$). Kaplan-Meier estimates of disease-free survival in patients with negative PET findings versus those with positive PET findings demonstrated a significant difference between the 2 curves (log-rank test = .001). Kaplan-Meier estimates of disease-free survival stratified by CI findings revealed a marginally significant difference between patients who were CI-positive and those who were CI-negative (log-rank test = 0.04).

Conclusions.—When used in combination with CI modalities, ^{18}F-FDG PET added accuracy to the prediction of outcome in patients with breast cancer who were reassessed after primary treatment.

▶ In the evaluation of the performance and imaging study, assessment groups want to know more than the sensitivity, specificity, and accuracy of the study. The impact of the imaging study on outcome is now being sought as an indicator of the usefulness of the study. This study demonstrates that FDG-PET imaging is superior to conventional imaging in predicting outcome of patients who have previously been treated for breast cancer.

R. E. Coleman, MD

Fluorodeoxyglucose Positron Emission Tomography for Detection of Recurrent or Metastatic Breast Cancer

Kim T-S, Moon WK, Lee D-S, et al (Seoul Natl Univ, Korea)
World J Surg 25:829-834, 2001   2–12

Background.—Locally recurrent disease and distant metastases are sought in the follow-up examinations performed after primary surgery for breast cancer patients. With early detection, treatment options are maximized, which influences overall survival. Whole-body FDG PET offers an especially useful technique for detecting recurrent disease and screening for occult distant metastases. The diagnostic accuracy of PET imaging was tested in patients who were suspected of having recurrent or metastatic breast cancer after undergoing primary surgery.

Methods.—Twenty-seven patients (aged 28 to 62 years; mean age, 46 years) suspected of having recurrent breast carcinoma had whole-body FDG-PET scans. The resulting images were assessed for each patient and lesion in a qualitative manner.

Results.—The 27 patients had 61 reference sites of malignant or benign lesions; 17 patients had confirmed recurrent or metastatic breast cancer and 10 had no evidence of recurrence. Sixteen of the 17 and 8 of the 10 were correctly identified on FDG-PET scans. The sensitivity was 94%, specificity was 80%, accuracy was 89% and positive and negative predictive values were 89%. The lesion-based analysis confirmed that 48 sites were recurrent or metastatic and 13 were not. FDG-PET scans showed 46 of 48 lesions and 11 of 13 lesions correctly.

For lesion sites, the sensitivity was 96%; specificity was 85%; accuracy was 93%; and the predictive values were positive, 96% and negative, 85%. For local recurrences, the sensitivity was 88%, specificity was 100%, and accuracy was 92%. Regional lymph node recurrences showed a sensitivity of 95%, specificity of 67%, and accuracy of 91%. For bone metastases, the sensitivity was 100%, specificity was 83%, and accuracy was 93%. FDG PET had a relatively high sensitivity for detecting distant metastatic lesions, an acceptable specificity, and a high degree of accuracy.

Conclusion.—Local recurrences, lymph node metastases, and distant metastases were all detected by the FDG-PET technique with high levels of sensitivity and accuracy and acceptable levels of specificity. Whole-body FDG-PET imaging allows a more reliable estimate of the true extent of disease, which has an impact on the choice of treatment.

▶ FDG-PET imaging is now covered by Medicare for staging, restaging, and monitoring the effect of therapy. This study confirms the high accuracy of FDG-PET scanning in restaging of patients after surgery. Almost 50% of the patients had their management changed based on the results of the PET scan.

R. E. Coleman, MD

Positron Emission Mammography-Guided Breast Biopsy
Raylman RR, Majewski S, Weisenberger AG, et al (West Virginia Univ, Morgantown; Jefferson Lab, Newport News, Va)
J Nucl Med 42:960-966, 2001   2–13

Introduction.—The use of positron emission mammography (PEM) in conjunction with x-ray mammography has been suggested for guiding biopsy of the breast. This approach relies on the use of a standard stereotactic x-ray mammogram–based system to determine the position of suggestive lesions also identified with PEM. This reliance on the ability to identify the lesion with x-ray screenings may restrict the versatility of this approach. The dual-image approach may by suboptimal in situations in which PEM imaging suggests a suspicious lesion and standard x-ray mammography produces indeterminate findings because of cystic or radiodense breast tissue.

A previously proposed approach for calculating the stereotactic coordinates of photon-emitting objects was adapted to the guidance of breast biopsy using PEM images. The capabilities of this new approach for guiding the biopsy of suspicious radiotracer-avid breast lesions were examined by means of simulated breasts.

Methods.—The PEM system includes 2 square (10 × 10-cm) arrays of discrete scintillator crystals. Detectors were placed on a stereotactic biopsy table. The stereotactic approach used 2 PEM images acquired at ±15° and a new trigonometric algorithm. The accuracy and precision of the guidance approach were evaluated by placement of small point sources of ^{18}F at known locations. Additionally, simulated stereotactic biopsies were performed of a breast phantom consisting of a 10-mm–diameter gelatin sphere with a concentration of ^{18}F-FDG consistent with that for breast cancer.

The simulated lesion was placed in a 4-cm–thick slab of gelatin containing a commonly reported concentration of FDG, simulating a compressed breast (target-to-background ratio, nearly 8.5:1). An anthropomorphic torso phantom was used to simulate tracer uptake in the organs of a patient 1 hour after administration of a 370-MBq injection of FDG. Five trials of the biopsy procedure were performed to evaluate repeatability. A method for verifying needle positioning was examined.

Results.—The positions of the point sources were successfully determined to within 0.6 mm of their true positions with a mean error of ±0.4 mm. The biopsy procedures, including the technique for verification of needle position, were successful in all 5 trials in acquiring samples from the simulated lesions.

Conclusion.—The success of the new PEM-guided breast biopsy approach has potential for guiding the biopsy of breast lesions optimally identified by PEM.

▶ Specialty devices for PET imaging are being developed. Several groups now have PEM available for evaluation. I am familiar with 1 group that is developing a specific prostate-imaging device. We need more data on the accuracy of PEM in the characterization of breast lesions. If the accuracy is good, its use in guiding breast biopsy could be important.

R. E. Coleman, MD

Impact of Whole-Body ^{18}F-FDG PET on Staging and Managing Patients With Breast Cancer: The Referring Physician's Perspective
Yap CS, Seltzer MA, Schiepers C, et al (Univ of California, Los Angeles; Northern California PET Imaging Ctr, Sacramento)
J Nucl Med 42:1334-1337, 2001   2–14

Introduction.—Several trials have shown that FDG PET identifies and stages breast cancer with a high diagnostic accuracy. It has been used to monitor the effects of treatment in patients with breast cancer. The impact of whole-body FDG-PET imaging on the staging and management of breast cancer was evaluated from the referring physician's perspective.

Methods.—Standardized questionnaires were mailed to the referring physicians of 160 patients with breast cancer. Physicians were asked if and how PET findings influenced patient stage and clinical management decisions. Management changes were classified as intermodality if the change was from 1 modality to another or as intramodality if the change was within the same modality.

Results.—Fifty of 160 surveys were returned (31% response rate). The clinical stage was changed by PET in 36% of patients (28% were upstaged and 8% were downstaged). Intermodality and intramodality changes were made in 28% and 30% of patients, respectively, as a result of FDG PET.

Conclusion.—Referring physicians reported that FDG PET has a important influence on the management of patients with breast cancer. Clinical stage and treatment approach were altered in 36% and 60% of patients, respectively.

▶ This article is one of several from the UCLA School of Medicine and the Northern California PET Imaging Center evaluating the impact of PET imaging on patient management. The results of several studies have documented the fact that PET does have a major impact on staging patients and on the subsequent management of the patients.

R. E. Coleman, MD

Positron Emission Tomography for the Evaluation of Metastases in Patients With Carcinoma of the Cervix: A Retrospective Review
Kerr IG, Manji MF, Powe J, et al (King Faisal Specialist Hosp and Research Ctr, Riyadh, Saudi Arabia)
Gynecol Oncol 81:477-480, 2001   2–15

Background.—Carcinoma of the cervix is one of the most frequently occurring cancers in women throughout the world. The treatment for this cancer is based on the International Federation of Gynecology and Obstetrics (FIGO) staging, but this clinical staging system can fail to detect the presence of pelvic and para-aortic node metastases. In addition to FIGO staging, the presence and size of pelvic and para-aortic (PA) lymph node metastases are important prognostic indicators. The identification of PA or more distant disease not only changes the prognosis but also alters the selection of treatment strategies. Surgical approaches have been considered the gold standard for the detection of PA disease, but a need exists for the use of other accurate noninvasive techniques. The utility of PET scanning for the evaluation of nodal and distant metastases for patients with carcinoma of the cervix was investigated.

Methods.—A retrospective review was conducted of 13 patients with carcinoma of the cervix who underwent FDG-PET scanning as part of their workup between 1997 and 1999. For 10 patients, the FDG-PET scan was performed during the initial workup, and the remaining 3 patients underwent FDG-PET scanning at relapse. Ten patients also underwent a fine-needle aspiration (FNA) under imaging guidance for verification.

Results.—The 10 patients with positive findings for carcinoma of the cervix on FDG-PET scanning who underwent an FNA were all positive for cancer. In the remaining 3 patients, the FDG-PET scanning identified cancer sites that were negative on other imaging studies.

Conclusions.—FDG-PET scanning is a useful modality for the evaluation of patients with carcinoma of the cervix. The findings of this study are supportive of other limited published data and indicative of the need for additional prospective studies.

▶ PET scanning is useful in evaluating patients with cervical cancer. This small study of the use of PET in staging and restaging cervical cancer demonstrates the potential utility of the modality. Other studies have documented the prognostic significance of the FDG-PET scan for patients with cervical cancer.

R. E. Coleman, MD

2-[Fluorine-18]-Fluoro-2-Deoxy-D-Glucose Positron Emission Tomography in the Diagnosis of Recurrent Ovarian Cancer
Zimny M, Siggelkow W, Schröder W, et al (Aachen Univ of Technology, Germany)
Gynecol Oncol 83:310-315, 2001   2–16

Background.—In up to 75% of patients with ovarian cancer, advanced disease is present at diagnosis because of a lack of previous symptoms. Those treated often have a relapse, which is indicated by a progressive rise in the tumor marker CA-125. However, imaging, usually CT, must be used to complete the diagnosis. The use of FDG PET can obtain relevant information for the primary diagnosis and staging of advanced ovarian cancer, but data are limited concerning its applicability in the detection of recurrent cases. The role of FDG PET was assessed in a population of patients being followed up after treatment for ovarian cancer.

Methods.—Of 106 FDG-PET scans (54 patients) assessed, 58 were done in patients suspected to have recurrent disease and 48 were done in patients deemed disease free based on clinical findings. PET scans were done a median of 7 months after the last cycle of chemotherapy, and the results were retrospectively re-evaluated without reference to findings on physical examination, imaging modalities, tumor marker levels, or other clinical information. Receiver operating characteristic curve analysis was carried out to determine the diagnostic accuracy for FDG PET.

Results.—On histologic or cytologic evaluation, a tumor relapse was detected in 34 patients and ruled out in 3. On follow-up, 51 cases of recurrent disease were noted, and a tumor relapse was excluded in 15. Of 88 cases assessed, 73 cases of recurrent disease were correctly identified by FDG PET (Fig 1). False-positive results were noted in 1 patient with cystic alterations of an ovarian ligament and in 2 with nonspecific bowel activity. Both conventional diagnosis and PET found 12 of 15 false-negative cases. The sensitivity and specificity of FDG PET were both 83%. When patients were suspected of having recurrent disease, the sensitivity of PET was 94%; when patients were considered disease free, the sensitivity was only 65%. When a recurrence was suspected on the basis of a rise in the CA-125 level only, PET's sensitivity was 96%. Twelve patients who were clinically disease free had a recurrence correctly identified by PET, and these results were obtained

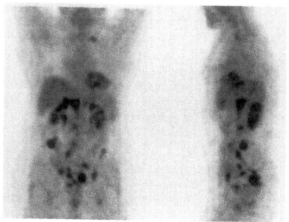

FIGURE 1.—Coronal (**left**) and sagittal (**right**) views of a widespread recurrence of poorly differentiated ovarian cancer 15 months after initial treatment. Multiple hypermetabolic lesions in pelvis and abdomen indicating peritoneal spread. A lymph node metastasis is shown in the left supraclavicular region. (Courtesy of Zimny M, Siggelkow W, Schröder W, et al: 2-[Fluorine-18]-fluoro-2-deoxy-D-glucose positron emission tomography in the diagnosis of recurrent ovarian cancer. *Gynecol Oncol* 83:310-315, 2001.)

a median of 6 months before conventional diagnosis. When the PET scan finding was negative, the median relapse-free interval was 20 months; when it was positive, the median relapse-free interval was 6 months.

Conclusions.—The use of FDG PET detected recurrent ovarian cancer with good sensitivity and specificity, especially in those suspected to have a recurrence. In addition, the PET scans were capable of detecting a recurrence before conventional methods. Patients whose PET scan findings are negative have a longer interval without a relapse than do those whose PET scan findings are positive.

▶ More studies are needed on the utility of FDG-PET imaging in recurrent ovarian cancer. Two or 3 studies have now demonstrated that PET is useful in detecting recurrent ovarian cancer. The prognostic information that is provided is important information.

R. E. Coleman, MD

The Clinical Impact of ¹⁸F-FDG PET in Patients With Suspected or Confirmed Recurrence of Colorectal Cancer: A Prospective Study
Kalff V, Hicks RJ, Ware RE, et al (Peter MacCallum Cancer Inst, East Melbourne, Australia)
J Nucl Med 43:492-499, 2002
2–17

Background.—Patients suspected of having colorectal cancer recurrence can be evaluated using ¹⁸F-FDG PET scanning, which is superior to conventional staging techniques, generally including CT, especially in detecting extrahepatic disease. The clinical impact of ¹⁸F-FDG PET scanning on the man-

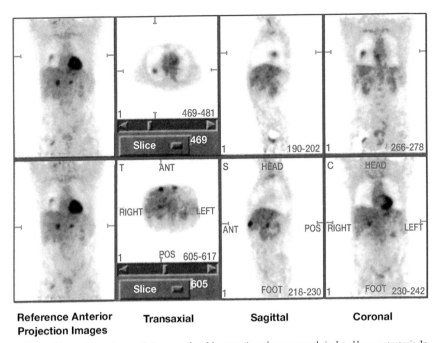

Reference Anterior Projection Images   **Transaxial**   **Sagittal**   **Coronal**

FIGURE 2.—This patient was being considered for resection of an apparently isolated lung metastasis. In addition to lung lesion shown in **upper panel**, PET found additional multiple liver metastases not apparent on CT, as shown in **lower panel**. Surgery was avoided, and abdominal metastases were subsequently confirmed by serial imaging. (Reprinted by permission of the Society of Nuclear Medicine from Kalff V, Hicks RJ, Ware RE, et al: The clinical impact of ^{18}F-FDG PET in patients with suspected or confirmed recurrence of colorectal cancer: A prospective study. *J Nucl Med* 43:492-499, 2002.)

agement of recurrent colorectal cancer in routine oncologic practice was assessed, as well as the validity of PET-induced changes in management. Because PET results were unlikely to change the management of patients who had confirmed disseminated metastases, these patients were not evaluated.

Methods.—A treatment plan was prospectively assigned for 102 consecutive patients undergoing PET for suspected or confirmed colorectal cancer recurrence. None had evidence of unresectable disease as shown by conventional methods. The treatment plan was compared with one based on incremental information obtained on the PET scan, and changes in management were validated on follow-up.

Results.—Overall, PET results led to the alteration of management decisions in 59% of the patients evaluated. Ninety-eight percent of the findings in the 50 evaluable patients with positive PET findings were confirmed as having a relapse. Variation in the active treatment planned was the change made most frequently. Surgery and local radiotherapy management choices were prevented correctly in 31 patients and initiated in 18 patients; 60% of the 43 patients who were supposed to undergo surgical intervention did not do so, based on PET scans. Ten of those with apparently limited metastases underwent surgery, with 2 cases detected by PET to be inoperable being confirmed. Among the 19 patients identified on CT as having solitary liver metastases, 2 had more hepatic metastases, 8 had extrahepatic disease, and 3 had more extensive intrahepatic spread and extrahepatic disease on PET. In 9 patients, PET was clearly correct for the presence and extent of relapse, but it was ignored inappropriately; in 2 patients, PET found that relapse was present but it underestimated the disease's extent. Generally, using PET led to correct management decisions (Fig 2).

Conclusion.—[18]F-FDG PET proved useful in determining the appropriate management of patients with suspected or confirmed colorectal cancer recurrence. Underestimation of disease can occur when there is a single PET ^{18}F-FDG–positive lesion that is believed to be suitable for surgery or when structural lesions that are less than 1 cm in size and are PET negative are found.

► Several studies have documented the impact of PET on patient management, and these studies have shown an average of approximately 30% of the patients have their management changed. In this study of patients with suspected or confirmed recurrence of colorectal cancer, 59% of the patients had their management directly influenced by the result of the PET scan. The impact that PET has in patient management is impressive. On a daily basis in a PET reading room, PET identifies a previously unidentified disease. It is nice to see the clinical impressions from the reading room documented by studies such as this.

R. E. Coleman, MD

Evaluation of (Pre-)Malignant Colonic Abnormalities: Endoscopic Validation of FDG-PET Findings
Drenth JPH, Nagengast FM, Oyen WJG (Univ Med Ctr St Radboud, Nijmegen, The Netherlands)
Eur J Nucl Med 28:1766-1769, 2001   2–18

Background.—Most colorectal cancers are thought to develop from adenomatous polyps, and their early detection should allow prevention of progressive malignant disease. The use of FDG PET has detected many tumor foci and may be superior to CT for assessing patients with recurrent colorectal cancer. Whether FDG-PET imaging can detect possibly premalignant colorectal lesions was investigated.

Methods.—The study included 13 women and 26 men (mean age, 62.3 years) who were selected to undergo both FDG PET and endoscopy during 2 years with a maximal interval between examinations of 3 months. Twenty-four patients had colorectal malignancies, 9 had other malignancies, and 6 had other disorders. FDG-PET results were compared with those of sigmoidoscopic or colonoscopic examinations, which were usually performed as a component in the follow-up of resected colorectal cancer. Carcinoembryogenic antigen (CEA) measurements were also taken.

Results.—The sensitivity of FDG PET was 74%, and its specificity was 84%; its positive predictive value was 78%, and its negative predictive value was 81%, with an odds ratio of 19.7. FDG PET and endoscopy found significant lesions of the colon in 14 (35.8%) patients, and the site of FDG accumulation corresponded with the site of the lesion. PET did not find small polyps in 4 patients. The abnormal accumulation of FDG prompted endoscopy in 9 patients without any other indications; large adenomatous polyps with mild-to-moderate dysplasia were found in 4 patients and carcinomas in 2, but 3 patients had no abnormalities on endoscopy.

Conclusions.—The accumulation of FDG usually corresponded to the site of carcinomas or large adenomatous polyps. Thus, FDG PET was useful in detecting the colorectal cancers but missed small adenomatous polyps. Two thirds of the cases where FDG PET indicated an abnormality showed significant pathology on endoscopy, so that clinical management was altered.

▶ The differentiation of physiologic and pathologic accumulation within the bowel is not easy. The determination of when focal accumulation is too much and suggests disease is very subjective. However, all of us who read many PET scans do identify focal areas of accumulation that are greater than expected. It is not surprising that PET misses small polyps. It is interesting that when the endoscopy was performed in 9 patients because of findings on the PET scan, 4 of these patients had large adenomas and 2 had carcinomas. Abnormal focal accumulation in the bowel should not be ignored.

R. E. Coleman, MD

Value of Positron Emission Tomography With [F-18]Fluorodeoxyglucose in Patients With Colorectal Liver Metastases: A Prospective Study
Ruers TJM, Langenhoff BS, Neeleman N, et al (Univ Med Ctr Nijmegen, The Netherlands)
J Clin Oncol 20:388-395, 2002   2–19

Background.—Patients with colorectal carcinoma can undergo supposedly curative resection; however, 50% may develop liver metastases within 5 years. Even after resection of metastases, 60% to 65% of patients develop recurrent disease, suggesting that tumor foci are not being detected. FDG-PET scans may offer an improved modality for staging, providing information on tumor growth that is based on increased glucose uptake and metabolism in malignant cells. The clinical significance of FDG PET in an adjunct role with conventional diagnostic modalities (CDM) was assessed prospectively for its possible utility with candidates for resection of colorectal liver metastases.

Methods.—A complete workup was performed with CDM in 51 patients being assessed for resection of colorectal liver metastases, and the management decisions were recorded. FDG-PET scans were then done, and changes in clinical management on the basis of the PET analysis were noted. Discrepancies between CDM and FDG-PET findings were documented and compared with the final diagnosis using histopathologic, intraoperative, and follow-up data.

Results.—The extrahepatic findings of CT in 40 (78%) patients reflected the FDG-PET findings and were confirmed. In 8 (16%) patients, CDM found no evidence of more extrahepatic lesions, but such evidence was found by FDG-PET scans, which proved to be accurate for 7 (88%) patients. In 3 patients, CDM indicated additional extrahepatic metastases, but FDG PET found 1 false-negative (lung metastasis), 1 true-negative (benign lung lesions), and 1 local recurrence on CT that was not confirmed by either FDG PET or follow-up. FDG PET found 43 (65%) of the 66 liver metastases. Lesions whose diameter was 1.5 cm or less were best visualized on spiral CT; 64% of those measuring 1.5 cm were found on CT, but only 14% on FDG PET. Lesions between 1.5 and 3 cm in diameter were seen with comparable sensitivity by FDG PET and CT, and those greater than 3 cm were seen with 100% accuracy by both methods. FDG-PET scans indicated that 12 patients should be upstaged (11 correctly) and 7 downstaged (5 correctly). For 26 patients, the combined CDM and FDG-PET work-up indicated no need for surgical exploration. For 25 patients, laparotomy was performed, which found unresectable lesions in 10 patients; the causes were extensive liver involvement, diaphragmatic and intestinal tumor involvement, or a retroperitoneal/peritoneal metastasis. Ten patients (20%) had their clinical management decisions changed when the FDG-PET findings were available. In addition, retrospective analysis showed that choices for 15 patients (29%) could have been altered.

Conclusions.—The information offered by FDG PET led to radical management decision changes in 20% of patients who were analyzed for resection of colorectal liver metastases. Thus, FDG PET provided significant information not obtained on CDM and may be appropriately included in staging algorithms.

▶ Several studies have documented that FDG-PET results in a change in patient management in as many as 50% of patients with a mean change of 30%. In this prospective study in which FDG PET was performed after the conventional diagnostic workup, 20% of the patients had their management changed on the basis of the PET findings. Studies continue to show that PET does have a major impact on patient management.

R. E. Coleman, MD

Detection of Hepatic Metastases From Cancers of the Gastrointestinal Tract by Using Noninvasive Imaging Methods (US, CT, MR Imaging, PET): A Meta-analysis

Kinkel K, Lu Y, Both M, et al (Geneva Univ Hosp; Univ of California, San Francisco; Christian-Albrechts-Universität zu Kiel, Germany)

Radiology 224:748-756, 2002

2–20

Background.—Numerous noninvasive methods are used to detect hepatic metastases from cancers of the gastrointestinal (GI) tract. This meta-analysis compares the accuracy and sensitivity of US, contrast-enhanced CT, MRI, and FDG PET in identifying hepatic metastases from colorectal, gastric, and esophageal cancers.

Methods.—The authors searched the MEDLINE database from December 1985 to December 2000 and relevant reference lists to identify trials that compared the sensitivities of these 4 methods in diagnosing hepatic metastases from GI cancers. To be included, the trial had to involve histopathologic confirmation at 1 site or more of hepatic metastasis or follow-up for 6 months or more, and all images had to have been interpreted by investigators blinded to the histopathologic findings. The authors also searched their own institutional records to identify patients who met the inclusion criteria. Two authors independently abstracted data to ensure their integrity. Summary-weighted estimates of sensitivity were calculated, and only those data sets reporting a specificity of 85% or more were compared. The influence of patient or study factors on sensitivity was examined in covariate analyses.

Results.—A total of 54 data sets fulfilling the inclusion criteria were extracted from 32 published articles and the authors' institutional records. The data included 9 US data sets involving 509 patients, 25 contrast-enhanced CT data sets involving 1747 patients, 11 MRI data sets involving 401 patients, and 9 FDG PET data sets involving 423 patients. Within the studies reporting a specificity of 85% or more, US had a mean weighted sensitivity of 55%; the mean weighted sensitivity of CT was 72%, that of MRI was 76%, and that of PET was 90%. In pairwise comparisons, PET was significantly more sensitive than any of the other 3 modalities, whereas the sensitivities of US, CT, and MRI did not differ significantly from each other. Covariate analyses indicated that the sensitivity of all 4 studies increased as the prevalence of metastasis increased. PET was significantly more sensitive than US, CT, or MRI in these analyses as well.

Conclusion.—This meta-analysis indicates that, at equivalent specificity, the most sensitive noninvasive modality for identifying hepatic metastases caused by GI cancers is FDG PET. However, protocols for the use of FDG PET in imaging hepatic metastases need to be standardized before this methodology can be widely and reliably incorporated into clinical practice.

▶ In studies that have directly compared PET with the anatomical imaging modality in patients with suspected hepatic metastases from cancers of the GI tract, PET has been demonstrated to have the better accuracy. This meta-analysis confirms the higher sensitivity of PET at an equivalent specificity of the modalities.

R. E. Coleman, MD

The Role of F-18 FDG Positron Emission Tomography in Preoperative Assessment of the Liver in Patients Being Considered for Curative Resection of Hepatic Metastases From Colorectal Cancer
Rohren EM, Paulson EK, Hagge R, et al (Duke Univ, Durham, NC)
Clin Nucl Med 27:550-555, 2002   2–21

Background.—FDG PET is more sensitive than CT in identifying extrahepatic metastases of colorectal cancer. The accuracy of FDG PET in diagnosing intrahepatic metastases of colorectal cancer, however, is less well established. The sensitivity and specificity of FDG PET in the diagnosis of hepatic metastases of colorectal cancer were examined, along with its accuracy in determining the number and distribution of hepatic metastatic lesions.

Methods.—The medical records of 23 patients (15 men and 8 women; mean age, 62 years) with colorectal cancer who were being evaluated for surgical resection of possible hepatic metastasis were reviewed. All patients underwent preoperative FDG PET and intraoperative CT. The results of FDG PET were retrospectively compared with those of CT and surgical exploration.

Results.—Hepatic metastasis was confirmed at surgery in 22 of the 23 patients. FDG PET accurately excluded hepatic metastasis in the 1 patient who did not have metastasis (specificity, 100%) and was positive in 21 of the 22 patients with hepatic metastasis (sensitivity, 95%). These 21 patients had a total of 48 metastatic lesions in the liver. PET identified 38 of these 48 lesions (79%). The lesions not detected by PET were significantly smaller than those

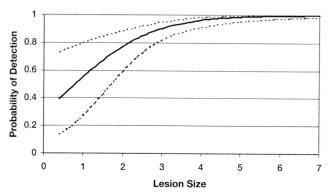

FIGURE 2.—The probability curve for detection of colorectal metastases by PET as a function of lesion size. Mean values (*solid line*) and 95% confidence intervals (*dashed lines*) are shown. Logistic regression analysis with a generalized estimating equation adjustment was used for clustering of lesions within patients. (Courtesy of Rohren EM, Paulson EK, Hagge R, et al: The role of F-18 FDG positron emission tomography in preoperative assessment of the liver in patients being considered for curative resection of hepatic metastases from colorectal cancer. *Clin Nucl Med* 27(8):550-555, 2002.)

that were detected by PET (mean size, 1.6 vs 3.2 cm) (Fig 2). The determination of the distribution of lobar disease with PET was discordant with surgical findings in 3 of the 23 patients evaluated (13%). These 3 cases included 1 patient with a negative PET scan who had 2 lesions in the right lobe, 1 patient with bilobar disease whom PET indicated had disease only in the right lobe, and 1 patient with disease confined to the right lobe whom PET indicated had bilobar disease.

Conclusion.—FDG PET accurately predicted the presence and absence of hepatic metastasis in patients with colorectal cancer. PET performed less well when lesions were small, and it was not as accurate in detecting individual hepatic lesions. Thus, intraoperative US is a better method for determining the number and distribution of metastatic hepatic lesions in patients with colorectal cancer.

▶ This article is written by my colleagues from Duke. The results demonstrate the high accuracy of FDG PET in detecting hepatic metastases in patients with colorectal cancer. However, it also points out the limitations of detecting individual hepatic metastases, particularly lesions less than 2 cm in size.

R. E. Coleman, MD

Whole-Body PET With FDG for the Diagnosis of Recurrent Gastric Cancer
De Potter T, Flamen P, Van Cutsem E, et al (Univ Hosp Leuven, Belgium)
Eur J Nucl Med 29:525-529, 2002   2–22

Background.—The prognosis of gastric cancer is extremely poor, with at least 80% of patients with a more advanced tumor stage initially suffering recurrence and the development of recurrence nearly always fatal. The timing, or when the recurrence develops (within 1 year of diagnosis or after 5 years of disease-free survival), appears to be predictive of the prognosis, with extent of lymph node metastasis serving as an independent factor that predicts timing of recurrence and death. Simple clinical surveillance has proved as useful as biochemical and radiological studies in confirming relapse. While FDG PET has been able to accurately identify primary and recurrent gastrointestinal tumors, few data document its usefulness in gastric cancer. The accuracy of FDG PET in diagnosing recurrent gastric cancer, its sensitivity in predicting recurrent disease related to histologic type of the primary lesion, and its prognostic significance were assessed in patients with recurrent gastric cancer.

Methods.—A PET database provided data for 23 men and 10 women (mean age, 60) who had undergone surgery with curative intent for gastric cancer, then had been evaluated with FDG-PET scan for a suspected recurrence. Results were compared with those obtained through histologic confirmation or radiologic and clinical follow-up, which constituted the gold standard.

Results.—Thirteen patients had signet ring cell carcinoma or mucinous adenocarcinoma, 19 had other adenocarcinomas, and 1 was unknown. A recurrent disease prevalence of 61% was determined using the gold standard (20 of 33 patients). FDG-PET scan achieved a sensitivity of 70%, finding 14 of 20 cases, and a specificity of 69%, or 13 of 20 cases. Its positive and negative predictive values were 78% and 60%, respectively. All 6 false-negative cases had intra-abdominal lesions, and 3 had a signet cell differentiation of their primary tumors. Among those with signet cell differentiation, FDG-PET scan had a sensitivity of 63% and a specificity of 60%; these values were 75% and 75%, respectively, for nonsignet cell primary tumors. Those who were negative on PET scan had a longer survival than those who were positive (18.5 vs 6.9 months).

Conclusions.—A significant correlation was found between FDG-PET uptake and patient survival, with patients who were positive on FDG-PET scan having a significantly shorter survival. Accuracy in detecting recurrent disease was moderate for the FDG-PET scan technique.

▶ A paucity of literature exists on the use of FDG-PET imaging in gastric cancer. One of the problems with the use of FDG-PET imaging in the diagnosis of gastric cancer is the variable accumulation in the stomach. In this study of PET in recurrent gastric cancer, the sensitivity was 70% and specificity 69%. The patients who were PET positive had a significantly shorter survival than those who were PET negative. More studies are needed to determine the role of FDG-PET imaging in gastric cancer.

R. E. Coleman, MD

Fluorine-18 Fluorodeoxyglucose Positron Emission Tomography, Gallium-67 Scintigraphy, and Conventional Staging for Hodgkin's Disease and Non-Hodgkin's Lymphoma
Wirth A, Seymour JF, Hicks RJ, et al (Peter MacCallum Cancer Inst, East Melbourne, Victoria, Australia)
Am J Med 112:262-268, 2002   2–23

Background.—Patients with Hodgkin's disease or non-Hodgkin's lymphoma are treated and their prognoses determined on the basis of staging. Thus the accuracy of staging is critical. The abilities of CT are limited, but the addition of gallium scanning improves staging, response assessment, and confirmation of relapse studies. Another alternative, FDG PET, offers improved spatial resolution, reduced nonspecific abdominal uptake, and a shorter time for imaging. PET and gallium scanning were both used to stage patients with Hodgkin's disease or non-Hodgkin's lymphoma and the results compared with those of conventional assessment.

Methods.—PET, gallium scanning, and conventional staging were available for 50 patients who ranged in age from 17 to 80 years (median age, 48 years). Retrospective analysis focused on disease sites, stage, and subsequent treatment plans.

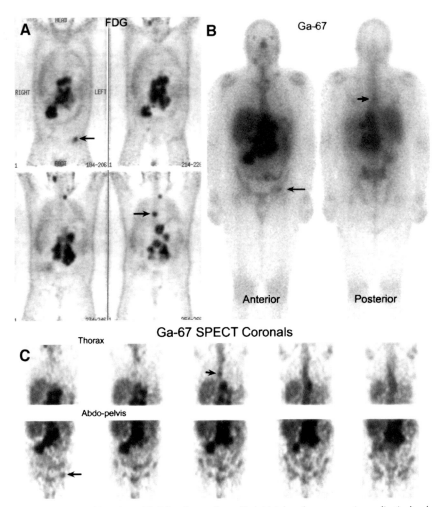

FIGURE 2.—In this patient with diffuse large-cell non-Hodgkin's lymphoma, posterior mediastinal and left inguinal disease (*arrows*) are evident on PET (**A**), but cannot be distinguished from marrow activity on gallium scanning planar (**B**) or SPECT (**C**). (Reprinted from the *American Journal of Medicine* courtesy of Wirth A, Seymour JF, Hicks RJ, et al: Fluorine-18 fluorodeoxyglucose positron emission tomography, gallium-67 scintigraphy, and conventional staging for Hodgkin's disease and non-Hodgkin's lymphoma. *Am J Med* 112:262-268, 2002. Copyright 2002, with permission from Excerpta Medica Inc.)

Results.—Seven cases were upstaged by both PET and gallium scanning in comparison with conventional staging. PET results altered treatment plans in 9 cases; gallium scanning did so in 7 cases. A total of 117 sites and 42 cases were positive. Conventional staging identified 90% of cases as positive, PET identified 95%, and gallium scanning identified 88%. The site positivity rates were 68% for conventional staging, 82% for PET, and 69% for gallium scans. When conventional assessment was combined with either of the other methods, site and case positivity rates exceeded 90%. Of the 13 extranodal positive sites, PET detected 6, gallium 11, and conventional methods 8.

Marrow involvement was not detected on either PET or gallium scanning but was present in 4 patients. Conventional techniques missed 3 cases of Hodgkin's disease in supradiaphragmatic lymph nodes and 1 case of follicular lymphoma in a groin node; PET missed 1 small lymphocytic lymphoma in abdominal nodes and 1 Hodgkin's disease in para-aortic nodes in an extremely obese patient; and gallium missed both of the PET cases plus another case of Hodgkin's disease and 2 large cell lymphomas. Concordance between PET and gallium was present in 31 patients at all positive sites; PET results were positive in an additional 25 nodal sites (Fig 2) and gallium results were positive in an additional 10 sites. Four sites were out of the PET field of view but were detected on gallium scanning.

PET results were positive for 29 sites that were negative or equivocal on conventional methods, and gallium scanning results were positive for 27 sites found negative or equivocal by conventional methods. Of the 50 patients, 2 had at least 1 false-positive site on conventional assessment, 1 on PET, and 2 on gallium scanning.

Conclusion.—PET had a higher site positivity rate than gallium scanning and the case positivity rates were similar between the 2 techniques. Thus PET would be an appropriate alternative to gallium scanning for the staging of Hodgkin's disease or non-Hodgkin's lymphoma in terms of accuracy and it offers several advantages. Its drawbacks are greater cost and lack of availability.

▶ Gallium imaging has been an excellent modality for staging Hodgkin and non-Hodgkin lymphoma. This study is one of many that demonstrate the superiority of FDG PET over gallium scintigraphy and conventional imaging in staging lymphoma. If both FDG-PET and gallium scintigraphy are available, I cannot think of 1 reason why a gallium scan would be performed instead of an FDG-PET scan in a patient with lymphoma.

R. E. Coleman, MD

Comparison of Fluorine-18 Fluorodeoxyglucose Positron Emission Tomography and Ga-67 Scintigraphy in Evaluation of Lymphoma
Kostakoglu L, Leonard JP, Kuji I, et al (Cornell Univ, New York)
Cancer 94:879-888, 2002   2–24

Background.—In the management of patients with lymphomas, it is important to identify the anatomical extent of disease and responses to therapy. CT is the modality of choice for staging lymphomas, but it misses normal-sized lymph nodes that are involved, cannot differentiate between enlarged lymph nodes caused by various mechanisms, and mistakes fibrosis for viable disease. MRI provides better morphological detail than non–contrast-enhanced CT but shows no advantages in disease site identification. The response to therapy and predictions of response early in treatment have been assessed in high-grade lymphomas with use of ⁶⁷Ga imaging. Another modality that can be used in oncology is FDG PET. The accuracy of these newer tools in identifying disease sites in Hodgkin disease (HD) and non-Hodgkin lymphoma (NHL) was compared both at initial staging and with a recurrence before chemotherapy.

Methods.—The 51 consecutive patients (31 male, 20 female; age range, 15-83 years; mean age, 50.7 years) had histologically confirmed lymphomas. Each underwent FDG-PET and ⁶⁷Ga scintigraphy for NHL (35 intermediate grade and 3 high grade) or HD (13). Disease sites were correlated on

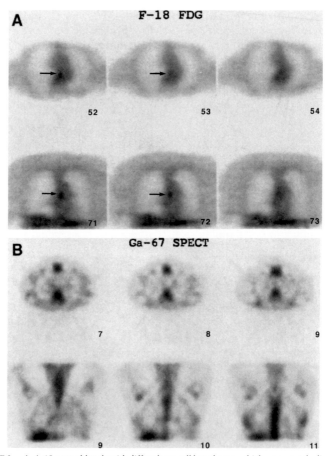

FIGURE 2.—**A,** A 65-year-old male with diffuse large cell lymphoma, which was recently diagnosed, underwent FDG-PET and ⁶⁷Ga imaging for the assessment of extent of disease before the initiation of chemotherapy. FDG PET images demonstrate intense FDG uptake in the chest in the paravertebral area consistent with active lymphoma. **B,** ⁶⁷Ga SPECT images of the chest demonstrate no appreciable uptake in the corresponding region. CT scan revealed a 0.7-cm lymph node in the corresponding region. Posttherapy FDG PET images revealed complete resolution of disease (not shown). Note the nonspecific hilar and bone marrow uptake. (Courtesy of Kostakoglu L, Leonard JP, Kuji I, et al: Comparison of fluorine-18 fluorodeoxyglucose positron emission tomography and Ga-67 scintigraphy in evaluation of lymphoma. *Cancer* 94(4):879-888, 2002. ©2002 American Cancer Society. Reprinted by permission of Wiley-Liss, Inc., a subsidiary of John Wiley & Sons, Inc.)

a site-by-site basis, and tumor-to-background ratios were determined. Any FDG-PET or ^{67}Ga findings that seemed discordant were compared with CT findings or clinical assessments.

Results.—[67]Ga scintigraphic findings (SPECT or planar) were positive in 41 patients at 113 sites, whereas FDG-PET findings were positive for all patients at 158 sites. None of the patients had completely negative findings on ^{67}Ga planar images. Forty-four patients had complete ^{67}Ga SPECT data available; in these patients, FDG-PET findings were positive at 126 sites and ^{67}Ga SPECT findings were positive at 81 sites. At 45 sites, ^{67}Ga SPECT did not detect any disease, and in 10 patients, ^{67}Ga SPECT found no disease at 22 sites and only partially identified 23 sites (Fig 2). The tumor site and histologic features did not correlate with any of these failures. CT showed that the lesions in these patients measured 0.7 to 14.0 cm. Disease at a higher stage than found with ^{67}Ga imaging was identified on FDG PET. No cases had a positive ^{67}Ga SPECT finding and a negative FDG-PET finding. The 2 techniques had statistically different tumor-to-background ratios; FDG PET had higher ratios.

Conclusions.—FDG PET was better than ^{67}Ga scintigraphy in detecting disease sites in patients with intermediate- and high-grade NHL and HD because it was more accurate: FDG PET had a site and a patient sensitivity of 100% compared with a site sensitivity of 71.5% and a patient sensitivity of 80.3% for ^{67}Ga scintigraphy. CT was also surpassed by FDG PET in terms of sensitivity. FDG-PET findings may influence management decisions, and this tool is recommended as a part of the routine staging algorithm for lymphomas.

▶ These results demonstrating the superiority of FDG PET over gallium-67 SPECT imaging were obtained with camera-based PET. The use of a dedicated PET scanner would likely make the discrepancy between the PET and SPECT imaging even greater. Despite the previously wide use of gallium-67 imaging for lymphomas, every article that I have seen comparing PET and SPECT has demonstrated superiority by PET. One must remember that low-grade lymphomas are less sensitive to FDG than are high-grade lymphomas.

R. E. Coleman, MD

Somatostatin-Receptor Scintigraphy for Staging and Follow-up of Patients With Extraintestinal Marginal Zone B-Cell Lymphoma of the Mucosa Associated Lymphoid Tissue (MALT)-Type
Raderer M, Traub T, Formanek M, et al (Univ of Vienna; KH Lainz, Vienna)
Br J Cancer 85:1462-1466, 2001   2–25

Background.—Lymphoma of the mucosa-associated lymphoid tissue (MALT) is a distinct clinicopathologic entity with characteristic histologic features and has been incorporated into the REAL-classification under the term "extranodal marginal zone B-cell lymphoma of MALT-type." Most MALT-type lymphomas begin in the stomach, but extragastric locations are frequently encountered. Previous findings have indicated that somatostatin receptor (SSTR)-expression distinguishes gastric from extragastric MALT-type lymphoma. The role of SSTR-scintigraphy for staging and for follow-up of patients with extragastric MALT-type lymphoma was assessed.

Methods.—The study included 30 consecutive patients with histologically verified MALT-type lymphoma who were prospectively evaluated. Twenty-four patients had primary extragastric MALT-type lymphoma, 5 patients had dissemination to extragastric sites after an initial gastric MALT-type lymphoma, and 1 patient had dissemination to the stomach, lung, and lymph nodes after parotid lymphoma. All of the patients underwent SSTR scintigraphy with ^{111}In-DPTA-D-Phe1-Octreotide (^{111}In-OCT) before chemotherapy or radiotherapy, and 13 patients had a second scan after treatment.

Results.—Findings were compared with conventional staging. No positive scans were obtained in patients with dissemination after gastric lymphoma, while all patients with primary extragastric lymphoma had positive scans at the site of a histologically documented involvement before the initiation of therapy. In the patient with secondary spread to the stomach, lung, and lymph nodes, SSTR-scintigraphy scans were positive in all documented lymphoma sites. In the posttherapy scans, focal tracer accumulation in the left orbit indicated persistence of disease after irradiation in 1 patient with an otherwise negative workup, which was verified by MRI and biopsy 6 months later. In another patient, a positive scan indicated disease relapse in the lacrimal gland 9 months before clinical verification by US.

Conclusions.—^{111}In-OCT is an excellent modality for the staging and noninvasive monitoring of extragastric MALT-type lymphoma, and earlier findings that gastric MALT-type lymphomas do not express relevant amounts of respective SSTR are confirmed. In addition, this study demonstrated that SSTR scanning can distinguish gastric from extragastric MALT-type lymphomas.

▶ Somatostatin-receptor scintigraphy using indium-111 octreotide appears to be an accurate method for staging and follow-up of MALT lymphoma. Previous studies using FDG have shown it to be less accurate in these low-grade lymphomas than most other types of lymphoma. Somatostatin-receptor scintigraphy also appears to be able to restage these patients accurately after therapy.

R. E. Coleman, MD

Head and Neck Imaging With PET and PET/CT: Artefacts From Dental Metallic Implants
Goerres GW, Hany TF, Kamel E, et al (Univ Hosp Zurich, Switzerland)
Eur J Nucl Med 29:367-370, 2002   2–26

Background.—PET has been found to be a reliable imaging method for the staging of patients with malignant disease, including head and neck cancers.

The lesions usually present with high uptake of FDG. However, several anatomic structures in the head and neck can manifest physiologic FDG uptake, which may impair the clear distinction between normal tissue and pathology. Germanium-68 based attenuation correction (PET_{Ge68}) is performed in PET imaging for quantitative measurements. The recent introduction of combined in-line PET/CT scanners has enabled the use of CT data for attenuation correction. Because dental implants can cause artefacts in CT images, CT-based attenuation correction (PET_{CT}) may cause artefacts in PET images. The influence of dental metallic artwork on the quality of PET images by comparison of noncorrected images and image attenuation corrected by PET_{Ge68} and PET CT was evaluated.

Methods.—Imaging in this study was performed with a newly developed in-line PET/CT system using a 40-mAs scan for PET_{CT} in 41 consecutive patients with high suspicion of malignant or inflammatory disease. Additional PET_{Ge68} images were acquired in 17 patients in the same imaging system. Visual analysis of FDG distribution in several regions of the head and neck was scored on a 4-point scale in comparison with normal grey matter of the brain in the corresponding PET images. Artefacts adjacent to dental metallic artwork were also evaluated.

Results.—The only significant difference in image quality scoring was found for the lips and the tip of the nose, which appeared darker on noncorrected than on corrected PET images. Artefacts were seen on CT in 33 patients, and in 28 of these patients the artefacts were also seen on PET imaging. In 8 patients without implants, artefacts were not seen on CT or on PET images. A direct comparison of PET_{Ge68} and PET_{CT} images revealed a different appearance of artifacts in 3 of 17 patients. Malignant lesions were equally well visualized with both transmission correction methods.

Conclusions.—Dental implants can cause artefacts in attenuation-corrected images obtained with either a conventional [68]Ge transmission source or the CT scan obtained with a combined PET/CT camera. It is recommended that the non-attenuation–corrected PET images should also be evaluated in patients who are undergoing PET of the head and neck.

▶ Attenuation correction for PET imaging is performed using either a germanium-68–based correction or, more recently, a CT-based correction. The anatomic information from the CT scan in a combined PET/CT scan is very useful, particularly in evaluating abnormalities in the head and neck. However, artefacts on the attenuation scan may result in artefacts on the attenuation corrected images. Fortunately, the non-attenuation corrected images are quite accurate in evaluating head and neck lesions.

R. E. Coleman, MD

Positron Emission Tomography in the Evaluation of Stage III and IV Head and Neck Cancer

Teknos TN, Rosenthal EL, Lee D, et al (Univ of Michigan, Ann Arbor)
Head Neck 23:1056-1060, 2001   2–27

Background.—The accurate evaluation of distant disease for head and neck squamous cell carcinoma patients is vital to the determination of the appropriate therapeutic approach and prognosis. It is common for distant disease to escape detection in this patient population during conventional preoperative evaluation. The detection of distant disease can radically alter treatment options for these patients, because surgical management is reserved for patients with locoregional disease. Conventional radiographic modalities, such as CT and MRI, can provide excellent anatomical detail but do a poor job of identifying unenlarged lymph nodes that harbor metastatic disease. The utility of ^{18}F FDG-PET detection of metastatic disease in patients with advanced-stage head and neck cancer was evaluated.

Methods.—The study included 12 consecutive patients who underwent prospective total body FDG-PET imaging. All of the patients had a new diagnosis of stage III or IV mucosal squamous cell carcinoma of the head and neck. These patients also underwent chest CT. Histopathologic confirmation of disease was obtained for all patients found to have metastatic disease on either CT or PET imaging.

Results.—FDG-PET scans demonstrated metastatic disease in 3 patients (25%). Two of these patients had no disease on chest radiograph or chest CT but were found to have positive FDG-PET images within the mediastinal lymphatics (Fig 1). For these patients, mediastinoscopy was performed to confirm metastatic disease. The third patient had a peripheral lung lesion detected on chest radiograph, CT and FDG PET. On CT-guided biopsy, this nodule was diagnosed as squamous cell carcinoma.

Conclusions.—FDG-PET scanning detected mediastinal disease in 2 (17%) of patients with advanced head and neck squamous cell carcinoma not identified with conventional imaging techniques. These findings indicate

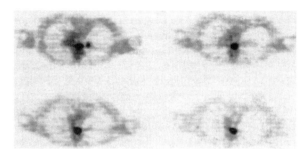

FIGURE 1.—Panels from FDG-PET scan of patient, showing multiple foci of increased uptake in the mediastinum. The patient's CT scan of the chest was entirely normal. (Courtesy of Teknos TN, Rosenthal EL, Lee D, et al: Positron emission tomography in the evaluation of stage III and IV head and neck cancer. *Head Neck* 23:1056-1060, 2001. Copyright 2001. Reprinted by permission of John Wiley & Sons, Inc.)

significant potential exists for PET imaging in the detection of occult metastatic disease, particularly, in the mediastinal lymphatics.

▶ This study of 12 consecutive patients with a new diagnosis of stage III or IV mucosa squamous cell carcinoma of the head and neck provides additional data on the utility of PET imaging in head and neck cancer. A cost analysis performed in this study suggests that the savings by having a PET scan are greater than $17,000 for the patients in this study. As has been shown by previous studies, the avoidance of surgery that will not benefit the patient does result in cost savings.

R. E. Coleman, MD

The Use of Lymphoscintigraphy and PET in the Management of Head and Neck Melanoma
Kokoska MS, Olson G, Kelemen PR, et al (St Louis Univ Health Sciences Ctr; Mayo Clinic Found, Rochester, Minn; Pennsylvania State Univ, Hershey)
Otolaryngol Head Neck Surg 125:213-220, 2001   2–28

Objectives.—Lymphoscintigraphy with sentinel node dissection and 18 fluoro-2-deoxyglucose PET are being used independently in the management of many intermediate and thick melanomas of the head and neck. We report a series of patients with melanoma of the head and neck with Breslow depths greater than 1.0 mm and clinically negative regional nodes that were evaluated prospectively with PET and lymphoscintigraphy.

Study Design and Setting.—Between July 1, 1998, and December 30, 2000, PET scans were obtained preoperatively on 18 patients undergoing resection of head and neck melanoma. Lymphoscintigraphy and sentinel node dissection were performed. Resection of the primary lesion was then carried out with adequate margins, and the defects were reconstructed.

Results.—Sentinel node(s) were found in 17 of 18 patients (94.4%); 5 of the 18 (27.8%) patients had metastases. PET detected nodal metastasis preoperatively in 3 patients (16.7%), 1 of which had a positive sentinel node dissection.

Conclusion.—PET and lymphoscintigraphy offer complementary ways of evaluation for metastatic melanoma.

▶ Sentinel lymph node studies are more sensitive for detecting lymph node involvement than is PET imaging. This finding is not surprising because microscopic disease is detected pathologically by the use of lymphoscintigraphy. PET should not be used in an attempt to avoid lymphoscintigraphy in the evaluation of patients with melanoma.

R. E. Coleman, MD

Initial Results in the Assessment of Multiple Myeloma Using ^{18}F-FDG PET

Schirrmeister H, Bommer M, Buck AK, et al (Univ of Ulm, Germany; J W Goethe Univ of Frankfurt, Germany)
Eur J Nucl Med 29:361-366, 2002   2–29

Background.—The clinical course of multiple myeloma (MM) varies widely, and survival can range from under 1 month to over 10 years. Differentiating MM from a solitary plasmacytoma (PC) or monoclonal gammopathy of unknown significance can be difficult. Using PET with FDG allows nodal and extranodal manifestations of lymphoma to be viewed in a single examination and is highly accurate in depicting infiltration of the bone marrow. The appearance and distribution pattern of PC and MM were evaluated by FDG PET, and the accuracy of FDG PET in detecting MM lesions was assessed with respect to its impact on staging and clinical management decisions.

Methods.—Twenty-eight patients with known MM and 15 with solitary PC were assessed by FDG PET, and the results were checked against findings on radiographs, MRI, CT, and clinical assessment. Bone marrow involvement was defined as intense FDG uptake in the complete skeleton.

Results.—All 5 of the extramedullary PC lesions and 9 of the 10 bone PC lesions were detected on FDG PET. In addition, among patients who were assumed to have solitary PC, FDG PET found additional lesions in 1 patient who had vertebral PC and 1 who had extravertebral PC. MM was detected in 19 patients who had the multifocal pattern of disease. Three patterns of FDG uptake in 37 patients with active PC or MM were observed; PET scans were negative in 3 patients with active disease. PET detected 31 of 31 patients who had focal lesions. A positive predictive value for active disease of 75% was found in patients who exhibited diffuse bone marrow uptake.

FDG PET had a sensitivity of 83.8%, specificity of 100%, and accuracy of 86% when using focal lesions as the criterion for active disease. Using both focal lesions and diffuse tracer uptake in bone marrow as criteria, the sensitivity was 91.9%, specificity was 83.3%, and accuracy was 90.7%. True positives were found in 92.7% of MM lesions, and 5 previously unknown lesions were found in 2 patients. The diagnosis of PC was changed to MM based on FDG-PET findings in 2 patients.

Conclusion.—While diffuse bone marrow uptake did not prove to be a reliable predictor of active disease, although active disease is not excluded, focal uptake reliably predicted active disease. PET scans achieved a sensitivity of 83.8% to 91.9% and specificity of 83.3% to 100% in these cases. FDG PET was able to detect lesions not always identified by other imaging modalities. The clinical management of patients with MM or solitary PC can be improved by using FDG PET when greater sensitivity than that achieved with radiographs is required.

▶ The data in the literature on the role of PET in MM are sparse. We have performed PET scans on a few patients with MM at our medical center, and the results of the study have been rewarding. The results from this article demonstrate that PET will be useful in evaluating patients with MM. More data on larger numbers of patients will be published in the near future, but low-prevalence MM appears to be another of the malignancies that PET will be useful in evaluating.

R. E. Coleman, MD

Evaluation of High-Risk Melanoma: Comparison of [^{18}F]FDG PET and High-Dose ^{67}Ga SPET
Kalff V, Hicks RJ, Ware RE, et al (Peter MacCallum Cancer Inst, East Melbourne, Victoria, Australia)
Eur J Nucl Med 29:506-515, 2002   2–30

Background.—The triple peaked gamma cameras led to a greater sensitivity of single-photon emission tomographic (SPET) imaging, when combined with higher gallium-67 (^{67}Ga) doses, in finding locoregional and disseminated melanoma, whereas the multiple imaging sessions required and the questionable clinical usefulness of ^{67}Ga SPET limit its availability. PET imaging that uses fluorine F 18 FDG has demonstrated sensitivity and specificity exceeding 90% in melanoma cases. [^{18}F]FDG PET and high-dose ^{67}Ga SPET techniques were compared.

Methods.—The 121 patients (122 cases of melanoma, most stage II or III, with 9 cases stage IV) were all at high clinical risk for occult metastatic disease and underwent the 2 scans in less than 6 weeks. Forty-nine patients (40%) had an abnormality that suggested metastatic disease on at least 1 functional image. When scan findings did not match, an analysis was carried out to see which technique most accurately reflected the patient's actual disease status.

Results.—While the overall agreement between the 2 techniques was good, some patients whose disease status was graded as the same showed variations in extent of disease. Two of the 20 patients who had equivocal findings on both methods were found to have disease at that site, so equivocal findings were generally considered negative. Nine patients had more abnormalities on ^{67}Ga scans than on PET scans, 6 of which were truly positive for disease, but only 2 led to a change in staging. In 14 patients, FDG PET found more or larger abnormalities than ^{67}Ga scans, and in 5 cases the discrepancy led to a change in clinical stage. Of the 23 cases when PET and SPET results differed, if 3 cases of incidental malignancies are taken as important additional information, PET accurately predicted melanoma stage in 17 and ^{67}Ga in 6. No change in clinical management would have occurred in response to ^{67}Ga findings in 2 of these cases, and none would have been made in 3 of the PET cases. Of the 18 patients for whom management would have been altered, 14 were identified by PET and 4 by ^{67}Ga SPET.

Conclusions.—A higher detection rate and more accurate disease staging in melanoma patients was achieved by using FDG PET than high-dose ^{67}Ga SPET imaging. PET also demonstrated a greater sensitivity in the detection of synchronous or metachronous primary malignancies. Because the added information can lead to changes in management in approximately 10% of patients at a slightly higher cost, FDG PET would be a cost-effective alternative to the ^{67}Ga SPET technique.

▶ Very few nuclear medicine services are performing ^{67}Ga imaging in high-risk melanoma patients. This study, using a sodium iodide detector-based 3-dimensional PET scanner, demonstrated that PET provides more accuracy in detecting recurrent disease than did ^{67}Ga imaging. A bismuth germinate-dedicated PET scanner would be even better. This study confirms the superiority of PET imaging over gallium imaging in melanoma, and we are seeing similar results in lymphoma.

R. E. Coleman, MD

Gamma-Detecting Probe Used Intraoperatively to Locate the Sentinel Lymph Node in Patients With Malignant Melanoma
Sugrañes G, Vidal-Sicart S, Piulachs J, et al (Univ of Barcelona)
Eur J Surg 167:581-586, 2001   2–31

Background.—Only 3% of all neoplasms are malignant melanomas, but every 10 years the incidence increases 2-fold, so 1 of 90 people may eventually be affected by this neoplasm. Metastases follow the route of the lymphatics of the regional nodes, so regional lymphadenectomy is generally indicated when the lymph nodes are involved. The considerable morbidity that attends this radical operation prompted investigations into the use and feasibility of a lymphoscintigram with an intraoperative gamma ray–detecting probe to find the sentinel lymph node. Evidence indicating whether the histologic evaluation of this node can predict the status of the rest of the regional lymph nodes was also sought.

Methods.—Of the 40 patients with malignant melanoma who were evaluated, 24 were stage I/II (11 men and 13 women; mean age, 47 years) and 16 were stage III (8 men and 8 women; mean age, 42 years). Each had a lymphoscintigram with ^{99m}Tc-nanocolloid taken the day before surgery, and the first lymph node that was found was presumed to be the sentinel node. Intraoperative mapping was carried out using a hand-held gamma probe.

Results.—Sentinel nodes were detected in all but 1 patient. In 16 patients, the regional lymph nodes were palpable; 22 sentinel lymph nodes were identified. In 24 patients whose regional lymph nodes could not be palpated, 34 sentinel lymph nodes were noted. Ninety-eight percent of the sentinel nodes were identified preoperatively using the gamma-ray detecting probe. Of the 161 regional lymph nodes harvested, none had been invaded by melanoma. Of the 89 regional lymph nodes excised in patients with invaded sentinel nodes, 44 showed melanomatous invasion and 45 were clear of disease. All 41 lymph nodes excised from patients whose sentinel nodes were not invaded showed no evidence of melanoma.

Conclusion.—Use of the lymphoscintigram and gamma-ray detecting probe allowed the identification of sentinel lymph nodes in all but 1 patient. Patients who had metastases were identified reliably.

▶ The surgical literature continues to be supportive of the use of sentinel lymph node studies in patients with malignant melanoma. This prospective study further documents the utility of the technique and that sentinel node identification seems to work with different radiopharmaceuticals (nanocolloid, filtered sulfur colloid, unfiltered sulfur colloid) and at different times after injection (same day vs next day).

R. E. Coleman, MD

Fluorinated Deoxyglucose Positron Emission Tomography Imaging in Progressive Metastatic Prostate Cancer

Morris MJ, Akhurst T, Osman I, et al (Mem Sloan-Kettering Cancer Ctr, New York; Cornell Univ, New York; New York Univ; et al)
Urology 59:913-918, 2002   2–32

Background.—Metastatic prostate cancer can be difficult to follow accurately, with bone scans not reliably indicating progression or acute changes and few patients having soft tissue disease detectable on standard imaging modalities. Even the prostate-specific antigen (PSA) levels can be misleading in patients with high-grade tumors. While FDG PET has shown limited usefulness in prostate cancer, the mixed patient populations that were used may produce too much heterogeneity to give a clear measure of PET abilities. FDG PET was evaluated in a population of patients with metastatic disease who met standardized biochemical and radiographic criteria for disease progression to see whether it was comparable with standard imaging modalities in detecting osseous and soft tissue lesions.

Methods.—CT, MRI, or bone scan results were compared with those of FDG PET. The 17 patients' PSA levels were all increasing, and their disease was determined to be progressing. Four patients had androgen-dependent and 13 had androgen-independent disease. Standard uptake value (SUV) changes were compared with PSA changes in patients undergoing serial scans after being treated.

Results.—Bone scan, PET, or both found 132 osseous lesions in 14 patients, with 71% proving to be FDG-avid as well as evident on bone scan. All lesions found on PET alone became areas of active disease in 2 to 4 months, whereas all but 1 of those noted only on bone scan were stable up to 1 year after imaging. CT/MRI or PET or both found 23 soft tissue lesions, with 6 patients having none found. The 18 lesions found on CT/MRI were all new or enlarging relative to previous studies. The sample size was not large enough to detect any difference between PET and standard modalities. Twelve cases were evaluated for correlations between changes in PSA and mean SUV after treatment, and 9 showed parallel changes in the 2 parameters. Two showed rises in both and 7 showed falls in both.

Conclusions.—While limited in detecting soft tissue metastases, FDG PET was able to discriminate active osseous lesions from stable ones and showed new lesions before they were detectable on bone scans. Further analysis is required before recommendations regarding the use of FDG PET in prostate carcinoma can be made.

▶ Previous studies on the use of FDG PET in patients with bone metastases from prostate cancer have demonstrated that only a small percentage of the sites that are abnormal on a radionuclide bone scan are FDG avid. These studies have been primarily performed in patients who were responding to hormonal therapy or who had stable disease. In this study, patients who had progressive metastatic prostate cancer had their active bony metastatic disease detected by FDG-PET imaging. PET is limited in detecting soft tissue metastases. The patient population studied can certainly influence the results.

R. E. Coleman, MD

2-[^{18}F]Fluoro-2-deoxyglucose and Glucose Uptake in Malignant Gliomas Before and After Radiotherapy: Correlation With Outcome
Spence AM, Muzi M, Graham MM, et al (Univ of Washington, Seattle)
Clin Cancer Res 8:971-979, 2002
2–33

Background.—Whether quantitative FDG PET has a role in evaluating the response to treatment of patients with malignant glioma or how accurately FDG-PET studies determine long-term outcome is not established. FDG and 1-[^{11}C]glucose have been used as tracers but behave differently in transport, phosphorylation, and glycolysis. Radiotherapy (RT) should kill tumor cells and thus reduce metabolic rate; when tumor cells are not killed, a higher metabolic rate should result. Whether this held true was investigated in adults with malignant gliomas.

Methods.—Thirty patients all had supratentorial malignant gliomas and were evaluated within 2 weeks before and/or 1 to 3 weeks after RT except 1 (assessed 6 weeks after RT). Four patients had imaging performed only before RT, 12 only after RT, and 14 both before and after. Arterial plasma sampling was included in each study. An optimization program was employed in assessing kinetic parameters, glucose metabolic rate (MRGIc), and FDG metabolic rate (MRFDG). The 14 patients who had imaging performed before and after scanning were used to assess changes in MRGIc or MRFDG. In addition, overall survival and survival relative to historical controls were evaluated.

Results.—Higher pre-RT values for MRGIc or MRFDG were associated with a shorter survival time; longer survival was linked to lower values on the parameters before RT was performed. In contrast to the expected findings, increased metabolism determined with either 1-[^{11}C]glucose or FDG from the time RT was begun until the end of treatment was linked to longer survival times and a fall in metabolism with shorter survival. No correlation was found between MRGIc and MRFDG measured shortly after RT and survival. Histology was a significant predictor of survival, and chemotherapy was linked to a 65% lower risk of death.

MRFDG was not as useful as MRGlc in relationship to pre-RT assessments. Comparison of pre-RT with post-RT findings showed a significant relationship between change in MRGlc and survival, with a 10% decline in MRGlc translating to a 75% increase in the risk of death. A 1-unit increase in MRFDG reduced the risk of death by 10%, although this did not become a significant relationship.

Conclusion.—Less aggressive disease was indicated by low MRFDG or MRGlc values before RT, with more aggressive disease accompanying higher values on these parameters. A longer survival is related to an increase in MRFDG or MRGlc between pre-RT and post-RT. This unexpected finding may be attributed to a decrease in tumor cell density that leaves cells with higher metabolism, by infiltration of inflammatory cells that take up either 1-[^{11}C]glucose or FDG where tumor cells are dying, or by the consumption of energy for apoptosis of tumor cells induced by RT. Quantitative PET determinations with either FDG or 1-[^{11}C]glucose showed no correlation with survival.

▶ This study was not an easy one to do. Performing a patient study that includes both arterial blood sampling and administration of 2 radiopharmaceuticals is a major accomplishment. It is good to have the quantitative data, but I am not sure the conclusions would have been changed if the studies were not performed quantitatively. The authors note that they are evaluating their data to determine that absolute quantification was necessary.

It is well known that low levels of glucose or FDG uptake into tumors before therapy portends a good prognosis. The improved prognosis in patients who showed an increase in the accumulation of glucose or FDG after therapy is not expected. The authors provide an excellent discussion of the potential reasons for this unexpected finding.

R. E. Coleman, MD

Localisation of Motor Areas in Brain Tumour Patients: A Comparison of Preoperative [^{18}F]FDG-PET and Intraoperative Cortical Electrostimulation

Schreckenberger M, Spetzger U, Sabri O, et al (Aachen Univ of Technology, Germany)
Eur J Nucl Med 28:1394-1403, 2001   2–34

Background.—One of the most important components of presurgical planning for patients with intracranial tumors is the exact estimation of the spatial relationship of the tumor to adjacent, functionally relevant areas of the brain. The utility of a preoperative ^{18}F FDG-PET activation protocol for patients with tumors near the central area was assessed, and the question of whether this noninvasive preoperative PET imaging protocol can provide results equivalent to those obtained with the "gold standard," an invasive neurosurgical approach, was investigated.

Methods.—The study included 20 patients with various tumors in the central area who underwent 2 PET scans, each after IV injection of 134 to 341 MBq ^{18}F FDG. The first scan was a resting baseline scan, and the second scan was an activation scan performed using a standardized motor task, such as finger tapping or foot stretching. PET/MRI realignment and normalization to the whole brain counts were done, after which parametric images of the activation versus the rest study were calculated. Pixels above categorical threshold values were projected to the individual MRI scan for bimodal assessment of morphology and function (PET/MRI overlay). A Viking IV probe was used to obtain intraoperative direct cortical electrostimulation, with findings documented using a dedicated neuronavigation system. The results were then compared with preoperative PET findings.

Results.—Significant activation of the contralateral primary motor cortex was seen on PET in 95% of the brain tumor patients, with a mean increase in normalized ^{18}F FDG uptake of 20.5% for the hand activation task and 17.2% for the foot activation task. Additionally detected activation of the ipsilateral primary motor cortex was considered a metabolic indication of interhemispheric compensational processes.

Conclusions.—The evaluation of PET findings by cortical stimulation yielded a 94% sensitivity and a 95% specificity for the identification of motor-associated brain areas. These findings suggest that ^{18}F FDG PET activation provides an accurate assessment of the local relationship between an intracranial tumor and the adjacent motor cortex areas. This relatively simple and clinically available protocol may facilitate the presurgical planning for patients about to undergo tumor resection.

▶ Those persons who do FDG-PET imaging of brain tumors will find this a very fascinating study. I have tried to do stimulation on a patient or 2 and was not as successful as the authors in this carefully performed study. Attention to detail must be used for these studies. Image registration is mandatory.

R. E. Coleman, MD

Cancer Research UK Procedures in Manufacture and Toxicology of Radiotracers Intended for Pre-Phase I Positron Emission Tomography Studies in Cancer Patients
Aboagye EO, Luthra SK, Brady F, et al (Imperial College of Science, Technology and Medicine, London)
Br J Cancer 86:1052-1056, 2002   2–35

Background.—The use of PET allows the noninvasive evaluation of anticancer agents' pharmacokinetics and pharmacodynamics in humans even before conventional phase I clinical testing. Compounds labeled with positron-emitting isotopes (radiotracers) are given IV, but no guidelines have been published outlining the process for safety testing of radiopharmaceutical agents before use in clinical trials for patients with cancer. Minimum requirements for product quality, animal toxicology, and initial clinical studies at tracer doses for PET radiopharmaceutical agents used for oncology patients were proposed on the basis of the experience of Cancer Research UK.

Methods.—Only cancer patients and tracer dose studies were assessed; these latter included pharmacokinetic evaluation of new anticancer agents using PET in humans and the evaluation of new PET radiotracers for use in assessing the physiology of human tumors or for use as either pharmacodynamic or mechanistic end points.

Results.—The performance of PET studies using radiolabelled anticancer agents at tracer doses before phase I clinical trials was deemed feasible. This was based on the ability to produce radiopharmaceuticals with high specific radioactivity but in extremely small amounts of stable compound and on the inherent sensitivity of PET scans. The recommended formulation preferred is [^{11}C]N-[2-(dimethylamino) ethyl]acridine-4-carboxamide ([^{11}C]DACA) that contains less than 1 of 1000 of the proposed phase I starting dose of DACA. This allows the assessment of metabolism and mode of action before the phase I trial.

Because positron emitters have a short half-life, few quality control tests can be performed before the radiopharmaceuticals are used for clinical studies, so the quality assurance system takes on special significance and requires compliance with all relevant rules and guidance for pharmaceutical manufacture and development. Because only a low dose of radiolabelled drug is required for detection by tracer PET studies and each patient receives few doses (generally 1), single-dose toxicology studies of the radiopharmaceutical agent in the same formulation to be used in humans is recommended.

Tests are needed even if toxicology data for unlabeled compounds are available because of differences in the synthetic routes, impurity profiles, and even the vehicle used. The levels of other components in the formulation should also be considered, for example, anti-oxidants and residual solvents. Immunogenicity must also be evaluated. The overall goals are to confirm that the stable compound linked to the radiopharmaceutical is the same as the nonradiolabelled compound, that animal toxicity studies are performed at a rate of at least 10 times (or typically 100 times) the tracer dose to be used in humans, and that patients are carefully monitored during tracer PET studies.

Conclusion.—The minimum studies required for all candidate compounds are chemical identity and purity, animal toxicology, and clinical trial. Pre–phase I studies allow pharmacokinetic and pharmacodynamic evaluations to be done early in the clinical development of anticancer agents. Meeting the goals outlined should ensure safety in the use of radiopharmaceutical agents.

▶ The PET community and the Food and Drug Administration (FDA) are struggling to develop recommendations for the development of PET radiopharmaceuticals. The Radioactive Drug Research Committee (RDRC) is a mechanism for the initial evaluation of the distribution of PET tracers. The FDA does not like this approach for testing new PET tracers and wants the investigator to submit an Investigative New Drug (IND) application. The development of new PET tracers in the United States is too complicated and expensive using the present IND to New Drug Application (NDA) mechanisms. Fortunately, the National Cancer Institute has developed some programs that facilitate getting an IND. A United Kingdom expert committee has made the recommendations that are included in this article. Hopefully, we will be able to develop appropriate guidelines for developing new PET radiopharmaceuticals in the near future.

R. E. Coleman, MD

Influence of OSEM and Segmented Attenuation Correction in the Calculation of Standardised Uptake Values for [18F]FDG PET
Visvikis D, Cheze-LeRest C, Costa DC, et al (Royal Free and University College, London; Université de Bretagne Occidentale, Brest, France)
Eur J Nucl Med 28:1326-1335, 2001   2–36

Background.—Standardized uptake values (SUVs) are widely used in PET to provide a semiquantitative index of fluorine-18 FDG uptake ([18F]FDG). The potential for bias in the calculation of SUVs because of the use of ordered subsets-expectation maximization (OSEM) image reconstruction and segmented attenuation correction (SAC) was investigated.

Methods.—A variety of emission and transmission times were investigated, using a phantom and clinical evaluation of the bias with software implemented in the GE Advance PET scanner. The phantom studies involved simulation of tumor imaging conditions. A variable count rate may influence the results obtained using OSEM, so similar acquisitions were performed at total count rates of 34 kcps and 12 kcps. The clinical data were obtained from 100 patient studies. Emission data sets of 5 and 15 minutes' duration were combined with 15-minute, 3-minute, 2-minute, and 1-minute transmission data sets for the reconstruction of both phantom and patient studies. Two SUVs were estimated using the average (SUVavg) and maximum (SUVmax) count density from regions of interest that were placed inside the structures of interest. The percentage bias of these SUVs was then compared with the values obtained using a reference image; that is, the image produced by filtered back-projection (FBP) image reconstruction with measured attenuation correction, using the 15-minute emission and transmission data sets for each phantom and patient study.

Results.—The bias ranged from 5% to 20% for the SUVavg and SUVmax for FBP with SAC using variable transmission times. For OSEM with SAC, the bias increased to 10% up to 30%. The use of SUVmax resulted in an overall increase of 5% to 10%. Use of the 5-minute emission data set led to an increase in the bias of 25% to 100%, and the largest increase was recorded for the SUVmax.

Conclusions.—The findings suggest that OSEM and SAC with transmission times of 3 minutes and 2 minutes are effective in reducing the overall data acquisition time without compromising the accuracy of SUVs.

▶ This study nicely characterizes the effects of using OSEM and SAC on SUVs, and their comparison with filtered back-projection image construction. The authors conclude that the 5-minute emission scan using OSEM and a 2-minute or 3-minute transmission scan using SAC will not compromise the accuracy of SUVs. The results were based on phantom and patient studies. We have attempted to develop a method for varying the transmission scan time based on the size of the patient. For example, very large patients need longer transmission scans than very small patients if the image noise is to be kept constant. Perhaps large patients need 4- or 5-minute transmission scans, and thinner patients need only 1- or 2-minute transmission scans. Hopefully, in accordance with some description of the patient, we will be able to develop a method for predicting appropriate transmission scan times on the basis of the patient's size.

R. E. Coleman, MD

PET-CT Image Co-Registration in the Thorax: Influence of Respiration
Goerres GW, Kamel E, Heidelberg T-NH, et al (Univ Hosp, Zurich, Switzerland)
Eur J Nucl Med 29:351-360, 2002   2–37

Background.—FDG PET is superior to CT or MRI in identifying the appearances of various tumors, in defining their biological behavior, and in evaluating the response to therapy. However, anatomical information gleaned through FDG-PET whole-body images is limited, so the combination of PET and CT has been used. The breathing protocol needed for the CT images to best match the PET images is yet to be determined. Patients with tumors who were undergoing routine FDG-PET examinations were assessed for information leading to a determination of this important aspect of combined imaging.

Methods.—For 10 patients, the PET and CT studies were done using a combined high-performance in-line PET-CT camera that did not require patient repositioning. For 18 patients, the PET and CT scans were done on separate scanners situated close to each other. Four respiration levels were used for the CT examinations: free breathing (FB), maximal inspiration (MaxInsp), maximal expiration (MaxExp), and normal expiration (NormExp). The differences in CT and PET images were compared at 4 distances: between a reference point at the anterior superior edge of the intervertebral disk space T10-11 and the apex of the lung; from the lung apex to the diaphragm's top; from the lung apex to the costodiaphragmatic recess; and from the reference point to the lateral thoracic wall. Changes in the tumor's position between the PET and CT examinations were also noted.

Results.—The least comfortable breathing position for patients, which many could not maintain during CT scanning, was MaxExp, so the data observed by this method were not reliable. Difficulty was also noted with MaxInsp; NormExp was acceptable, but some patients preferred FB. Greater attentiveness and compliance were achieved during NormExp.

Measurements showed greater agreement between observers for the CT scans (80%) than for the PET scans (20%). In the 18 patients evaluated on separate scanners, the 4 breathing protocols resulted in small differences in measurements and between left and right sides.

Best and second-best matches between PET and CT were found in 80.5% during NormExp and 47.2% during FB. Worst matches occurred during MaxInsp in 88.9% of cases. In the 10 patients evaluated on the combined scanner, best and second-best matches were found with NormExp in 83.3% of patients and FB in 40.5%. Worst matches were again with MaxInsp.

The probability of a good fit between the PET and CT images increased during NormExp for image co-registration, and the range of measured values was smallest with this protocol. Only slight differences were found among the 4 respiration protocols and a small discrepancy between right and left values. Movement of the tumors depended on their position in the lung, with those in the lower parts showing a larger range of movements. Best and second-best matches were noted during NormExp.

Conclusion.—Using a normal expiration breath-hold protocol for CT acquisition achieves the best match with PET values whether the scans are performed on separate or combined systems. The next-best alternative is the free breathing approach.

▶ This article provides information on the best method for performing imaging of the chest on a PET-CT device. If the emission and transmission images are not obtained at the same level of chest expansion and diaphragmatic position, artifacts will be present on the attenuation-corrected image. The authors have performed a quantitative study to address the state of the patient's breathing for performing the CT scan. We will have to see whether other investigators find similar results using PET-CT.

R. E. Coleman, MD

CT vs ^{68}Ge Attenuation Correction in a Combined PET/CT System: Evaluation of the Effect of Lowering the CT Tube Current

Kamel E, Hany TF, Burger C, et al (Univ Hosp, Zürich, Switzerland; GE Med Systems)

Eur J Nucl Med 29:346-350, 2002   2–38

Background.—When performing PET, it is necessary to include attenuation correction. Disadvantages of performing attenuation correction using rotating ^{68}Ge pin sources include the long acquisition times needed, the poor transmission scan imaging quality, and the lack of anatomical information, as well as the need for an extended imaging time when doing a whole-body scan. This leads to patient discomfort and the inability to see as many patients. Combining CT with PET in a PET-CT system allows higher resolution and greater contrast achieved in a shorter time. To address questions that have arisen, 1 group of patients underwent evaluation to see how much the CT current can be lowered and still give adequate attenuation maps. The quantified FDG uptake in lesions and lesion size were compared in these patients. In a second group of patients, measurements were made of tumor FDG uptake and tumor size using CT_{80} and comparisons were carried out against ^{68}Ge attenuation-corrected scans.

Methods.—Multidetector CT scans were acquired in 26 patients by 10, 40, 80, and 120 mA and then used to perform attenuation correction for a single FDG PET emission scan. FDG uptake and lesion size were measured on scans at the 4 levels in 60 tumorous lesions. Another 18 patients had 1 CT scan at 80 mA and a standard transmission scan using ^{68}Ge sources for attenuation correction of the FDG emission scan. Comparisons were made between uptake values and lesion size.

Results.—While the CT_{10} scan was of poorer quality than the CT_{80} scan, a Gaussian filter nearly eliminated the differences. CT current was demonstrated to exert no significant influence on tumor FDG uptake or size of the lesion in the first group of patients. In the second group, a slightly higher FDG uptake by the tumor was shown by CT than by ^{68}Ge attenuation correction. Lesions with high FDG uptake were particularly affected. The 2 scans showed essentially the same lesion sizes.

Conclusion.—The use of low-current CT was acceptable for attenuation correction in the PET scans of these patients. The 10 mA CT scan achieved quantified uptake values equal to those obtained with higher-current CT scans. A slightly higher tumor FDG uptake was noted with CT attenuation correction than with ^{68}Ge correction.

▶ The combination of PET and CT scanners will be the standard instrumentation a few years from now. At this time, we have a lot to learn about the quality of the CT scanner needed for PET imaging. Furthermore, the mode in which the CT scanner should be operated is to be determined. This article evaluates the effect of lowering the CT tube current on lesion size and standardized uptake values. Anyone using a combined PET/CT scanner should read this article.

R. E. Coleman, MD

---

^{99m}Tc Sestamibi Breast Imaging for the Examination of Patients With Dense and Fatty Breasts: Multicenter Study
Khalkhali I, Baum JK, Villanueva-Meyer J, et al (Univ of California, Los Angeles, Torrance; Beth Israel Hosp, Boston; Univ of Texas, Galveston; et al)
Radiology 222:149-155, 2002   2–39

Background.—The reduced sensitivity of mammography in dense breasts presents a challenge to the early detection of breast cancer. Scintimammography with technetium-99m (^{99m}Tc) sestamibi has been suggested as a useful adjunct to physical examination and mammography for the diagnosis of breast cancer. The accuracy of scintimammography in women with dense and fatty breasts was assessed.

Methods.—This prospective study included 558 women at 42 centers in North America. Scintimammographic images obtained from these subjects were interpreted by readers blinded to the clinical history, mammographic findings, and other test results of the subjects. The Breast Imaging Reporting and Data System classification was used to describe breast density. Dense breasts were classified on the basis of parenchymal patterns of "heterogeneously dense" and "extremely dense," while fatty breasts were classified on the basis of being "almost entirely fat" or having "numerous vague densities." Differences between the groups were evaluated with the χ^2 test for categorical variables and the Student t test for continuous variables. The accuracy of scintimammography was assessed against the standard of the core laboratory histopathologic evaluation. The 95% CIs around point estimates of sensitivity, specificity, and positive and negative predictive values were calculated with the normal approximation to the binomial distribution.

Results.—The final analyses were based on 580 breasts with an abnormality. There were 276 (48%) dense breasts and 22 breasts with a malignant lesion. The diagnostic properties for scintimammography of fatty versus dense breasts were as follows: sensitivity, 72% versus 70%; specificity, 80% versus 78%; positive predictive value, 72% versus 67%; negative predictive value, 81% versus 81%; and accuracy, 77% versus 75%. None of these differences were statistically significant.

Conclusions.—Scintimammography yielded similar and significant changes in the posttest probability of cancer in both dense and fatty breasts; the results of this study indicate that breast density does not affect the diagnostic accuracy of scintimammography.

▶ The reported studies on scintimammography continue to be quite positive. However, I have never been asked to do a clinical sestamibi scan at our institution. Although the accuracy of sestamibi is quite good and not affected by breast density, the impact of scintimammography on patient management when breast biopsy is readily available is not clear to me.

R. E. Coleman, MD

High-Resolution Scintimammography: A Pilot Study
Brem RF, Schoonjans JM, Kieper DA, et al (George Washington Univ, Washington, DC; Johns Hopkins Insts, Baltimore, Md; Thomas Jefferson Natl Accelerator Facility, Newport News, Va)
J Nucl Med 43:909-915, 2002   2–40

Background.—^{99m}Tc-sestamibi scintigraphy is a useful method for detecting malignant lesions of the breast. However, current general-purpose gamma cameras have limited ability to detect small, nonpalpable breast lesions. A new, high-resolution, breast-specific gamma camera (HRBGC) was tested to determine its performance in detecting breast cancer.

Methods.—The subjects were 50 women 30 to 80 years old who were referred for ^{99m}Tc-sestamibi scintimammography because of indeterminant clinical and mammographic findings. All patients underwent repeat mammography and scintigraphy with both a conventional gamma camera and a prototype HRBGC. Two radiologists independently rated the results of each evaluation as negative (normal tissue or benign lesions) or positive (suggestive of disease or malignant). A biopsy specimen from each lesion was then obtained, and the accuracy of the diagnostic methods was calculated on the basis of the histologic findings.

Results.—Fifty-eight lesions were examined histologically: 30 were benign and 28 were malignant. The conventional gamma camera detected 18 of the 28 malignant lesions (sensitivity, 64.3%), whereas the HRBGC detected 22 of these lesions (sensitivity, 78.6%). In comparison, mammography detected 24 of these 28 lesions (sensitivity, 85.7%). The HRBGC detected 4 lesions that the conventional gamma camera missed. Both scintigraphic methods missed 6 malignant tumors; however, the general-purpose gamma camera detected 2 lesions that were not detected by mammography and the HRBGC detected 3 such lesions. Each of the scintigraphic systems accurately ruled out malignancy in 28 of the 30 benign lesions (specificity, 93.3%). Specifically, 18 of the malignant lesions were nonpalpable; the conventional gamma camera identified 10 of these lesions (55.6%), whereas the HRBGC detected 13 of them (72.2%). Fifteen of the lesions were 1 cm or smaller; the general-purpose gamma camera identified 7 of these lesions (46.7%), whereas the HRBGC detected 10 of them (66.7%).

Conclusion.—For the evaluation of patients with indeterminate breast lesions, a HRBGC was more sensitive than a conventional gamma camera in detecting breast malignancy, without adversely affecting specificity. HRBGC was particularly more sensitive for detecting nonpalpable lesions and lesions 1 cm or smaller, although the small sample size precluded determinations of statistical significance. These preliminary results suggest that a new approach to scintimammography can overcome the intrinsic limitations of general-purpose gamma cameras in imaging nonpalpable or smaller lesions.

▶ Scintimammography performed with a higher-resolution system results in greater sensitivity. Other high-resolution systems are being developed and evaluated. I have yet to have a single clinical scintimammography study requested at my institution.

R. E. Coleman, MD

Estrogen Receptor Status in Primary Breast Cancer: Iodine 123–Labeled *cis*-11β-Methoxy-17α-Iodovinyl Estradiol Scintigraphy
Bennink RJ, Rijks LJ, van Tienhoven G, et al (Academic Med Ctr, Amsterdam; Eindhoven Univ, The Netherlands)
Radiology 220:774-779, 2001   2–41

Background.—Several investigators have studied the possibility of in vivo imaging of estrogen receptors with receptor-specific radioligands at PET or SPECT. The sensitivity of ^{123}I-labeled *cis*-11β-methoxy-17α-iodovinyl estradiol (Z-MIVE) scintigraphy for detecting estrogen receptors in patients with primary breast cancer was determined.

A   B

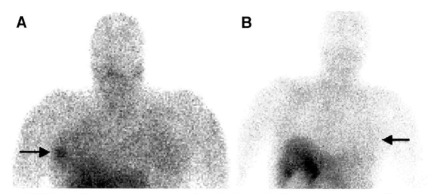

FIGURE 1.—Planar anterior scintigrams obtained 4 hours after the injection of 185 Mbq ^{123}I-labeled Z-MIVE. **A,** Image in a 54-year-old woman (patient 11) with a T2 infiltrating ductal carcinoma of the right breast is a clear example of strong uptake of tracer in the tumor (*arrow*). **B,** Image in a 76-year-old woman (patient 20) with a T2 infiltrating ductal carcinoma of the left breast is a clear example of no detectable uptake in the tumor (*arrow*). (Courtesy of Bennink RJ, Rijks LJ, van Tienhoven G, et al: Estrogen receptor status in primary breast cancer: Iodine 123–labeled *cis*-11β-methoxy-17α-iodovinyl estradiol scintigraphy. *Radiology* 220:774-779, 2001. Radiological Society of North America.)

Methods.—Estrogen receptor status in 22 patients was assessed by planar scintigraphy and SPECT 4 hours after ^{123}I-labeled Z-MIVE injection (Fig 1). Breast cancer tissue was obtained by biopsy or primary tumor resection for histologic and estrogen receptor immunohistochemical analysis.

Findings.—Breast cancer was diagnosed histologically in all patients. Immunohistologic staining for estrogen receptors yielded negative findings in 4 patients and positive findings in 18. Planar ^{123}I-labeled Z-MIVE scintigraphic results were negative in 5 and positive in 17 patients, with 1 false-negative finding. On ^{123}I-labeled Z-MIVE SPECT, findings were negative in 4 patients and positive in 18. The sensitivities of ^{123}I-labeled scintigraphy for estrogen receptors with SPECT and planar scintigraphy were 100% and 94%, respectively. Immunohistologic and planar scintigraphic estrogen receptor status scores had a 0.72 correlation.

Conclusion.—The sensitivity of ^{123}I-labeled Z-MIVE scintigraphy for detecting estrogen receptor–positive primary breast carcinoma is high. The strong association between the amount of ^{123}I-labeled Z-MIVE uptake and the level of estrogen receptor expression shows that conventional scintigraphy is a reliable method for assessing estrogen receptor status in breast carcinoma.

▶ PET imaging of estrogen receptors using F-18 fluoroestradiol has been available for several years. An I-123 agent is now available for use with SPECT imaging. Although PET and SPECT approaches appear able to accurately characterize the estrogen receptor status of the tumors, it is unclear where this technique will be used in patient management.

R. E. Coleman, MD

Subareolar Injection of [99m]Tc Facilitates Sentinel Lymph Node Identification

Tuttle TM, Colbert M, Christensen R, et al (Park Nicollet Clinic, Minneapolis; Univ of Minnesota, Minneapolis; Univ of Louisville, Ky)

Ann Surg Oncol 9:77-81, 2002   2–42

Introduction.—Sentinel lymph node (SLN) biopsy with the standard intraparenchymal injection is an alternative to routine axillary dissection in patients with breast cancer. The detection and false-negative rates with this approach can vary greatly among surgeons. The subareolar area has a rich lymphatic network and is a potential site of injection for SLN identification. Patients underwent an intraparenchymal injection of blue dye and a subareolar injection of [99m]technetium (Tc) in a large single-institution investigation to determine whether ^{99m}Tc facilitates detection of SLN.

Methods.—Between August 1, 1999 and December 31, 2000, 158 patients with breast cancer underwent 159 SLN biopsy procedures. During the procedure, ^{99m}Tc-labeled sulfur colloid was injected into the subareolar site, and 1% isosulfan blue dye was administered as an intraparenchymal injection.

Results.—In all procedures, a minimum of 1 radioactive SLN was detected with the subareolar injection of technetium, and a blue SLN was identified in 97% of cases. The blue SLN was radioactive in 98% of cases, indicating that the blue dye injected around the tumor and the technetium injected into the subareolar site drained to the same SLN.

Conclusion.—Subareolar injection of technetium can improve the SLN detection rates for breast cancer. The simplicity and accuracy of this method may also decrease the variable results reported with the standard intraparenchymal approach.

▶ The technique used in this study was administering 0.75 mCi of filtered ^{99m}Tc-labeled sulfur colloid with a 27-gauge needle. The radiolabeled colloid was administered below the nipple at the 6 o'clock subareolar location regardless of tumor location. The volume injected was 0.5 mL. The blue dye was injected around the tumor. Excellent identification of lymph nodes was obtained. The issue is whether the subareolar lymphatics correspond to tumor lymphatics elsewhere in the breast. The subareolar injection of all patients certainly simplifies the procedure compared with peritumoral injection, injection subcutaneously over the lesion, or if the lesion is not palpable, injection localized with ultrasound guidance. The evidence does appear to be mounting to confirm that the subareolar injection does work well for lymphoscintigraphy in breast cancer.

R. E. Coleman, MD

Multicentre Study of Detection and False-Negative Rates in Sentinel Node Biopsy for Breast Cancer

Bergkvist L, Frisell J, Liljegren G, et al (Uppsala Univ, Sweden; Central Hosp, Västerås, Sweden; Huddinge Univ Hosp, Stockholm; et al)
Br J Surg 88:1644-1648, 2001   2–43

Background.—In sentinel node biopsy, the status of the sentinel node predicts that of the other nodes in that basin. Patients with breast cancer may have sentinel node biopsy with vital blue dye, lymphoscintigraphy with an intraoperative γ probe, or a combination of these methods. Training is required for surgeons to use these methods efficaciously. Factors that affect the rate of detecting the sentinel node and the false-negative rate during the learning phase were assessed prospectively.

Methods.—Seventeen participating hospitals in Sweden contributed data on 498 sentinel node biopsies in patients who had operable unifocal breast cancer and no palpable lymph nodes suggestive of cancer in the axilla but who were undergoing axillary dissection. Lymphoscintigraphy was performed preoperatively, the dissection was done, and the sentinel node was evaluated histopathologically.

Results.—For 450 (90%) of the patients, a sentinel node was identified, and the median number of sentinel nodes retrieved was 2.0. In 83% of the patients, lymphoscintigraphy revealed at least 1 sentinel node. The γ probe detected 39% of those not revealed on lymphoscintigraphy and missed 8%. Nodes were detected at a higher rate in patients who had the isotope injection on the same day as the operation (96%) than in those who received it on the previous day (86%). When the dye was injected more than 5 minutes but less than 30 minutes before beginning the operation, 65% of the patients had visual identification of the sentinel node; this fell to 60% when the dye was injected less than 5 minutes or more than 30 minutes before operation. A statistically insignificant trend was noted toward a lower detection rate with increasing age: the detection rate was 95% in those younger than 50 years, 90% in those aged 50 to 69 years, and 87% in those older than 69 years. Detection rates for different surgeons ranged from 61% to 100%. Once 30 operations had been performed, surgeons detected sentinel nodes in 90% of cases overall. An 11% false-negative rate was found for the entire group. Factors contributing to the false-negative rate included the hospital in which the operation was performed, the S-phase fraction, and the presence of multiple foci. Only the S-phase fraction and the presence of multiple tumor foci were statistically significant risk factors for false-negative results on multiple logistic regression analysis.

Conclusions.—The surgeon's training and the timing of the tracer and dye injection significantly influenced the ability to detect sentinel lymph nodes. Specific biological factors (ie, S-phase fraction and multiple tumor foci) were linked to the false-negative rate attending sentinel lymph node biopsy.

▶ At our institution, we prefer injecting the radiopharmaceutical the day before the study rather than on the same day. We find that we can better identify the lymph nodes and differentiate the axillary lymphatics from axillary lymph nodes in the 2-day study.

R. E. Coleman, MD

Expression of Multidrug Resistance Protein and Messenger RNA Correlate With ⁹⁹ᵐTc-MIBI Imaging in Patients With Lung Cancer

Zhou J, Higashi K, Ueda Y, et al (Kanazawa Med Univ, Ishikawa, Japan)
J Nucl Med 42:1476-1483, 2001   2–44

Background.—Multidrug resistance (MDR) is the most significant barrier to efficient chemotherapeutic treatment of cancer. MDR has been closely associated with altered expression of MDR phenotype, and in lung cancer the MDR phenotype has been defined on the basis of the cellular drug targets involved, specifically P-glycoprotein (Pgp), MDR-associated protein (MRP), lung resistance protein (LRP), and atypical MDR (mediated through altered expression of topoisomerase type II). In vitro studies have shown that ⁹⁹ᵐTc-

FIGURE 1

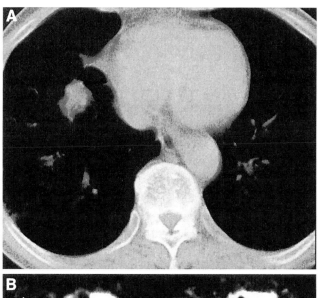
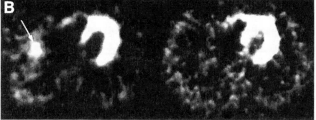

(Continued)

FIGURE 1 (cont.)

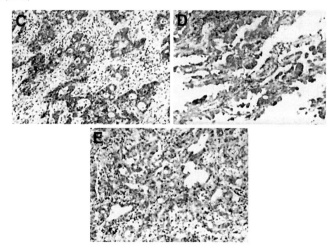

FIGURE 1.—Patient 1, 73-year-old man with 2.8 × 2.8 cm lung adenocarcinoma. **A,** CT scan shows nodule in right lung. **B,** Early ^{99m}Tc-MIBI SPECT scan (**left**) shows intense uptake (*arrow*) of ^{99m}Tc-MIBI in tumor (L/Ne = 3.81). Delayed scan (**right**) shows faint ^{99m}Tc-MIBI uptake in tumor (L/Nd = 1.00), suggesting rapid washout of ^{99m}Tc-MIBI from tumor (L/Nwr = 73.8%). Immunohistochemistry (×200) reveals strong Pgp expression (**C**), strong MRP expression (**D**), and weak LRP expression (**E**) in corresponding tumor tissue. (Reprinted by permission of the Society of Nuclear Medicine from Zhou J, Higashi K, Ueda Y, et al: Expression of multidrug resistance protein and messenger RNA correlate with ^{99m}Tc-MIBI imaging in patients with lung cancer. *J Nucl Med* 42:1476-1483, 2001.)

sestamibi (MIBI) is a transport substrate for the Pgp pump and the MRP pump. Whether MRP and LRP affect tumor accumulation and efflux of ^{99m}Tc-MIBI in lung cancer was investigated.

Methods.—The study group comprised 34 patients with lung cancer who underwent surgery. Before surgery, ^{99m}Tc-MIBI SPECT was performed 15 minutes and 180 minutes after injection. Early uptake, delayed uptake (L/Nd), and washout rate (L/Nwr) were obtained. Immunohistochemical analysis was used to investigate the expression of Pgp, MRP, and LRP. Real-time reverse transcription polymerase chain reaction (RTPCR) was used to determine the messenger RNA (mRNA) level of Pgp, MRP, and LRP. The lung cancer ^{99m}Tc-MIBI images were then correlated with protein and mRNA expression.

Results.—The mean L/Nd of the Pgp (−) group was significantly higher than that observed in the Pgp (++) group, which had a higher L/Nwr than did the Pgp (−) group (Fig 1). The mean L/Nd of the Pgp mRNA low-expression group was significantly higher than that of the Pgp mRNA high-expression group. The Pgp mRNA high-expression group had a higher L/Nwr than did the Pgp mRNA low-expression group. No significant correlation was noted between the lung cancer ^{99m}Tc-MIBI imaging and the expression of MRP or LRP on the level of protein or mRNA.

Conclusions.—An increased level of Pgp expression is correlated with a low accumulation on delayed scans and a high delayed washout rate of

⁹⁹ᵐTc-MIBI in patients with lung cancer. No correlation was found of MRP or LRP expression on the level of either protein or mRNA and the tumor accumulation or efflux of ⁹⁹ᵐTc-MIBI in lung cancer.

▶ Multidrug resistance is a problem in treating cancer. Technium-99m MIBI has been demonstrated to be a marker of the P-glycoprotein efflux pump. MIBI washout does correlate with increased levels of P-glycoprotein levels in lung cancer and does not correlate with the expression of MRP-associated protein or lung resistant protein. Beware of delayed imaging using MIBI for diagnosis of lung cancer!

R. E. Coleman, MD

Diagnostic 131-Iodine Whole-Body Scan May Be Avoided in Thyroid Cancer Patients Who Have Undetectable Stimulated Serum Tg Levels After Initial Treatment
Pacini F, Capezzone M, Elisei R, et al (Univ of Pisa, Italy)
J Clin Endocrinol Metab 87:1499-1501, 2002   2–45

Background.—Recommended treatment for differentiated thyroid cancer involves near-total thyroidectomy and ¹³¹I ablation of residual thyroid tissues, followed by a ¹³¹I whole-body scan (WBS) and serum Tg measurement within 1 year. Usually local or distant metastases are detected better with Tg measurements than with WBS, so the question arises as to whether it is necessary to perform WBS in all patients as part of the follow-up protocol. Those who perhaps could be excluded are those no longer taking L-T₄ therapy and whose Tg levels are undetectable. The usefulness of the first control WBS after initial treatment was assessed, with the focus in particular on its impact on subsequent outcome.

Methods.—Of 662 patients having their initial control ¹³¹I WBS and serum Tg measurements, 315 (54 men and 261 women) had no detectable serum Tg levels. These patients ranged in age from 12 to 76 years (mean age, 40.9 years); 272 had papillary thyroid carcinoma and 43 had follicular thyroid carcinoma. Follow-up examinations were carried out for 9 to 19 years (mean, 12 years).

Results.—At thyroid ablation, all patients had thyroid bed uptake, 33 had cervical node metastases, and 4 had lung metastases. For 225 patients, 6 to 12 months after ablation, the ¹³¹I WBS was negative; for 90 patients, it was positive. Neither local nor distant metastases were present at 6 to 12 months. Fifty-four of the 90 patients with positive results had a second course of radioiodine therapy and 7 patients had 2 additional courses; no treatment was carried out in 29 patients. After 9 to 19 years, 281 patients had undetectable serum Tg and negative ¹³¹I WBS results and 29 were free of disease, although thyroid bed uptake and undetectable Tg levels remained. Two patients had recurrent disease of the cervical lymph nodes. Three patients died of nonthyroid causes.

Conclusion.—Finding an undetectable serum Tg level once the patient has completed L-T$_4$ therapy was highly predictive of complete remission. Thus the need for ^{131}I WBS is minimal, although follow-up of such patients is advisable, using the serum Tg measurements.

▶ I am always in a quandary as to what to do with low-level uptake in the thyroid bed that is present after surgery or even after an initial ^{131}I ablative dose. It should be noted that all of the patients in this study underwent thyroid ablation with ^{131}I using doses of 30 to 100 mCi soon after surgery. From the results of this study, if the Tg levels are negative, these patients need no further therapy even if there is low uptake in the thyroid bed region. The recommended approach seems reasonable to me.

R. E. Coleman, MD

Sensitivity of [123]I Whole-Body Scan and Thyroglobulin in the Detection of Metastases or Recurrent Differentiated Thyroid Cancer
de Geus-Oei L-F, Oei H-Y, Hennemann G, et al (Univ Hosp Rotterdam, Dijkzigt, The Netherlands; Univ Med Ctr St Radboud, Nijmegen, The Netherlands)
Eur J Nucl Med 29:768-774, 2002   2–46

Background.—The primary treatment of differentiated thyroid carcinoma is total thyroidectomy with postoperative radioactive iodine therapy to destroy the remaining thyroid tissue and possible metastases. Subsequent recurrence or metastasis can be detected by measuring serum levels of thyroglobulin (Tg) and by scintigraphy. The sensitivity of serum Tg measurements was compared with that of ^{123}I scintigraphy in the detection of thyroid cancer recurrence or metastasis.

Methods.—The subjects were 55 patients (15 men and 40 women; median age, 54 years) with differentiated thyroid carcinoma who had initially been treated with total thyroidectomy and postoperative ^{131}I radiotherapy. L-thyroxine was administered to all patients, and serum Tg levels were measured during therapy. All patients had recurrent (n = 36) or metastatic (n = 19) disease develop 3 to 6 months after the initial treatment. When recurrence or metastasis was suspected, L-thyroxine therapy was discontinued for 4 to 6 weeks and serum Tg levels during L-thyroxine discontinuation were measured. Then patients underwent a diagnostic whole-body scan with 111 to 370 MBq of [123]I. Within 24 hours afterward, patients received a therapeutic dose of 1850 to 5550 MBq of ^{131}I and a posttherapeutic ^{131}I scan was obtained. The sensitivities of the diagnostic ^{123}I scan and of serum Tg measurements during L-thyroxine therapy and after its discontinuation were compared. In addition, findings from the diagnostic ^{123}I scan were compared with those from the posttherapeutic ^{131}I scan.

Results.—The sensitivity of the diagnostic ^{123}I scan (75%) was lower than that of either serum Tg measurement (82% during L-thyroxine therapy, 98% after its discontinuation). Combining the results of the diagnostic ^{123}I scan with serum Tg measurements improved the sensitivity somewhat (95%

during L-thyroxine therapy, 100% after its discontinuation). The mean serum Tg levels after L-thyroxine discontinuation were significantly higher than those during L-thyroxine therapy (4991 vs 1501 ng/mL, respectively). In 12 of 51 patients for whom the diagnostic ^{123}I scan was available, serum Tg measurements during and/or after L-thyroxine therapy were elevated, but the diagnostic ^{123}I scan was negative. Diagnostic ^{123}I scans could be visually compared with posttherapeutic ^{131}I scans for 36 patients. In 21 patients the results of these 2 studies were equivocal, but in 13 of the remaining 15 patients, more lesions were visible on the posttherapeutic ^{131}I scan than on the ^{123}I scan.

Conclusion.—Serum Tg measurements during L-thyroxine withdrawal were significantly more sensitive for the detection of recurrent or metastatic differentiated thyroid cancer than either ^{123}I scintigraphy or serum Tg measurements during L-thyroxine therapy. [131]I therapy is indicated for patients whose serum Tg levels during L-thyroxine withdrawal are clearly above levels during L-thyroxine therapy. In this setting, diagnostic ^{123}I scanning does not provide substantial additional diagnostic information and is not warranted.

▶ Patients who have had a total thyroidectomy for well-differentiated thyroid cancer appear to benefit from ^{131}I ablation if the Tg levels are elevated and the ^{123}I scan is negative. This study found that more lesions were detected on the posttherapeutic ^{131}I scan than on the ^{123}I scan.

R. E. Coleman, MD

The Role of ^{123}I-Diagnostic Imaging in the Follow-up of Patients With Differentiated Thyroid Carcinoma as Compared to ^{131}I-Scanning: Avoidance of Negative Therapeutic Uptake Due to Stunning
Siddiqi A, Foley RR, Britton KE, et al (St Bartholomew's Hosp, London)
Clin Endocrinol (Oxf) 55:515-521, 2001   2–47

Background.—Increased thyroglobulin (Tg) levels may be observed in some patients with relapsed differentiated thyroid cancer despite a lack of ^{131}I uptake on routine whole body imaging. Many of these patients may show positive ^{131}I uptake with a subsequent fall in serum Tg after therapeutic doses of ^{131}I, implying a therapeutic effect. Attempts to identify these patients, however, by increasing the dose of diagnostic ^{131}I tracer may result in inhibition of subsequent uptake after the therapeutic dose. This effect is referred to as "stunning" and is associated with a reduction in therapeutic effect. [123]I is a short half-life γ-emitter and is thought to be unlikely to cause stunning. The safety and efficacy of ^{123}I for diagnostic imaging of thyroid cancer was assessed and compared with the same characteristics of [131]I.

Methods.—This longitudinal study included 12 patients who were selected because they showed elevated serum Tg levels and a negative diagnostic ^{131}I whole body study before therapy with [131]I.

Results.—Concordance was nearly complete between ^{123}I diagnostic imaging and the final scans performed after ^{131}I therapy (therapy studies) in 11 of 12 patients at the first evaluation, in 4 patients who received ^{123}I at their second evaluation, and in 1 patient who received ^{123}I at a third evaluation (Fig 1). One patient had a positive ^{123}I study but a negative ^{131}I therapy study. After therapy, Tg levels declined from 5.5 pg/L to undetectable levels, a result that implied a therapeutic effect and suggested that the negative uptake

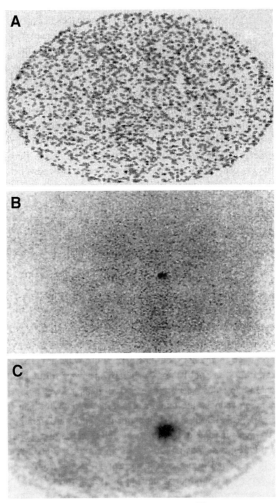

FIGURE 1.—Patient 1. Posterior views of the thoracic spine. **A**, ^{131}I tracer imaging (100 MBq). No focal uptake is seen in the spine. **B**, ^{123}I imaging at 24 hours (185 MBq). Focal and diffuse uptake is seen in the thoracic spine. **C**, ^{131}I therapy (5.5 GBq) imaging at 4 days. Similar uptake is seen at the same site in the thoracic spine. (Courtesy of Siddiqi A, Foley RR, Britton KE, et al: The role of ^{123}I-diagnostic imaging in the follow-up of patients with differentiated thyroid carcinoma as compared to ^{131}I-scanning: Avoidance of negative therapeutic uptake due to stunning. *Clin Endocrinol (Oxf)* 55:515-521, 2001. Reprinted with permission from Blackwell Science, Inc.)

was not the result of stunning. ^{123}I correctly identified disease in the 9 patients with metastases in the lungs, mediastinum, and bone at the first evaluation, in all 4 patients at the second evaluation, and in the solitary patient at the third evaluation. At the conclusion of the study, patients had received up to 3 therapy doses of ^{131}I. Tg had increased in 4 patients, decreased in 8 patients, and decreased to undetectable levels in 1 patient.

Conclusions.—These findings show that ^{123}I is quite sensitive in the diagnosis of local recurrence and metastatic disease and produces scintigraphic evidence that is in good concordance with uptake after ^{131}I therapy. It is proposed that ^{123}I imaging in combination with serum Tg assay should replace ^{131}I tracer imaging as an indicator of the potential efficacy of ^{131}I therapy. Such a practice would avoid the detrimental effects of stunning.

▶ Perhaps we should be doing our follow-up imaging with 5 mCi of ^{123}I. It may be more sensitive than ^{131}I and avoid the potential problem of stunning.

R. E. Coleman, MD

---

^{123}I Isotope as a Diagnostic Agent in the Follow-up of Patients With Differentiated Thyroid Cancer: Comparison With Post ^{131}I Therapy Whole Body Scanning

Alzahrani AS, Bakheet S, Mandil MA, et al (King Faisal Specialist Hosp and Research Ctr, Riyadh, Saudi Arabia)
J Clin Endocrinol Metab 86:5294-5300, 2001   2–48

Background.—Radioactive iodine-131 (^{131}I) is used postoperatively for patients with differentiated thyroid cancer (DTC) for diagnostic whole body scanning to monitor for the recurrence of disease, for ablation of remnant thyroid tissue, and for the treatment of recurrent and metastatic disease. ^{131}I emits both β- and γ-radiation, and the β-radiation has a lethal effect on follicular thyroid cells; for this reason it is used in large administered therapeutic activities for ablation and treatment of DTC. Concern is growing, however, that the use of ^{131}I in diagnostic scanning has a sublethal effect that may produce "stunning," a condition in which the tumor tissue is less avid for subsequent ^{131}I treatments. The use of ^{123}I may minimize this stunning effect, but data are limited. The utility of ^{123}I posttherapy scanning was assessed by comparing it with ^{131}I posttherapy scanning in 3 clinical situations: the first ^{131}I therapy, the second ^{131}I therapy, and in patients with elevated thyroglobulin and a negative diagnostic scan.

Methods.—A total of 238 diagnostic whole body scans performed 24 hours after oral ingestion of 185 to 555 MBq ^{123}I were compared with corresponding ^{131}I whole body scans obtained 4 to 5 days after ^{131}I therapy. The scans were studied in the 3 clinical situations described above.

Results.—Of 177 pairs of scans obtained with the first ^{131}I therapy, complete concordance between pretreatment and posttreatment scans was obtained in 166 pairs, for a concordance rate of 93.8%. With the second ^{131}I therapy, 34 pairs of scans were obtained and showed complete concordance in 28 pairs, for a concordance rate of 82.4%. In the 27 pairs of scans in patients with elevated thyroglobulin and negative pretreatment scans, 15 posttreatment scans remained negative, 6 showed an uptake in the thyroid bed, and 3 showed lung uptake in patients whose chest CT scans indicated only bronchiectasis (n = 2) and lung scarring (n = 1) with no evidence of lung metastases. In 56 pretreatment scans, the ^{123}I diagnostic activity was 185 MBq, and the results demonstrated complete concordance in 54 pairs.

Conclusions.—These findings indicated that pretreatment scanning with ^{123}I is highly comparable with ^{131}I posttreatment scanning. [123]I is an excellent diagnostic agent for use in differentiated thyroid cancer.

▶ This study of a large number (238 pairs) of scans demonstrates the utility of using [123]NaI in the follow-up for patients with differentiated thyroid cancer. These investigators administered between 5 and 12.5 mCi of [123]NaI, and scanned 24 hours later. Other studies seem to be presenting similar results (see Abstract 2–47).

R. E. Coleman, MD

Preoperative Diagnostic Value of [¹⁸F] Fluorodeoxyglucose Positron Emission Tomography in Patients With Radioiodine-Negative Recurrent Well-Differentiated Thyroid Carcinoma
Frilling A, Tecklenborg K, Görges R, et al (Univ Hosp Essen, Germany; Univ Hosp Hamburg, Germany)
Ann Surg 234:804-811, 2001   2–49

Introduction.—Most patients with well-differentiated thyroid carcinoma (WDTC) who are surgically treated and undergo iodine-131 (^{131}I) whole-body scintigraphy and serum thyroglobulin determination have an excellent long-term prognosis. In the event of tumor dedifferentiation, reduced or lost iodine-accumulating ability may lead to false-negative ^{131}I scanning results. The poor prognosis in this patient subgroup is due to diagnostic and therapeutic delay. Efforts have been focused on searching for suitable imaging modalities capable of early detection of recurrent thyroid carcinoma. The utility of 2-^{18}F FDG PET in identifying recurrent disease in the follow-up of 24 patients with WDTC who have negative diagnostic ^{131}I scans and abnormal thyroglobulin levels was prospectively analyzed.

Methods.—The study included all patients who had negative results of whole-body ^{131}I scintigraphy and had elevated serum thyroglobulin concentrations. Patients underwent attenuation-corrected whole-body FDG-PET scans from the neck to the upper legs. They also underwent cervical US. Imaging and histologic findings were compared. When no resection of the suspicious lesion was performed, data from CT were used.

Results.—Thirty-eight hot spots were identified by FDG PET. Sensitivity, specificity, and diagnostic accuracy were 94.6%, 25.0%, and 87.8%, respectively. There were 3 false-positive findings in 2 patients with benign cervical lymph nodes (Fig 4). Two false-negative findings were observed in 1 pa-

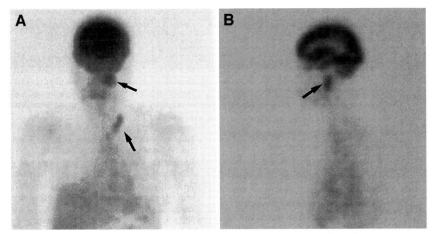

FIGURE 4.—Coronal (A) and sagittal (B) PET study in a 33-year-old patient with papillary carcinoma. Increased accumulation of FDG was obvious in the left cervical region and in the parapharyngeal region. At the first operation, left lateral lymphadenectomy and a biopsy of the parapharyngeal mass were carried out. Although histologic examination of the cervical lymph nodes showed no evidence of malignancy (false-positive FDG-PET result), the parapharyngeal tumor was classified as a metastasis of a papillary carcinoma. As expected, only the parapharyngeal hot spot was demonstrable in the postoperative FDG-PET slice. Consequently, the tumor was removed transorally and histologically confirmed as a metastasis of the primary tumor. (Courtesy of Frilling A, Tecklenborg K, Görges R, et al: Preoperative diagnostic value of [18F]fluorodeoxyglucose positron emission tomography in patients with radioiodine-negative recurrent well-differentiated thyroid carcinoma. *Ann Surg* 234(6):804-811, 2001.)

tient with regional lymph node metastases. US classified both of these findings as malignant. Because of unexpected findings, FDG PET indicated potential modification of the surgical management in 9 patients. Distant metastases were detected using FDG PET in 3 patients.

Conclusion.—FDG PET should be used as the whole-body imaging method of choice in the follow-up of patients with thyroid cancer suspected of tumor recurrence, as indicated by ^{131}I scanning results. FDG PET appears to be superior to other whole-body imaging techniques when used for this purpose.

▶ Medicare is presently considering covering FDG-PET scans in thyroid cancer, particularly for this indication. From this study, 3 patients had false-positive results, with 2 patients having benign cervical lymph nodes that were considered positive on FDG PET. The sensitivity of 95%, however, was quite high.

R. E. Coleman, MD

Clinical Relevance of Thyroid Fluorodeoxyglucose-Whole Body Positron Emission Tomography Incidentaloma

Van Den Bruel A, Maes A, De Potter T, et al (Universitaire Ziekenhuizen Gasthuisberg, Leuven, Belgium)
J Clin Endocrinol Metab 87:1517-1520, 2002   2–50

Background.—Thyroid incidentalomas, which occur in 19% to 46% of persons, can be detected by US or CT. Generally, 1.5% to 10% prove to be carcinoma. FDG PET detects glucose metabolism in the lesions. While it has been used effectively in the follow-up of thyroid cancers, the highly prevalent cold thyroid nodules have not been studied by this technique for diagnosis. When performing whole-body FDG PET for a nonthyroid malignancy or paraneoplastic occurrence, a hot spot within the thyroid region may be detected (thyroid incidentaloma). The first 8 cases of thyroid FDG PET incidentaloma referred to 1 institution were described.

Subjects.—All had been referred to the endocrine department to evaluate thyroid "hot spots" found on whole body FDG PET scans. US, fine needle aspiration cytology (FNAC), and histologic assessments were carried out to determine the pathologic condition responsible for the thyroid incidentalomas. On FNAC, all cases required surgery, which was performed in 7 of the 8 patients.

Results.—Five patients had malignancies, 2 of which were medullary thyroid carcinomas and 3 of which were papillary thyroid carcinomas. One of the medullary thyroid carcinomas had invaded the lymph nodes; 2 of the papillary thyroid carcinomas invaded through the thyroid capsule. In 2 patients for whom the FDG-PET results were positive, FNAC indicated a follicular neoplasm which was confirmed histologically in 2 cases to be follicular adenoma. Surgery was yet to be performed in the third case.

Conclusion.—Malignancy occurs at a high rate among thyroid FDG-PET incidentalomas.

▶ Focal areas of abnormal accumulation in the thyroid have been associated with thyroid malignancy. Several reports have noted that most of these focal areas of accumulation are proven to be papillary thyroid cancer. In our experience, we have also seen metastatic melanoma and cellular adenoma cause focal uptake in the thyroid. Focal areas of abnormal accumulation of FDG in the thyroid should be pursued.

R. E. Coleman, MD

Bone and In-111 Octreotide Imaging in Oncogenic Osteomalacia: A Case Report

Garcia CA, Spencer RP (Univ of Connecticut, Farmington)
Clin Nucl Med 27:582-583, 2002   2–51

Background.—Osteoporosis associated with aging is the most frequent cause of bone mineral loss, but other causes do exist. A case of abnormal bone loss with excessive osteoid formation caused by osteomalacia is described.

>*Case Report.*—A 46-year-old man presented with chronic hip and lower extremity pain. Five years earlier he had experienced inflammation of the knees and prostatitis, which was attributed to Reiter's syndrome and which was successfully treated with drainage of the knees. Since that time, he had begun experiencing increasing pain in the pelvis and right hip that was attributed to spondyloarthropathy. He did not respond to sulfasalazine, prednisone, indocin, or methotrexate, which promoted his referral to the authors. His previous laboratory tests revealed normal free androgen and serum calcium levels, a slightly low phosphate level (2 mg/dL), and elevated levels of serum alkaline phosphatase (300 U/L) and intact parathormone (69 pg/mL). The patient underwent a bone scan of the hip and pelvis, which revealed numerous sites of uptake. A scan performed with ^{111}In octreotide revealed a focus in the right humeral head (Fig 2). The patient underwent surgery, at which time a phosphaturic tumor of mesenchymal origin was partially resected. The patient had an incomplete chemical response to resection and thus was referred for additional surgery and chemotherapy. After additional treatment, his condition improved markedly.

Conclusion.—[111]In octreotide identified the site of a phosphaturia-inducing mesenchymal tumor. This is an uncommon cause of osteomalacia that is related to the secretion of phosphaturic material from a fibroblast growth

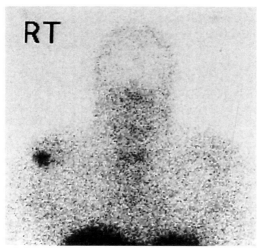

FIGURE 2.—The anterior [111]In OctreoScan showed accumulation in the right humeral head. (Courtesy of Garcia CA, Spencer RP: Bone and In-111 octreotide imaging in oncogenic osteomalacia: A case report. *Clin Nucl Med* 27(8):582-583, 2002.)

factor and should be considered in patients with osteomalacia for whom there are atypical laboratory findings.

▶ I do not generally consider case reports for inclusion in this book. During the last several years, I have been asked to perform an OctreoScan in patients with suspected oncogenic osteomalacia. I have had 1 patient who had a positive scan that was documented to be a phosphaturic tumor of mesenchymal origin. The FDG-PET scan also demonstrated the abnormality.

This syndrome is one that I was not aware of, and radionuclide imaging may be important in evaluating the site of the tumor causing the osteomalacia.

R. E. Coleman, MD

Phase II Trial of Murine ^{131}I-Labeled Antitenascin Monoclonal Antibody 81C6 Administered Into Surgically Created Resection Cavities of Patients With Newly Diagnosed Malignant Gliomas
Reardon DA, Akabani G, Coleman RE, et al (Duke Univ, Durham, NC; Univ of California at Davis, San Rafael)
J Clin Oncol 20:1389-1397, 2002   2–52

Background.—The poor prognosis of patients with malignant glioma, especially glioblastoma multiforme (GBM), has not been improved with current treatments, carrying a median survival for patients newly diagnosed of only 40 to 60 weeks and that for patients with recurrent disease of 16 to 24 weeks. Because 90% of recurrences are linked to the failure to eradicate local tumor growth, adjuvant therapies that improve local control are particularly needed. Phase I clinical trials were performed using ^{131}I-labeled murine 81C6 (mu81C6) monoclonal antibodies (mAbs) injected directly into the patients' surgically created resection cavities (SCRCs). The results of a phase II study using 120 mCi of ^{131}I-labeled mu81C6 mAb injected into the SCRCs were evaluated in patients newly diagnosed and previously untreated with malignant gliomas.

Methods.—Of the 33 patients (10 women, 23 men), 27 had GBM, 4 had anaplastic astrocytoma, and 2 had anaplastic oligodendroglioma. Patients ranged in age from 19 to 68 years (median age, 50 years) and had been diagnosed a median of 1.3 months before treatment began. All had the 120 mCi of ^{131}I-labeled mu81C6 mAbs injected directly into the SCRC, then received conventional external-beam radiotherapy, and finally alkylator-based chemotherapy for 1 year. Follow-up extended for 49 to 220 weeks (median, 93 weeks).

Results.—Twenty-two patients have died, with a median survival of 86.7 weeks overall and 79.4 weeks for those with GBM. Reversible hematologic toxicity developed in 27% of patients, treatment-related neurologic toxicity developed in 15%, and radionecrosis that required reoperation developed in 3% (1 patient). In 2 patients, irreversible neurologic toxicity developed that was related to progressive tumor rather than treatment.

Conclusion.—The use of ^{131}I-labeled mu81C6 mAb injected into the SCRC of these patients with malignant glioma prolonged survival when compared with the results of conventional therapy or interstitial chemotherapy. Only 1 patient required reoperation for symptomatic radionecrosis, and hematologic and neurologic toxicities were within acceptable limits.

▶ Patients who have malignant gliomas have a poor prognosis. Chemotherapy and external beam radiotherapy have not been particularly effective in treating these tumors. We have been instilling radiolabeled mAbs into the cystic resection cavities of these patients in an attempt to prolong survival. The results of this phase II study suggest that the radiolabeled mAb therapy improves survival compared with historical controls and compares favorably with interstitial brachytherapy and stereotactic radiosurgery. We continue to modify the procedure in an attempt to improve patient outcome.

R. E. Coleman, MD

3 Musculoskeletal

Introduction

Many of the new and interesting articles on the role of nuclear medicine in musculoskeletal imaging are those evaluating PET techniques. PET does appear to have an increasingly important role in evaluating both primary and metastatic bone disease. Fluorine-18 fluoride PET bone imaging may become a standard of care in the future.

Some old topics—such as the frequency of metastatic disease in a solitary rib lesion and the relationships between prostate specific antigen levels and bone scan positivity—are revisited. And some new data on the use of bone scans for evaluating trauma are included.

R. Edward Coleman, MD

Prospective Evaluation of the Clinical Value of Planar Bone Scans, SPECT, and ^{18}F-Labeled NaF PET in Newly Diagnosed Lung Cancer
Schirrmeister H, Glatting G, Hertzel J, et al (Univ of Ulm, Germany)
J Nucl Med 42:1800-1804, 2001   3–1

Background.—Although 20% to 25% of lung cancers are of the small-cell type (SCLC), it is the non–small-cell lung cancer (NSCLC) that has no distant metastases that is potentially curable. Bone metastases occur in 20% to 30% of lung cancers when they are initially diagnosed and are found in 35% to 66% of the autopsies performed on these patients. The most commonly affected region is the vertebral column, and the most accurate imaging modality for detecting bone metastases in the vertebral column is MRI. Other methods include planar bone scintigraphy (BS), ^{18}F-labeled PET scans, and SPECT. These modalities were compared for their capability in detecting bone metastases in patients with newly diagnosed lung cancer.

Methods.—The 53 patients (42 men and 11 women; age range, 43-78 years; median, 63 years) had either SCLC (12 patients) or locally advanced NSCLC (41 patients). Planar BS, SPECT of the vertebral column, and ^{18}F PET were used; MRI, other imaging methods, and the clinical course were used as reference methods. A 5-point scale for receiver operating characteristic (ROC) curve analysis was developed to compare BS with and without SPECT and ^{18}F PET.

Results.—Metastatic bone disease was found in 12 patients. Planar BS found only 5 and also produced 6 false-negative and 5 equivocal results. BS gave the correct diagnosis in 35 patients free of bone metastases but also produced 2 false-positive results. SPECT imaging found vertebral bone metastases in 5 of the 6 false-negative results found on planar BS. ^{18}F PET correctly identified 52 patients. The findings for 1 patient who had a single rib metastasis were deemed equivocal on the basis of SPECT, BS, and ^{18}F PET. Planar BS had an area under the ROC curve of 0.779, BS plus SPECT had 0.944, and ^{18}F PET had 0.993. Tomographic methods showed significantly higher diagnostic accuracy than planar BS used alone. Because of the improved imaging offered by ^{18}F PET and MRI, 3 patients with SCLC and 3 with NSCLC were found to have bone metastases, which changed their staging and treatment. Instead of curative surgery, palliative chemotherapy was given to the patients with NSCLC; a different chemotherapy regimen was chosen for the 3 with SCLC. Seven of 12 cases showed an underestimation of the metastatic bone disease on BS plus SPECT imaging, although no change in management was required. The use of ^{18}F PET and MRI led to a management change in 50% of patients, and the use of complementary SPECT imaging changed it in 42%.

Conclusions.—The use of at least 1 tomographic modality would be warranted for patients with lung cancer who are at increased risk of having bone metastases. Whole-body imaging can be done with ^{18}F PET, but it is costly and not always available. Combining planar BS and SPECT complemented by MRI in select cases offers the most practical and cost-effective strategy for staging disease in these patients.

▶ I predict that ^{18}F-NaF PET imaging will become the standard of care in diagnosing bone metastases instead of the ^{99m}Tc-phosphate bone scan when an adequate number of dedicated PET scanners are available to accommodate these procedures. This transition will take several years to occur.

R. E. Coleman, MD

Quantitative Evaluation of Skeletal Tumours With Dynamic FDG PET: SUV in Comparison to Patlak Analysis
Wu H, Dimitrakopoulou-Strauss A, Heichel TO, et al (German Cancer Research Ctr, Heidelberg, Germany; Univ of Heidelberg, Germany; Univ of Zürich, Switzerland)
Eur J Nucl Med 28:704-710, 2001   3–2

Background.—FDG PET has been extensively studied in the past decade in experimental and clinical oncology and has been found to be a valuable imaging tool for the evaluation of a variety of tumors, primarily on the basis of the observations that malignant tumors have increased glucose metabolism in comparison with normal tissues and that more aggressive malignant lesions have higher rates of glucose use. FDG PET is reported to have been used in a small number of cases to evaluate skeletal tumors. Whether bone lesions could be assessed with FDG PET and whether dynamic and quantitative PET data might aid in the differentiation of benign lesions from malignant masses were determined.

Methods.—The study group included 40 patients with primary bone lesions, with the final diagnosis confirmed by histopathologic analysis. All of the subjects underwent a 60-minute dynamic FDG PET acquisition. From the dynamic PET images, indexes such as the average and maximal standardized uptake values (SUVs), the tumor SUV-to-muscle SUV ratio (T/M), and the SUV at 60 minute-to-SUV at 30-minute ratio were calculated. The sensitivity and specificity of each parameter in differentiating between malignant and benign lesions were evaluated on the basis of the receiver operator characteristic (ROC) curve.

Results.—Histologic findings revealed 21 malignant tumors and 19 benign tumors in the study group, representing a considerable overlap between benign and malignant lesions in each index. The average SUV correlated positively with the metabolic rate of FDG (MRFDG). A cutoff of 1.8 average SUV yielded a sensitivity and specificity for discrimination of malignancy from benign disease of 85% and 82.4%, respectively. MRFDG showed a similar sensitivity (82.4%) and a better specificity (92.9%).

Conclusions.—A detectable difference was noted in glucose metabolism between malignant and benign skeletal lesions. The static DG uptake indexes alone may not provide enough differentiation between benign and malignant lesions. Quantitative dynamic imaging can yield more helpful information but does not allow a definite diagnosis. The use of uptake indexes may provide an alternative and interesting approach to evaluating skeletal lesions.

▶ More studies on a large number of patients with sarcoma are appearing in the literature. This carefully performed study demonstrates the potential advantages of combining indices obtained from PET scans to obtain a more accurate diagnosis. As has been previously demonstrated, the SUV in this population correlates with the metabolic rate of FDG. The mean SUV had a sensitivity and specificity of 85% and 82% respectively. Some benign skeletal lesions are hypermetabolic, and some malignant lesions are less metabolic. Thus, the accuracy of FDG PET in skeletal tumors may be less than in other tumors.

R. E. Coleman, MD

Clinical Value of Grading the Scintigraphic Appearances of Tibial Stress Fractures in Military Recruits
Dutton J, Bromhead SE, Speed CA, et al (Addenbrooke's Hosp, Cambridge, England; ATR Bassingbourn, Bassingbourn Barracks, Herts, UK)
Clin Nucl Med 27:18-21, 2002   3–3

Background.—Tibial stress fractures reportedly occur in 4% to more than 31% of military recruits, with various individual outcomes, but a number of recruits are unable to continue their careers in the military. The appearance of these stress fractures on bone scintigraphy was correlated with clinical outcome, specifically, whether the recruit would be able to recover enough to complete the 11-week initial course and continue to the subsequent phase of military training.

Methods.—A retrospective review was conducted of 58 technetium-99m methylene diphosphate (^{99m}Tc-MDP) images of recruits with possible tibial stress fractures. Each was graded using the criteria of Zwas et al. (Figs 1 and 2). Clinical information was correlated with the appearance of the stress fracture.

Results.—Bone scans detected 37 tibial stress fractures, with 23 grade I or II and 14 of grades III or IV. These fractures were not seen on radiographs that were available for 24 patients. The duration of rehabilitation required ranged from 6 to 20 weeks, but the time required was equivalent between those with grade III or IV fractures and those with grade I or II fractures. Five recruits left the army for nonmedical reasons. Of the 21 remaining recruits with grade I or II fractures, 15 were medically discharged, whereas of the 11 remaining recruits with more serious grade III or IV fractures, only 4 were discharged. No difference in discharge frequency was related to unilateral

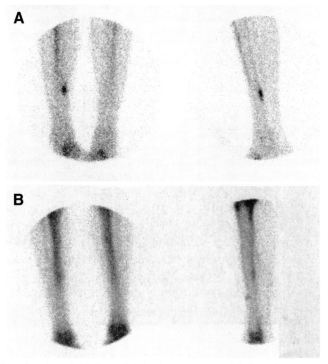

FIGURE 1.—Anterior and right leg medial Tc-99m MDP images of the lower legs in two recruits show low-grade focal abnormal uptake in the posteromedial aspect of the right tibia. These are examples of "low-grade" stress fractures included in the Zwas grade I-II group. (Courtesy of Dutton J, Bromhead SE, Speed CA, et al: Clinical value of grading the scintigraphic appearance of tibial stress fractures in military recruits. *Clin Nucl Med* 27(1):18-21, 2002.)

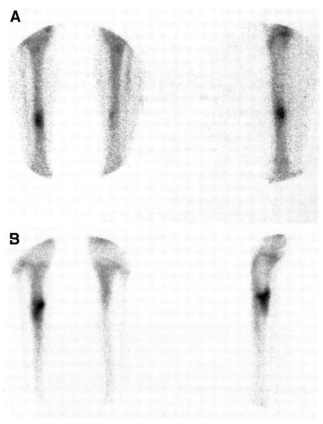

FIGURE 2.—Anterior and right leg medial Tc-99m MDP images of the lower legs in two recruits show relatively intense focal abnormal uptake in the posteromedial aspect of the right tibias. These are examples of "high-grade" stress fractures included in the Zwas III-IV group. Bilateral abnormalities are apparent in panel **A**. In addition to the uptake at the right tibial stress fracture, foci of less intense uptake are visible in the left tibia and proximal fibula that likely represent further sites of traumatic change. (Courtesy of Dutton J, Bromhead SE, Speed CA, et al: Clinical value of grading the scintigraphic appearance of tibial stress fractures in military recruits. *Clin Nucl Med* 27(1):18-21, 2002.)

versus bilateral stress fractures. Full recovery was made by 6 patients with upper-shaft fractures, but a significant trend was noted toward medical discharge when the fracture involved the mid-diaphyseal region rather than the upper or lower end of the shaft.

Conclusions.—Patients with more severe stress fractures had better clinical outcomes than those with less severe involvement. Stress fractures that occur in the upper-tibial shaft were of grade III to IV severity, and these recruits had complete recovery, completing the training program. Patients with middle- or lower-shaft fractures had a poorer clinical outcome and were more likely to be medically discharged.

▶ We evaluate several patients each week for possible stress fracture. I have included this article because there are not many articles appearing in the literature on the use of bone scanning in stress fractures. I think that it is useful to use grading of the abnormality from I to IV.

R. E. Coleman, MD

Distinguishing Scintigraphic Features of Spondylolysis
Van der Wall H, Storey G, Magnussen J, et al (Concord Hosp, Sydney, Australia; Prince of Wales Hosp, Sydney, Australia)
J Pediatr Orthop 22:308-311, 2002   3–4

Background.—The initial diagnosis and management of back pain in young athletes has been helped by using scintigraphy, but the proximity of the pars interarticularis to the facet joints of the lumbar spine is sometimes confusing. With multiheaded gamma cameras becoming available, high counts are routinely acquired in tomographic studies. These studies have shown increased uptake in the ipsilateral or contralateral pedicle of the segment with a pars fracture. These patterns were assessed to see whether they were specific to pars fractures.

Methods.—The 25 young athletes (15 patients with pars fractures and 10 patients with back pain of a nonspondylolytic etiology) ranged from ages 9

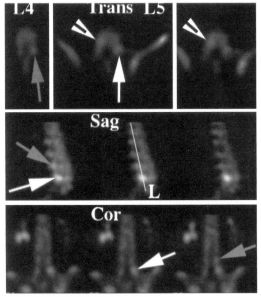

FIGURE 3.—Contralateral uptake in the pedicle. Cricketer with lower back pain. CT showed a pars interarticularis fracture at L5. The scintigraphic study shows increased uptake in the left pars interarticularis of L5 (*white arrow*) as well as increased uptake in the contralateral pedicle (*arrowhead*). There is also increased uptake in the left-sided facet joint of L4 (*gray arrow*). In the sagittal view, the triangular pattern of uptake is again evident, extending across the posterior aspect of the spinal canal, unlike the uptake from facet joint disease, which ends at the posterior margin. The posterior limit of the spinal canal is indicated by an oblique line (*L*). (Courtesy of Van der Wall H, Storey G, Magnussen J, et al: Distinguishing scintigraphic features of spondylolysis. *J Pediatr Orthop* 22(3):308-311, 2002.)

to 16 years. Their medical records were assessed retrospectively, with diagnoses confirmed using plain radiography, CT, and/or clinical outcome.

Results.—Twelve of the 15 patients had abnormal CT results; 3 who had pinpoint tenderness over the pars at L4 or L5 had normal findings. Five patients had abnormal results of plain radiographs consistent with pars fractures. Scintigraphy identified all 15 patients with spondylolysis as having increased uptake in the ipsilateral or contralateral pedicle (Fig 3). Eight had L5 pars involvement and in 7, the L4 pars was affected. Patients who had had back pain the longest had the contralateral pedicle involved. This characteristic pattern of uptake was not found in any of the patients with facet joint disease, intervertebral disk disease, or muscle insertion injury, nor did the triangular pattern of uptake seen in the sagittal view of those with pars fractures occur in patients with facet joint disease.

Conclusion.—Patients with a pars fracture are likely to have increased uptake in the pedicle, and those lacking this fracture will not exhibit this pattern. The biological and prognostic significance of these findings require assessment. A triangular pattern of uptake in the sagittal projection is probably the result of anatomical factors specific to the pars interarticularis.

▶ Bone scans at our institution are most frequently ordered for evaluating possible metastatic disease to bone. The second most common indication is evaluation of sport injuries. Young athletes often develop back pain, and stress fractures of the pars interarticularis are considered. Bone imaging has an important role in evaluating these patients. This study documents the accuracy of bone imaging in identifying spondylolysis. SPECT imaging demonstrates a triangular pattern of uptake on the sagittal view, a finding of which I was unaware.

R. E. Coleman, MD

Can Initial Prostate Specific Antigen Determinations Eliminate the Need for Bone Scans in Patients With Newly Diagnosed Prostate Carcinoma? A Multicenter Retrospective Study in Japan
Kosuda S, Yoshimura I, Aizawa T, et al (Natl Defense Med College, Tokorozawa, Japan; Tokyo Med College; Chiba Univ, Japan; et al)
Cancer 94:964-972, 2002   3–5

Background.—Among Japanese men, prostate carcinoma may soon become the second leading cause of cancer death, an increase probably attributable to increased detection with serum prostate specific antigen (PSA) measurements as well as the aging of the Japanese population. Those newly diagnosed undergo bone scintigraphy and serum PSA measurements, the results of which are used for staging and baseline values for later bone scans. To control costs, it would be helpful to avoid performing bone scintigraphy in all cases, but appropriate PSA levels must be set for eliminating the bone scans. Patients with newly diagnosed prostate carcinoma were evaluated to see if a serum PSA level of 10 ng/mL or less would allow the elimination of bone scanning.

Methods.—The 1294 patients were assessed retrospectively; 290 had well differentiated tumors, 629 moderately differentiated, and 328 poorly differentiated. Bone scans, serum PSA measurements, and a core needle biopsy of the prostate were performed. Identification of positive bone scan based on serum PSA level was evaluated using a receiver operating characteristic curve, and a decision tree was developed to assess expected 10-year cumulative cost and disease-specific survival rate. The 2 strategies adopted were PSA alone, in which only patients whose PSA level was more than 10 ng/mL had a bone scan, and PSA plus baseline bone scan.

Results.—Gleason scores were available for 614 patients and ranged from 2 to 10 (score of 2 in 22 patients, 3 in 44 patients, 4 in 42 patients, 5 in 130 patients, 6 in 73 patients, 7 in 179 patients, 8 in 48 patients, 9 in 70 patients, and 10 in 6 patients). Three hundred patients had PSA values of 10 ng/mL or less, and bone scans were positive for metastasis in 287 patients and negative in 1007 patients. Sensitivity and specificity curves for serum PSA levels in detecting bone metastasis crossed at 60 ng/mL. The area under the receiver operating characteristic curve was 0.870 for the detection of bone metastasis based on PSA value. The highest proportion of positive bone scans was found in patients with Gleason grade 5 primary tumors and the lowest for patients with grade 1 and 2 tumors; it was also lower for patients with grade 6 tumors or above. As serum PSA levels fell, cost saving gradually declined, as did the proportion of positive bone scans. By eliminating the bone scan in patients whose serum PSA levels were 10 ng/mL or less, the hospitals could realize a cost savings annually of $107.60 per patient newly diagnosed with prostate carcinoma. The decision-tree analysis showed PSA-alone strategy saved $16 in cumulative net cost per patient over the PSA plus bone scan strategy, based on 10 years of monitoring.

Conclusions.—The baseline bone scan could be eliminated in Japanese men who have been newly diagnosed with prostate carcinoma if their PSA levels are under 10 ng/mL and especially if their Gleason grade is 2 or less or 6 or over.

► Similar results have been obtained from studies in the United States. I do not remember seeing a newly diagnosed prostate cancer patient who has a PSA level less than 10 ng/mL and a positive bone scan.

R. E. Coleman, MD

Scintigraphy of Injuries to the Distal Tibiofibular Syndesmosis
Frater C, van Gaal W, Kannangara S, et al (Charles Sturt Univ, Wagga Wagga, Australia; Concord Hosp, Sydney, Australia)
Clin Nucl Med 27:625-627, 2002   3–6

Background.—Sprains of the ankle are generally considered to be benign and are rather common, occurring in approximately 75% of athletes (and in

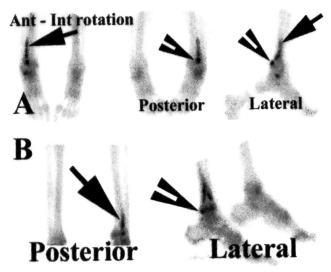

FIGURE 3.—These 2 examples show an extensive tear of the interosseous membrane (**A**, *arrow*) and the site of fracture-avulsion of the tibial plafond. More extensive tears of both the tibial and fibula insertions of the membrane (**B**, *arrow*) are shown, as is the fracture-avulsion of the plafond. (Courtesy of Frater C, van Gaal W, Kannangara S, et al: Scintigraphy of injuries to the distal tibiofibular syndesmosis. *Clin Nucl Med* 27(9):625-627, 2002.)

nonathletes as well). However, in approximately 5% of ankle sprains, the injury is more complex and has a rotational component. Forced rotational injury to the ankle can disrupt the tibiofibular syndesmosis and tear the tibiofibular ligaments and the interosseous membrane. This can compromise the integrity of the ankle mortice and lead to delayed healing. The scintigraphic features of 4 patients with such injuries are presented.

Methods.—The subjects were 3 male professional soccer players 18 to 24 years old and one 34-year-old female army officer undergoing basic training who incurred external rotation injuries to the ankle. All patients presented several weeks after trauma with a provisional diagnosis of distal tibial stress fracture. Standard anterior, medial, and lateral views were obtained with bone scintigraphy. In addition, anterior views were obtained with the feet internally rotated 25° to 35° to separate the tibia from the fibula.

Results.—In all cases, the posterior edge of the tibial plafond showed increased uptake, consistent with avulsion of the posterior-inferior tibiofibular ligament. All patients also showed an extensive tear of the interosseous membrane, characterized by either an elongated focus of uptake at the level of the fibula notch or as a tapered defect beginning at this level and extending superiorly (Fig 3).

Conclusion.—External rotational injuries to the ankle can tear the tibiofibular ligaments and the interosseous membrane and can fracture the tibial plafond. Scintigraphy with the feet internally rotated can help identify such injuries and facilitate specific treatment.

▶ Whenever I have a bone scan with an abnormality around the joint, I indicate that the abnormality is most likely resulting from trauma. This study suggests that we can be more specific about the type of trauma that the patient has undergone.

R. E. Coleman, MD

Clinical Significance of Solitary Rib Hot Spots on Bone Scans in Patients With Extraskeletal Cancer: Correlation With Other Clinical Manifestations
Wu P-S, Chiu N-T, Lee B-F, et al (Natl Cheng Kung Univ, Tainan, Taiwan)
Clin Nucl Med 27:567-571, 2002   3–7

Background.—In patients with extraskeletal cancer, bone scintigraphy has a low specificity in identifying the cause of a solitary area of increased radioactivity on a rib. To determine how often these rib hot spots are caused by metastatic disease and to examine the clinical correlates in such cases, a retrospective study was undertaken.

Methods.—The medical records of 93 patients (32 men and 61 women; mean age, 52 years) with a proven extraskeletal primary cancer but without evidence of skeletal metastasis were reviewed. Each case was characterized by the presence of a solitary hot spot in the ribs on scintigraphy. Follow-up radiographs and bone scans were examined to identify hot spots that represented metastatic disease. A metastatic hot spot was defined as scintigraphic evidence of bony destruction that showed progression on follow-up bone scans. The clinical characteristics of patients with metastatic hot spots were also assessed.

Results.—Of the patient cases reviewed, the solitary rib hot spot was malignant in 11 patients (11.8%) and benign in 82 patients (88.2%). The cases with a malignant rib hot spot included 3 of 48 patients (6.3%) with breast cancer, 3 of 12 patients (25%) with lung cancer, 2 of 7 patients (28.6%) with nasopharyngeal cancer, 2 of 3 patients (66.7%) with hepatic cancer, and 1 of 3 patients (33.3%) with prostate cancer. Of the 11 metastatic rib hot spots, 6 (54.5%) were in the posterior portion of the rib, 4 (36.4%) were in the lateral portion, 1 (9.1%) was in the anterior portion, and none were in the costochondral junction. Clinical manifestations did not differ significantly between patients with and without solitary malignant rib hot spots. Localized bone pain was reported by 9.1% of patients with malignant hot spots and by 2.4% of those with benign hot spots; 57.1% and 37.7% with malignant and benign hot spots, respectively, had elevated levels of tumor markers, 45.5% and 23.2% had concurrent extraskeletal metastases, and in 83.3% and 75.4%, the hot spot was concordant with the primary tumor (Fig 1).

Conclusion.—Only approximately 12% of the solitary rib hot spots found on bone scans represented metastatic disease. The clinical character-

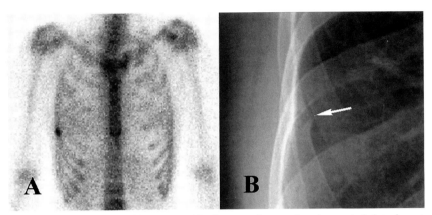

FIGURE 1.—In a patient with breast cancer (A), a bone scan shows a solitary hot spot in the lateral aspect of the right sixth rib. B) A subsequent chest radiograph shows bone destruction at the corresponding site. (Courtesy of Wu P-S, Chiu N-T, Lee B-F, et al: Clinical significance of solitary rib hot spots on bone scans in patients with extraskeletal cancer: Correlation with other clinical manifestations. *Clin Nucl Med* 27(8):567-571, 2002.)

istics of these patients were not particularly useful in differentiating malignant from benign hot spots. Patients with extraskeletal cancer who have a solitary rib hot spot should be followed up regularly with bone scintigraphy or radiography to identify changes in tumor activity.

▶ Single rib abnormalities in a patient with a known malignancy are problematic. I have not been impressed with the ability of radiographs to be accurate in clarifying the etiology of the lesion. The authors of this study have good follow-up and documentation of the etiology of the solitary rib lesions. The 10% likelihood of a solitary rib lesion being malignant that I have been quoting for years seems to still be appropriate. I am not convinced that plain films of the ribs help clarify the etiology of the solitary rib hot spot.

R. E. Coleman, MD

4 Inflammation and Infection

Introduction

Nuclear medicine imaging of inflammation and infection is not commonly performed in most institutions, but there are circumstances in which the nuclear medicine procedures do add value in patient management. The articles in this chapter further define the role of nuclear medicine imaging in orthopedics, fever of undetermined etiology, and spondylitis.

R. Edward Coleman, MD

FDG-PET, ^{99m}Tc-HMPAO White Blood Cell SPET and Bone Scintigraphy in the Evaluation of Painful Total Knee Arthroplasties

Van Acker F, Nuyts J, Maes A, et al (Katholieke Universiteit van Leuven, Belgium)

Eur J Nucl Med 28:1496-1504, 2001   4–1

Background.—Diagnosing an infection in a total knee arthroplasty (TKA) requires more than clinical evaluation, erythrocyte sedimentation rate, peripheral leukocyte count, and plain radiographs; the most useful single test is preoperative joint aspiration. Among the techniques explored in the search for more convenient, faster assessment tools are FDG PET, technetium-99m hexamethylpropyleneamine oxime–labeled white blood cell (WBC) scintigraphy, and bone scintigraphy. A comparison of these 3 techniques was carried out in patients with painful TKAs.

Methods.—Twenty-one patients (13 women and 8 men; age range, 33-78 years; mean, 66 years) and 17 asymptomatic control subjects (11 women and 6 men; age range, 48-76 years; mean, 67 years) all underwent TKAs. The 21 patients had 3-phase bone scans to exclude infection, followed by WBC scintigraphy and FDG PET.

Results.—Infections were confirmed by microbiological culture or clinical follow-up of at least 6 months in 6 TKAs of the patient group. Bone scans detected abnormal blood flow in 17 patients; a focal component was present in 8, and diffuse uptake was seen in 14. Of the patients with infected TKAs, only 1 showed focal nonpatellar tracer uptake of grade 2, 2 had grade 3, 2 had grade 4, and 1 had grade 4 with diffuse uptake. On WBC scans, focal uptake was found in 12 patients, and femoral bone marrow was clearly seen in 2 others. Focal lesions had a grade 2.6 uptake. Increased focal uptake was found in all scanned, infected TKAs. A specificity of 53% was found when focal uptake was the criterion for diagnosing infection. The FDG-PET scans showed focal FDG uptake in 11 patients; the intensity was 2.63. A specificity of 73% was achieved when focal FDG uptake at the bone–prosthesis interface was the criterion for diagnosing infection. With attenuation-corrected FDG PET, 18 focal lesions were found in 11 patients. The intensity of the FDG uptake visually was significantly less for focal lesions but the same for diffuse uptake as in non–attenuation-corrected images. The mean standardized uptake value for focal lesions on non–attenuation-corrected FDG was 3.72; nonpatellar focal lesions had a standardized uptake value of 3.29. Loosening of the TKA showed focal uptake at the tibial tip and/or prosthesis neck on bone scanning; focal uptake in 4 patients and diffuse uptake in 2 on WBC scanning; and diffuse uptake in 4 patients and focal uptake in 2 on FDG PET.

Conclusions.—Diffuse uptake (horseshoe pattern) in the dynamic and blood pool phases was found on bone scanning in all infected TKAs. WBC scans had a specificity of 93% for lesions also seen on bone scans but had only 53% specificity for focal uptake only. FDG-PET scans showed focal uptake at the bone–prosthesis interface with a sensitivity of 100% and a specificity of 73% on non–attenuation-corrected images. Comparing PET images with bone scan results allowed better detection of focal FDG uptake. Attenuation correction did not seem to be needed. Infected TKAs were detected with the highest specificity when WBC scanning was combined with bone scanning. FDG PET seemed to add no information to the process.

▶ FDG-PET imaging is infrequently performed for the evaluation of infection. Several studies evaluating FDG PET in painful arthroplasties have suggested that FDG PET may be useful in this condition. This article concludes that WBC scintigraphy in combination with bone scintigraphy is the best combination for evaluating these patients and that FDG-PET imaging does not add to the diagnosis in these patients. We will need more information to determine whether FDG PET has a role in this condition.

R. E. Coleman, MD

The Efficacy of Techetium-99m Ciprofloxacin (Infecton) Imaging in Suspected Orthopaedic Infection: A Comparison With Sequential Bone/ Gallium Imaging

Yapar Z, Kibar M, Yapar AF, et al (Cukurova Univ, Adana, Turkey; Numune Hosp, Adana, Turkey)
Eur J Nucl Med 28:822-830, 2001   4–2

Introduction.—^{99m}Tc ciprofloxacin (Infecton) is a new radiopharmaceutical for the imaging of infection. The value of Infecton imaging in identifying orthopedic infection was examined and results were compared with those of bone/gallium imaging.

Methods.—Twenty-two patients with suspected orthopedic infective conditions underwent 3 scintigraphic examinations in the following sequence: 740 MBq ^{99m}Tc–methylene diphosphonate 3-phase bone scintigraphy; at least 2 days later, 370 MBq Infecton scan at 1 to 4 hours; and 185 MBq ^{67}Ga scintigraphy. Four patients were not able to undergo ^{67}Ga imaging. Two blinded independent observers evaluated all images. The final diagnosis was made by consensus when findings were different. Interpretation of the early and late Infecton images was made separately. Visual findings were classified according to a 4-grade scale (0, +, + +, and + + +). Images graded 0 and + and those regions that demonstrated a reduction in uptake grade on late images, as compared with early images, were considered negative for infection; grades + + and + + + were considered positive. The bone/gallium images were considered positive when the images were spatially incongruent or when gallium uptake was more intense, compared with that of ^{99m}Tc–methylene diphosphonate. The diagnosis was verified by intraoperative microbiological or histologic findings, or by the presence of gross purulence.

Results.—The sensitivity, specificity, and accuracy of Infecton imaging were 85%, 92%, and 88%, respectively, compared with 78%, 100%, and 90%, respectively, for bone/gallium imaging.

Conclusion.—Infecton and bone/gallium imaging had similar clinical yield. The easy availability of Infecton and the short investigation time make Infecton imaging the better option for identifying infection.

▶ ^{99m}Tc–labeled ciprofloxacin is not routinely available in the United States. This agent for imaging infection does appear to have some advantages over the presently used agents. This article was selected to let the audience know that new agents are being developed for imaging infection.

R. E. Coleman, MD

Diagnostic Value of ^{111}In-Granulocyte Scintigraphy in Patients With Fever of Unknown Origin

Kjaer A, Lebech A-M (Univ of Copenhagen)
J Nucl Med 43:140-144, 2002   4–3

Background.—On the basis of studies performed more than 10 years ago, the sensitivity of scintigraphy using ^{111}In-granulocytes to assess patients with fever of unknown origin (FUO) has been estimated as 55% to 85%, and the corresponding specificity is between 74% and 94% for detecting infection as the cause. The diagnostic value of ^{111}In-granulocyte scintigraphy in patients with FUO defined under modern criteria was assessed, along with the usefulness of adding leukocyte count or C-reactive protein (CRP) evaluation to increase diagnostic performance.

Methods.—The files of 31 patients (17 females and 14 males), aged from 13 to 71 years, who had granulocyte scintigraphy were reviewed retrospectively to assess the ability of this modality to identify infection or chronic inflammatory bowel disease as the cause of the FUO. Elevated leukocyte counts and CRP levels were also analyzed.

Results.—For 22 (71%) of the patients, the following final diagnoses were obtained. Eight (36%) patients had an infection focus or chronic inflammatory bowel disease causing the FUO, 3 (10%) had neoplasms, 3 (10%) had Still's disease, 3 (10%) had cerebrally triggered fever, 1 (4%) had a lung embolism, 1 (4%) had subacute thyroiditis, 1 (4%) had polymyalgia rheumatica, 1 had other connective tissue disease, and 1 had hematoma fever. No cause was identified in 9 patients, of whom 6 (67%) recovered spontaneously. Scintigrams were true positive in 75% of the infectious cases and false negative in 25%. Scintigrams were true negative in 83% of the noninfectious cases and false positive in 17%. The sensitivity was determined to be 75%; specificity, 83%; positive predictive value, 60%; and negative predictive value, 90%. Leukocyte counts were increased in 39% of patients, and CRP levels were increased in 71%. Increased CRP levels were found in all patients with true-positive scintigrams and in half of those with true-negative scintigrams. Considering the 22 patients with increased CRP levels to evaluate test performance, sensitivity was 75%, specificity 71%, positive predictive value 60%, and negative predictive value 83%.

Conclusions.—The sensitivity and specificity of ^{111}In-granulocyte scintigraphy were high enough to make it an attractive adjunctive assessment. The high negative predictive value would definitely help rule out infection as causative of FUO. Peripheral leukocyte counts and CRP levels were not useful in determining which patients required scintigraphy.

▶ The evaluation of the patient who has a fever of unknown origin remains problematic. Most of these patients do not have an infectious process as the cause of the fever, but infection is still a primary consideration and is the cause of the fever in some of the patients. In this study of 31 patients, 8 had an infectious focus or chronic inflammatory bowel disease as the cause of the fever. My experience with Indium-111-labeled leukocyte imaging in fever of unknown origin has been that I have not found many patients with infections/inflammation as the cause of the fever. This article does suggest that Indium-111 leukocyte imaging is useful in identifying the patients who do have infection. In addition, it may be more useful in identifying the patients who do not have an infectious process as the cause of the fever.

R. E. Coleman, MD

---

¹⁸F-FDG Hybrid PET in Patients With Suspected Spondylitis
Gratz S, Dörner J, Fischer U, et al (Philipps Univ of Marburg, Germany; Georg August Univ of Göttingen, Germany)
Eur J Nucl Med 29:516-524, 2002   4–4

Background.—Infectious spondylitis presents a challenge in that it is marked by no specific clinical, laboratory, or radiologic findings. Complementary techniques performed in combination can be useful diagnostically. FDG imaging with a double-headed coincidence camera using a hybrid PET system was prospectively compared with conventional nuclear medicine imaging modalities (bone scan, ^{67}Ga citrate SPECT technique) and MRI in patients suspected of having infectious spondylitis. The FDG uptake in vertebral bodies that had degenerative changes was especially noted.

Methods.—The 9 male and 7 female patients (mean age, 59 years) underwent FDG hybrid PET (2 or 3 transverse scans) for suspected spondylitis. In addition, a ^{99m}Tc–methylene diphosphonate study was performed in 13 patients and a ^{67}Ga citrate assessment in 11 patients. Calculations were made of the ratios of infected to noninfected (target to background) vertebral bodies. Areas of interest were also imaged using MRI. Surgical intervention and histologic grading were performed for patients in whom spondylitis was found.

Results.—Twelve patients had spondylitis, and all were detected by MRI and/or FDG hybrid PET. FDG hybrid PET identified all of the known infected vertebrae, independent of grade of infection or spinal location. Infectious disease was indicated by target to background ratios above 1.45; degenerative change was found at ratios under this value. Patients who had a history of surgery and had high-grade infection plus paravertebral abscess formation and those who had low-grade spondylitis or diskitis were evaluated more accurately with FDG hybrid PET than with MRI.

Equal rates of detection were found for FDG hybrid PET and MRI in the evaluation of false-positive ^{67}Ga citrate or ^{99m}Tc–methylene diphosphonate SPECT images. The sensitivities of FDG hybrid PET, MRI, ^{67}Ga citrate, and bone scan were 100%, 82%, 73%, and 91%, respectively; the specificities were 87%, 85%, 61%, and 50%, respectively; and the diagnostic accuracies were 96%, 81%, 80%, and 80%, respectively.

Conclusion.—FDG hybrid PET successfully diagnosed vertebral osteomyelitis and helped in identifying mild infection and degenerative changes. In addition, manifestations outside of the spine were detected in several patients. The findings on FDG hybrid PET correlated with histologic findings indicating the infection's severity. FDG hybrid PET was easy to use, gave excellent imaging quality, and was diagnostically accurate.

▶ More articles on the use of FDG PET in imaging infection are beginning to appear in the literature. There are several ways of evaluating suspected infection in the spine, including MRI, ^{67}Ga-citrate imaging, and radionuclide bone imaging. Infectious spondylitis occurs with involvement with the disk and 2 adjacent vertebral bodies. This study demonstrates a high accuracy for detecting spondylitis. The results of the FDG-PET study were superior to the other imaging modalities, even with the use of hybrid PET.

R. E. Coleman, MD

5 Endocrinology

Introduction

As in previous years, a very large volume of work continues to be directed toward the role of nuclear medicine in endocrinology. The types of studies that are being reported are becoming increasingly sophisticated, and the majority of the work focuses on parathyroid, adrenal and thyroid imaging and therapy.

Although the techniques for parathyroid evaluation are relatively non-specific, the role of nuclear medicine in this area appears to be growing and becoming increasingly refined. Some of the molecular basis for the use of agents such as sestamibi is being studied with sophisticated in vitro investigations. We are also beginning to refine the interpretation criteria and to seek out a more important role for the intraoperative gamma probes, which have been a major advance in our diagnostic capabilities in many areas, especially breast and parathyroid. More importantly, we are beginning to see well thought out comparisons of the various diagnostic modalities to gain a better idea of the relative role of nuclear imaging in parathyroid disease and of its cost efficacy.

Adrenal lesions are reflected less in the literature than parathyroid with the expected lower prevalence of diseases of this organ. However, very importantly, the work that is beginning to appear with adrenal lesions is directed at PET where our diagnostic capability and potential for achieving high specificity is very optimistic. Although only a couple of articles are included in this year's YEAR BOOK, we will probably be seeing much more over the next several years.

Thyroid disease continues to be by far the most frequently encountered subject in the nuclear medicine literature in the field of endocrinology. This represents the very high prevalence of the diseases related to this organ. As with the parathyroid, we are beginning now to see more sophisticated analysis of radioiodine uptake by the thyroid as evidenced by investigations of the sodium iodide symporter and various other molecular investigations into iodine kinetics. It is remarkable that we are still discovering a variety of potentially confounding factors in our diagnostic studies of the thyroid and are continuing to debate over the optimal dose for treatment of benign thyroid disease.

In the field of thyroid cancer, the sodium iodide symporter has now been described and characterized and has received a considerable amount of attention during the past several years. Most importantly, the emerging role of

PET is becoming very apparent. We now have begun to appreciate the fact that in those patients who are positive on FDG scanning with PET and negative on ^{131}I whole body scans, there is need for more aggressive therapy because we are dealing with a potentially more malignant tumor. PET is having its role clearly defined and should play a role not only in diagnosis but also in helping us to refine therapeutic doses for thyroid cancer. Hopefully, this important role will be appreciated by third party insurance agencies, such as Medicare, and the indication for PET will be extended to the thyroid.

The diagnostic algorithm for both benign and malignant thyroid disease and for treatment for benign and malignant thyroid disease, continues to be refined and continues to be a fertile ground for investigation and productive contributions.

M. Donald Blaufox, MD, PhD

In Vitro Accumulation of Technetium-99m-Sestamibi in Human Parathyroid Mitochondria

Hetrakul N, Civelek AC, Stagg CA, et al (Yale Univ, New Haven, Conn)
Surgery 130:1011-1018, 2001   5–1

Introduction.—The imaging agent of choice for the preoperative localization of the parathyroid glands is technetium-99m-sestamibi (sestamibi). The subcellular localization of sestamibi uptake in enlarged parathyroid glands in patients with hyperparathyroidism has yet to be ascertained. The mechanism of retention of sestamibi by human parathyroid tissue was examined in 23 freshly harvested and 15 cryopreserved parathyroid glands excised from patients with primary or secondary hyperparathyroidism.

Methods.—The parathyroid tissue samples were examined for subcellular localization of Tc-99m-sestamibi. Tissues were incubated with 100 μCi of sestamibi, then isolated for mitochondria by differential centrifugation. The integrity of subcellular fractions was quantified using the mitochondrial enzyme marker, succinate dehydrogenase.

Results.—Ninety-two percent of sestamibi activity was correlated with mitochondria. After adding the mitochondrial uncoupler, carbonylcyanide m-chlorophenylhydrazone (CCCP), to the fresh parathyroid tissues, 84.96% and 73.86% of sestamibi was liberated from the mitochondrial components, respectively. Sestamibi activity in the mitochondrial component of cryopreserved human parathyroid tissue decreased to the same amount as that in the CCCP-treated group.

Conclusion.—Sestamibi uptake in abnormal human parathyroid tissues is clearly linked with mitochondrial functional integrity.

▶ It is remarkable how little is known about the actual mechanism of uptake of many of the radiopharmaceutical agents that we use every day. It is particularly true of agents whose uptake is relatively nonspecific but have been proven empirically to be of significant diagnostic value in clinical medicine. This may be especially true of technetium-99m-sestamibi, which is an excellent myocardial imaging agent and has also evolved into a valuable probe for the parathyroid glands. This study very nicely demonstrates the localization and uptake of technetium sestamibi in the mitochondria of human parathyroid tissue.

M. D. Blaufox, MD, PhD

The Efficacy of Sestamibi Parathyroid Scintigraphy for Directing Surgical Approaches Based on Modified Interpretation Criteria

Kim CK, Kim S, Krynyckyi BR, et al (New York Univ)
Clin Nucl Med 27:246-248, 2002   5–2

Introduction.—Improved localization of parathyroid adenomas with preoperative imaging allows more patients with primary hyperparathyroidism to undergo targeted surgery using unilateral neck exploration under local anesthesia, radioguided parathyroidectomy, and endoscopic parathyroidectomy. The efficacy of sestamibi parathyroid scintigraphy (SPS) for correctly directing surgical approaches was assessed in 80 consecutive patients.

Methods.—Patients were 65 women and 15 men with a mean age of 59 years. All had primary hyperparathyroidism and underwent SPS (based on modified interpretation criteria) before surgery, which was performed in all cases by the same surgeon. The SPS studies, both dual-isotope subtraction and Tc-99m-sestamibi dual-phase techniques, were reviewed. Final diagnoses were made based on histologic findings, the intraoperative parathyroid hormone assay, and clinical follow-up. Scintigraphic findings were classified as true-positive, false-negative, true-negative, or false-positive.

Results.—In the 75 patients with a solitary adenoma, SPS correctly identified a solitary abnormal focus on the correct side of the neck in 66 patients, and an abnormal focus in the correct quadrant in 63. The positive predictive value of SPS was thus 100% for side and 95.5% for quadrant. The re-

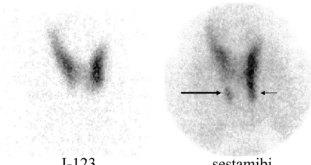

I-123   sestamibi

FIGURE 1.—Double parathyroid adenomas are shown. Comparison of the I-123 and early sestamibi images clearly shows 2 mismatched foci. Surgery revealed a 600-mg adenoma at the right lower pole (*long arrow*) and a 1400-mg adenoma at the left lower pole (*short arrow*). (Courtesy of Kim CK, Kim S, Krynyckyi BR, et al: The efficacy of sestamibi parathyroid scintigraphy for directing surgical approaches based on modified interpretation criteria. *Clin Nucl Med* 27(4):246-248, 2002.)

maining 9 patients had false-negative results: 2 studies failed to reveal abnormal foci, 5 were equivocal, and 2 showed 2 foci. Multiple-gland disease was found in 5 patients, 2 with double adenoma and 3 with 4-gland hyperplasia. In the cases of double adenomas, 1 study was equivocal and the other correctly identified the lesions (Fig 1). One of the remaining 3 studies in patients with multiple-gland disease was negative, 1 was equivocal, and 1 showed 2 lesions. All 5 studies were classified as true-negative, for results would not have led to unilateral or targeted surgery.

Conclusion.—By using modified interpretation criteria, SPS has a high predictive value when used to select patients for targeted parathyroidectomy. When findings are negative, equivocal, or show more than a single site, other imaging methods are recommended.

▶ The question of whether SPS should be performed before a first-time surgery on a patient with hyperparathyroidism has been debated for quite a while in the literature. The authors have modified the generally accepted criteria somewhat to determine more accurately whether a preoperative scan in a new patient can be helpful to the surgeon. They come down clearly on the side of using the scan. A very strong argument to support their contention is their statement that an increasing number of surgeons are using it in first-time patients as a guide to which side to operate on. Also, the increasing availability of minimally invasive surgery and intraoperative endoscopic localization further supports the movement toward using this test for first-time surgeries more often.

M. D. Blaufox, MD, PhD

Prospective Evaluation of Delayed Technetium-99m Sestamibi SPECT Scintigraphy for Preoperative Localization of Primary Hyperparathyroidism

Civelek AC, Ozalp E, Donovan P, et al (Johns Hopkins Med Institutions, Baltimore, Md; Yale Univ, New Haven, Conn)
Surgery 131:149-157, 2002   5–3

Introduction.—The advantages of SPECT over planar imaging for the preoperative localization of primary hyperparathyroidism (1°HPTH) include enhanced contrast 3-dimensional localization and estimation of lesion size. The ability to identify and localize abnormal parathyroid glands with technetium (Tc)-99m sestamibi-delayed SPECT images was assessed in a large series of patients with 1°HPTH.

Methods.—The study included 338 patients who underwent sestamibi SPECT for assessment of 1°HPTH. Prospective data were collected concerning preoperative demographics, clinical, sestamibi, operative findings, laboratory values, and pathologic and laboratory results.

Results.—Between 1994 and 2000, 287 unexplored patients (85%) and 51 re-explored patients (15%) were prospectively evaluated. Abnormal parathyroid glands were excised from 336 of 338 patients; 299 had single

TABLE 1.—The Sensitivity, Accuracy, and Positive Predictive Value of the Delayed Sestamibi-SPECT Scintigraphy for Localizing Abnormal Parathyroid Glands

Scintigraphic Results	Solitary Adenomas (299 Glands)	Double Adenomas (46 Glands)	Multiglandular Hyperplasia (55 Glands)*	Total (400 Glands)
No. of identified and lateralized lesions (Sensitivity)	286 (96%)	38 (83%)	25 (45%)	349 (87%)
No. of precise localization (Sensitivity)	269 (90%)	34 (73%)	25 (45%)	328 (82%)
Accuracy	96%	85%	60%	94%
Positive predictive value	85%	81%	100%	88%

*One hyperplastic gland was of normal size.
(Reprinted by permission of the publisher from Civelek AC, Ozalp E, Donovan P, et al: Prospective evaluation of delayed technetium-99m sestamibi scintigraphy for preoperative localization of primary hyperparathyroidism. *Surgery* 131:149-157. Copyright 2002 by Elsevier.)

adenomas (88%), 23 had double adenomas (7%), and 14 had multigland hyperplasia (4%). Sestamibi-SPECT correctly lateralized 349 of 400 abnormal parathyroid glands. The overall sensitivity, accuracy, and positive predictive values were 87%, 94%, and 86%, respectively (Table 1). Precise localization was possible in 82% of the abnormal parathyroid glands. Sestamibi was 87% for unexplored cases and 92% for reoperative cases; 286 of 299 (96%) solitary adenomas, 38 of 46 (83%) double adenomas, and 25 of 55 (45%) hyperplastic glands were detected. The mean weight of the true-positive glands was greater than that of the false-negative glands (1252 mg vs 297 mg; $P < .005$). The overall surgical cure rate was 98.5% (333/338); 5 patients (1.5%) experienced symptoms and signs of 1°HPTH after surgery. Three patients had persistent 1°HPTH, even with excision of sestamibi-detected lesions in 2 patients.

Conclusion.—Sestamibi SPECT is highly accurate for the localization of parathyroid adenomas in unexplored and re-explored cases, where it is frequently the only imaging needed. Its sensitivity is limited in the presence of multiglandular disease.

▶ This is a remarkably large study of the use of technetium-99m sestamibi in preoperative localization of primary hyperparathyroidism. The results seem to strongly support the use of delayed SPECT imaging at 2 ½ hours in this condition. The reported sensitivities in adenomas and multiglandular hyperplasia are in keeping with other reports and literature supporting the value of this technique. Our experience has generally been that SPECT has been useful in the delayed images to improve our confidence of a lesion, but we are usually able to identify suspicious areas on ordinary planar imaging.

M. D. Blaufox, MD, PhD

Presurgical Localization of Abnormal Parathyroid Glands Using a Single Injection of Tc-99m Sestamibi: Comparison of High-Resolution Parallel-Hole and Pinhole Collimators, and Interobserver and Intraobserver Variation

Arveschoug AK, Bertelsen H, Vammen B (Aalborg Hosp, Denmark)
Clin Nucl Med 27:249-254, 2002   5–4

Introduction.—Scintigraphy with Tc-99m sestamibi as a parathyroid imaging agent is sensitive in locating abnormalities in patients with hyperparathyroid disease (HPT). Methods used to increase the sensitivity of the single-tracer technique, such as SPECT, factor analysis of dynamic structures, and the addition of a pinhole collimator, may result in a loss of specificity. The sensitivity and specificity of the single-tracer technique with and without the addition of the pinhole collimator were compared in patients with primary and secondary HPT (pHPT and sHPT).

Methods.—Sixty-three patients, 47 with pHPT and 16 with sHPT, were evaluated with the Tc-99m sestamibi double-phase technique before surgery. After injection of Tc-99m sestamibi, 10-minute neck and mediastinum images acquiring 1000 K counts were obtained with the high-resolution (HR) parallel-hole collimator, and a neck image containing 500 K counts was obtained with the pinhole collimator. Within 2 to 3 hours, the same parallel-hole and pinhole collimator images were obtained with the same acquisition time as earlier images. To determine interobserver and intraobserver variation, 2 nuclear medicine specialists twice independently viewed all parallel-hole scintigrams, then all parallel-hole and pinhole scintigrams.

Results.—Bilateral neck surgery was performed in 36 patients and unilateral neck surgery in 27. A total of 121 sides in 63 patients were included in the analysis. A single adenoma was found in 38 patients (81%) with pHPT. The sensitivity and specificity for the correct side of localization were 54% and 89%, respectively, with the HR parallel-hole collimator, and 88% and 77%, respectively, with the addition of the pinhole collimator in all patients with pHPT. In those with sHPT, the sensitivity and specificity for the correct side of localization were 58% and 100%, respectively, with the HR parallel-hole collimator, and 85% and 100%, respectively, with the addition of the pinhole collimator. Interobserver agreement was acceptable (84% overall), and intraobserver agreement was even better (88% and 90% overall for the 2 observers). The degree of agreement and disagreement between observers was the same for pHPT and sHPT.

Conclusion.—Addition of the pinhole collimator to parathyroid scintigraphy in patients with pHPT or sHPT increases sensitivity and yields a high degree of precision. Specificity was lost only in patients with pHPT.

▶ It is not surprising that the use of a pinhole collimator improves diagnostic results in performing parathyroid scintigraphy. I have included this article to remind the readers of this very simple technique for improving the accuracy of our images. Unfortunately, on many cameras, it is not even possible to obtain a pinhole collimator anymore. It remains, however, a simple magnification technique based on very sound physics principles.

M. D. Blaufox, MD, PhD

Clinical Role of ⁹⁹ᵐTcO₄/MIBI Scan, Ultrasound and Intra-Operative Gamma Probe in the Performance of Unilateral and Minimally Invasive Surgery in Primary Hyperparathyroidism

Casara D, Rubello D, Pelizzo MR, et al (Regional Hosp of Padova, Italy; Univ of Padova, Italy; Univ of Michigan, Ann Arbor)

Eur J Nucl Med 28:1351-1359, 2001   5–5

Introduction.—The classical surgical approach to hyperparathyroidism (HPT) involves bilateral cervical exploration with the goal of visualizing all parathyroid glands and removing those that are enlarged. In many centers, biopsy specimens are obtained from all parathyroid glands to assess for possible multiglandular disease. Some reports have indicated that scintigraphy, alone or in combination with neck US, is able to accurately predict which patients with primary HPT may be sufficiently evaluated using a unilateral approach. Between September 1998 and June 2000, 143 consecutive patients with primary HPT were evaluated: (1) to determine the efficacy of an imaging protocol based on the combination of ⁹⁹ᵐTcO₄/MIBI scintigraphy and neck US in selecting patients with HPT for unilateral neck exploration, and (2) to determine the role of the intraoperative MIBI gamma probe (IMGP) approach in performance of minimally invasive radio-guided surgery (MIRS).

Methods.—A modified ⁹⁹ᵐTcO₄/MIBI scintigraphy procedure was used that included oral administration of potassium perchlorate to produce rapid ⁹⁹ᵐTcO₄ washout from the thyroid tissue, thereby allowing the acquisition of high-quality early MIBI images. A SPECT acquisition was obtained in 21 patients, 7 of whom had an enlarged parathyroid gland (EPG) in the mediastinum at plantar scintigraphy and 14 had discordant scan/US findings for the presence of a cervical EPG. Patients also underwent neck US during the same session using a small-parts high-resolution 10-MHz transducer. The PTH was measured intraoperatively via quick PTH assay to verify successful parathyroidectomy. For 91 patients with scan/US evidence of a solitary EPG and a normal thyroid gland, limited unilateral neck surgery or MIRS was planned. For the 21 patients with scan/US evidence of MGD, 24 patients with concomitant nodular goiter, and 7 patients with a negative scan/US evaluation, extensive bilateral neck exploration was planned (52 patients total).

Results.—In 87 of 91 patients (95.9%) for whom preoperative imaging revealed the presence of a solitary EPG and a normal thyroid gland, a single parathyroid adenoma was identified at surgery. These patients underwent unilateral neck exploration or MIRS. For the remaining 4 patients in this group, conversion to bilateral neck exploration was needed due to diagnosis of parathyroid carcinoma or MIRS (3 and 1 patients, respectively). For some patients, SPECT was the most useful in localizing the EPG. Specifically, in 5 of 21 patients evaluated, SPECT localized an EPG deep in the neck or mediastinum and at surgery a parathyroid adenoma was identified in the paratracheal or para-esophageal space. In 43 of 46 patients (93.5%) who were candidates for MIRS, the IMGP approach allowed parathyroidectomy to be performed through a small, 2- to 2.5-cm skin incision at a mean operative time of 34 min.

Conclusion.—The integrated scan/US imaging protocol seemed to be accurate in selecting patients with primary HPT for unilateral neck exploration. The most common reason for bilateral neck exploration was the coexistence of a nodular goiter. The SPECT examination can be useful when an EPG is located deep in the neck or mediastinum. The IMGP seems to be useful in the intraoperative evaluation of patients with solitary parathyroid adenomas and a normal thyroid gland because it is minimally invasive and saves time.

▶ This remarkably large series of patients with hyperparathyroidism helps to clarify the relative roles of the MIBI scan, intraoperative probe, and US in the localization of the abnormality. Only a small increase in sensitivity is gained by adding the US technique and it remains to be determined if this small increase in sensitivity justifies the added expense. It would not be practical to drop the MIBI scan because that would also make the concomitant use of the intraoperative γ probe uneconomical.

M. D. Blaufox, MD, PhD

Pre-Operative Localization of Parathyroid Adenomas: A Comparison of Power and Colour Doppler Ultrasonography With Nuclear Medicine Scintigraphy
Scheiner JD, Dupuy DE, Monchik JM, et al (Brown Univ, Providence, RI)
Clin Radiol 56:984-988, 2001   5–6

Introduction.—With the advent of minimally invasive parathyroid surgery and a rapid immunoassay for identifying circulating parathyroid hormone levels, the preoperative localization of parathyroid adenomas (PAs) is becoming increasingly more important. The efficacy of power and color Doppler US was compared with that of nuclear medicine scintigraphy (NM) in determining the preoperative localization of PAs in patients with primary hyperparathyroidism (PHPT).

Methods.—Between August 1998 and September 1999, 31 patients (mean age, 61 years) with PHPT underwent preoperative US (Fig 1) and NM for PA localization. Both tests were interpreted independently without prior knowledge of the other study's findings. All patients underwent surgical removal of the PA via standard neck exploration or minimally invasive unilateral surgical techniques. Rapid serum assays of circulating parathyroid hormone levels were used.

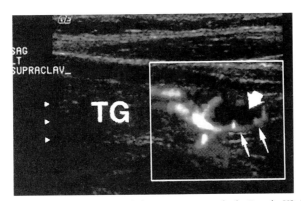

FIGURE 1.—Classic findings of parathyroid adenoma on power and color Doppler US. A sagittal image through the left supraclavicular region demonstrates the inferior thyroidal artery (*thin arrows*) draped around a hypoechoic mass (*thick arrow*), which is inferior to the left lobe of the thyroid gland (*TG*). This mass represents the parathyroid adenoma. (Courtesy of Scheiner JD, Dupuy DE, Monchik JM, et al: Preoperative localization of parathyroid adenomas: A comparison of power and color Doppler ultrasonography with nuclear medicine scintigraphy. *Clin Radiol* 56:984-988, 2001.)

Results.—Single parathyroid adenomas were observed at surgery in all patients. Prospective sensitivities for US, NM and both studies combined were 65%, 68%, and 74%, respectively (Table 1). All studies had a positive predictive value of 100%. The PA was localized by only 1 imaging modality in 16% of patients.

Conclusion.—Both US and NM offer complementary roles in the preoperative localization of PAs in patients with PHPT.

▶ Once again, when a careful comparison of apparently competing diagnostic modalities is carried out, it turns out that the 2 approaches combined yield better results than either 1 alone. In situations where sensitivities are in the 90s and specificities of similar high value are obtained by a single modality, there is little or no need for multiple testing and the single most effective approach should be used. However, a great many of the studies that we carry out yield sensitivities such as this one, ranging between 65% and 68%, and the com-

TABLE 1.—Prospective Sensitivity of US and NM for Parathyroid
Adenoma Localization

Imaging Result	Number of Cases
Not detected by US or NM	8
Detected only by US	2
Detected only by NM	3
Detected by US and NM	18
Sensitivity – NM	68%
Sensitivity – US	65%
Sensitivity – Combined NM and US	74%

Abbreviations: US, Power and color Doppler ultrasonography; *NM*, nuclear medicine scintigraphy.
(Courtesy of Scheiner JD, Dupuy DE, Monchik JM, et al: Preoperative localization of parathyroid adenomas: A comparison of power and color Doppler ultrasonography with nuclear medicine scintigraphy. *Clin Radiol* 56:984-988, 2001.)

bined procedures yield a higher sensitivity of 74%. Unfortunately, the study provides no statistical analysis of the results, so that the critical question of whether these findings are statistically significant or fall within the range of the error of the method cannot be answered. It would be nice if the authors or some future investigators carried out a study such as this with a careful statistical analysis.

M. D. Blaufox, MD, PhD

Effects of Preoperative Parathyroid Localisation Studies on the Cost of Operations for Persistent Hyperparathyroidism
Nilsson B, Fjälling M, Klingenstierna H, et al (Sahlgrenska Univ, Göteborg, Sweden)
Eur J Surg 167:587-591, 2001   5–7

Background.—The cost of medical care is a source of increasing concern not only in the medical community but also among the population at large. Diagnostic procedures can be evaluated not only for their efficiency but also for their costs. Preoperative parathyroid localization studies are often used before operations for previously missed parathyroid adenomas. Whether such preoperative localization studies are cost effective for these tumors was investigated retrospectively.

Methods.—The study was conducted at a university hospital in Sweden. The study included 3 groups of patients with persistent hyperparathyroidism (HPT) as follows: (1) 15 consecutive patients who underwent reoperation after localization studies; (2) 14 patients who had repeat operations for HPT without localization studies; and (3) 15 patients who had initial operations without localization studies. The localization procedures used ^{99m}Tc sestamibi scintigraphy and catheterization of the large cervical and mediastinal veins with measurements of serum concentrations of parathyroid hormone. The main outcome measures were operative time and the costs of operations, frozen section biopsy, and localization studies.

Results.—The mean duration of reoperation with localization studies was 124 minutes, and the mean duration of operations for the initial operation without localization studies was 135 minutes. In contrast, the mean duration of reoperations without studies was 269 minutes. The mean total cost of investigations, operating time, and frozen section biopsy was 28% less for patients who had localization studies before reoperation compared with patients who underwent reoperation without such studies.

Conclusions.—Localization studies before repeat operations for hyperparathyroidism are cost effective. The reduction in operating time and the decreased extent of dissection as determined by such studies are considered to have the potential to decrease morbidity.

▶ There can be little debate that preoperative parathyroid localization for patients with persistent hyperparathyroidism is cost effective. Numerous studies have now appeared documenting this fact. I am pleased that not only this, but several other studies have actually appeared in the surgical literature, so the nuclear medicine physician cannot be accused of presenting what could be biased data.

M. D. Blaufox, MD, PhD

---

^{18}F-FDG PET in Characterizing Adrenal Lesions Detected on CT or MRI
Yun M, Kim W, Alnafisi N, et al (Univ of Pennsylvania, Philadelphia)
J Nucl Med 42:1795-1799, 2001   5–8

Introduction.—Approaches for the diagnosis and management of adrenal lesions vary among institutions. Although most adrenal masses are likely to be benign, even in patients with cancer, it is important to differentiate benign and nonfunctioning lesions from those that are hormonally active or malignant, so that appropriate treatment strategies can be used. The ability of ^{18}F-FDG PET to characterize adrenal lesions was assessed in patients with proven or suspected cancers.

Methods.—Fifty adrenal lesions identified by CT in 41 patients were retrospectively examined. Thirteen lesions were detected in 10 patients with MRI. PET scans were performed in all patients to assess whether the disease was primary or metastatic. A proven malignancy was found in 34 patients (lung cancer, 28; thyroid cancer, 3; colorectal cancer, 2; and lymphoma, 1) and 7 had lung nodules. Of the 50 lesions, 18 (36%) were eventually determined to be malignant (histopathology, 7; follow-up, 11). The remaining 32 lesions were confirmed or assumed to be benign by histopathologic analysis (n = 4) or follow-up (n = 28). Unlike earlier reports, PET was considered positive if the uptake was equal to or greater than that of the liver.

Results.—No malignant lesions demonstrated a negative result on PET. Of the 18 malignant lesions, 13 (72.2%) demonstrated significantly higher FDG uptake compared with that of the liver. In the remaining 5 lesions (2 metastases from neuroendocrine tumor, 2 early metastases, and 1 necrotic metastasis), FDG uptake was equal to or slightly higher than that of the liver. Of the 32 benign lesions, 2 (6.2%) had uptake equal to or slightly higher than that of the liver, 3 (9.4%) had uptake less than the liver and more than the background, and 27 (84.4%) had uptake of the background. Three of the 13 false-positive lesions were identified by MRI; FDG PET correctly detected all 3 as benign. The other 10 adrenal lesions accurately diagnosed by MRI were also characterized by PET. The sensitivity, specificity, and accuracy of FDG PET were 100%, 94%, and 96%, respectively.

Conclusion.—The diagnostic performance of FDG PET in differentiating adrenal lesions identified on CT or MRI was excellent. Because FDG PET has the additional advantage of assessing both primary lesions and metastases, it might be cost effective and the modality of choice for the characterization of adrenal lesions, particularly in patients with malignancy.

▶ As I noted in my previous comments, I am always concerned when a study provides 100% sensitivity. My immediate reaction is that further experience will reduce that number. Anyone who has looked at adrenal uptake of FDG on PET scans realizes that this is not among the easier lesions to evaluate. Adrenal uptake of FDG is relatively common. This group has suggested different criteria that improve the results of imaging. This is a highly experienced PET center with great expertise. Hopefully, more widespread use of the criteria used here will confirm their results.

M. D. Blaufox, MD, PhD

6-[¹⁸F]Fluorodopamine Positron Emission Tomographic (PET) Scanning for Diagnostic Localization of Pheochromocytoma
Pacak K, Eisenhofer G, Carrasquillo JA, et al (NIH, Bethesda, Md)
Hypertension 38:6-8, 2001   5–9

Introduction.—The diagnosis of pheochromocytoma using imaging techniques necessitates specific localization of the tumor and a high sensitivity for tumor detection. Both CT and MRI have good sensitivity and poor specificity for identifying pheochromocytoma. Nuclear imaging approaches, including ¹³¹I-metaiodobenzylguanide scintigraphy, have limited sensitivity. Reported are initial results using 6-[¹⁸F]fluorodopamine PET scanning for the diagnostic localization of pheochromocytoma.

Methods.—Twenty-eight patients with known or suspected pheochromocytoma underwent PET scanning. They received 1 to 2 mCi of 6-[¹⁸F]-fluorodopamine intravenously over 3 min. Attenuation-corrected images were taken, starting immediately after injection (15 min/position), using a GE Advance scanner. The duration of emission scanning was 8 to 15 min for each level. A minimum of 1 transmission scan of 3 to 5 min duration was taken for each level. The MIRAGE program was used to reconstruct images. Two of 3 reviewers were blinded to the plasma metanephrine levels or CT and MRI findings.

Results.—Nine of 28 patients had surgical confirmation of the tumor; all 9 had 6-[¹⁸F]fluorodopamine PET scans that correctly identified the location of the tumor. All 8 patients with metastatic pheochromocytoma had 6-[¹⁸F]fluorodopamine scans that revealed ≥1 extraadrenal tumor. Nine of 11 patients with normal plasma levels of metanephrine had negative 6-[¹⁸F]fluorodopamine PET scans, 1 had extraadrenal localization of 6-[¹⁸F]fluorodopamine–derived activity medial to the left kidney and in the region of the tail of the pancreas (Fig 1), and 1 had essentially symmetric uptake of 6-[¹⁸F]fluorodopamine in the adrenal areas. Neither of the latter 2 patients had surgical verification of these sites of 6-[¹⁸F]fluorodopamine uptake.

Conclusion.—In patients with known disease, 6-[¹⁸F]fluorodopamine PET scanning can identify and localize pheochromocytomas with a high degree of sensitivity. In patients for whom the diagnosis of pheochromocytoma is considered, then excluded due to negative plasma metanephrine findings, 6-[¹⁸F]fluorodopamine PET scans are consistently negative. Thus, a clinical trial of 6-[¹⁸F]fluorodopamine is justified as a diagnostic tool.

Left Adrenal Pheochromocytoma

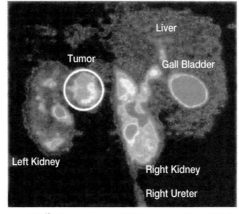

FIGURE 1.—Reprojected 6-[¹⁸F]fluorodopamine PET scan in a patient with left adrenal pheochromocytoma. The image was rotated ~20 degrees from coronal clockwise toward the viewer to delineate the tumor. The circle surrounds the tumor. (Courtesy of Pacak K, Eisenhofer G, Carrasquillo JA, et al: 6-[¹⁸F]fluorodopamine positron emission tomography (PET) scanning for diagnostic localization of pheochromocytoma. *Hypertension* 38:6-8, 2001.)

▶ ¹³¹I-labeled metaiodobenzylguanidine may be useful in the evaluation of patients with pheochromocytoma. However, it has significant limitations, not the least of which is the ¹³¹I label. It is encouraging to learn that 6-¹⁸F fluorodopamine also can be used to localize pheochromocytomas with a high sensitivity. Not only is the diagnosis of pheochromocytoma often challenging, but, because of the frequent occurrence of multiple lesions, it is particularly useful to have a reliable imaging technique for presurgical evaluation. Although this small study needs to be confirmed, the results are certainly very encouraging.

M. D. Blaufox, MD, PhD

Pheochromocytomas: Detection With ¹⁸F DOPA Whole-Body PET—Initial Results
Hoegerle S, Nitzsche E, Altehoefer C, et al (Albert-Ludwigs Univ, Freiburg, Germany)
Radiology 222:507-512, 2002   5–10

Introduction.—Several procedures have been established for the diagnostic imaging of pheochromocytomas. However, the assessment of pheochromocytomas remains challenging because of the potentially extra-adrenal and/or multifocal tumor sites. Fourteen consecutive patients with suspected pheochromocytomas underwent fluorine 18 (¹⁸F) dihydroxyphenylaline (DOPA) whole-body PET to determine its use as a biochemical imaging modality for these catecholamine-producing neuroendocrine tumors.

Methods.—Of 14 patients with pheochromocytoma, 5 had sporadic disease and 9 had von Hippel-Lindau disease. Patients underwent ¹⁸F DOPA

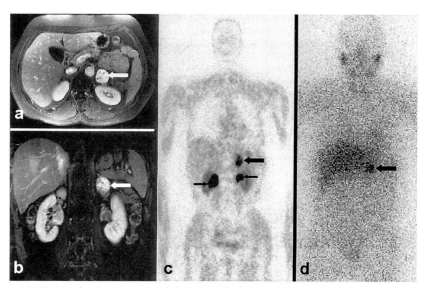

FIGURE 1.—Pheochromocytoma of the left adrenal gland (*large arrow*) in a 44-year-old woman (patient 12). Transverse (**a**) and coronal (**b**) contrast-enhanced MR (144/4), coronal ^{18}F DOPA PET (**c**), and planar MIBG scintigraphic (**d**) images show concordant findings. The small arrows in *c* point to the normal accumulation of ^{18}F DOPA in the renal collecting system. (Courtesy of Hoegerle S, Nitzsche E, Altehoefer C, et al: Pheochromocytomas: Detection with ^{18}F DOPA whole-body PET—Initial results. *Radiology* 222:507-512, 2002. Radiological Society of North America.)

PET and MRI. Twelve patients also underwent metaiodobenzyl-guanidine (MIBG) scintigraphy. The individual imaging findings were evaluated as a consensus by specialists in nuclear medicine and radiologists blinded to the results of the other studies. Functional imaging findings were compared with those of MR imaging, the reference standard. Histologic verification was possible in 8 patients with 9 tumors.

Results.—MRI identified 17 pheochromocytomas (11, solitary; 3, bifocal; 14, adrenal; 3, extra-adrenal). The ^{18}F DOPA PET and MR imaging findings in all 17 tumors were concordant (Fig 1). MIBG scintigraphy had 4 false-negative results for 4 patients, missing 3 adrenal tumors smaller than 2 cm and 1 extra-adrenal tumor with a diameter of 3.6 cm. On the basis of these data, sensitivities of 100% for ^{18}F DOPA PET and 71% for MIBG scintigraphy were demonstrated; specificity was 100% for both methods.

Conclusion.—^{18}F DOPA PET is a highly sensitive and specific biochemical imaging method for detection of pheochromocytomas. It has the potential to be the functional imaging approach of the future.

▶ It is encouraging that an ^{18}F-labeled pharmaceutical is reported here to be highly sensitive in the diagnosis of pheochromocytoma. Labeling with the ^{18}F radionuclide increases the potential availability of this agent. If the authors' observations are confirmed, then ^{18}F DOPA would certainly have many advantages over ^{123}I-labeled MIBG. I am concerned about any study where the sensitivity is reported to be 100%. This very often reflects the way in which the study subjects were chosen or some other confounding variable. Almost invariably, with further experience, this number falls below 100% and sometimes very much below that. Regardless, this is a very encouraging study, and the authors present many reasons why the use of ^{18}F DOPA would present an advantage over MIBG. However, all of these tumors were also imaged with MR, which certainly supports its role as a primary modality. The fact that both ^{18}F DOPA and MIBG yield a specificity of 100% is strong support for their role in identifying lesions that may be seen on MR, where the pathologic basis of the lesion may not be easily confirmed.

M. D. Blaufox, MD, PhD

Iodide Kinetics and Experimental [131]I Therapy in a Xenotransplanted Human Sodium-Iodide Symporter-Transfected Human Follicular Thyroid Carcinoma Cell Line
Smit JWA, Schröder-van der Elst JP, Karperien M, et al (Leiden Univ, The Netherlands; Wageningen Univ, The Netherlands)
J Clin Endocrinol Metab 87:1247-1253, 2002   5–11

Introduction.—The effectiveness of radioiodide therapy in thyroid cancer requires uptake of iodide, but loss of iodide uptake is often seen in patients with metastatic disease. In such cases, there appears to be diminished expression of the human sodium-iodide symporter (hNIS). A proposed strategy to restore iodide uptake in thyroid cancer is hNIS gene transfer into hNIS-defective tumors. Whether transfection of hNIS into the hNIS-deficient follicular thyroid carcinoma cell line FTC133 restores the in vivo iodide accumulation in xenografted tumors and their susceptibility to radioiodide therapy was investigated.

Methods.—Human thyroid tumors were established in BALB-c nu/nu mice. Four study protocols were designed to examine in vivo iodide kinetics and postmortem iodide accumulation. Two protocols followed a normal diet and 2 a low-iodide diet. In each diet group, mice were injected with the hNIS-transfected cell line FTC133-NIS30 or the empty vector transfected cell line FTC133-V4.

Results.—A high peak iodide accumulation was observed in tumors derived from FTC133-NIS30 (17.4% of administered activity compared with 4.6% with FTC133-V4). The half-life in FTC133-NIS30 tumors was 3.8 hours. Mice on the low-iodide diet exhibited reduced peak activity in FTC133-NIS30 tumors (8.1%), but thyroid iodide accumulation was increased. The half-life of radioiodide was markedly increased (26.3 hours) in thyroid-ablated mice on the low-iodide diet. Tumor development was postponed in thyroid-ablated, low-iodide diet mice treated with experimental radioiodide therapy (2 mCi).

Discussion.—In vivo iodide accumulation was restored with hNIS transfection into an hNIS-defective thyroid carcinoma. The short half-life of iodide can be improved to some degree by conventional conditioning with thyroid ablation and a low-iodide diet. In this animal model, the tumor dose required for tumor elimination could not be achieved.

▶ The sodium-iodide symporter hNIS made a sudden and dramatic appearance at the Society of Nuclear Medicine meeting this year. One entire session was devoted to the potential for this transporter both in terms of enhancing its expression as discussed in this article and as a possible approach to patients with otherwise intractable breast cancer where the symporter also is expressed. Given the remarkable effectiveness of radioactive iodine in the treatment of thyroid cancer, any successful genetic approach to increasing the presence of the symporter in thyroid cancer cells has very great and positive implications for its potential role in thyroid cancer. This is just 1 of many remarkable new approaches that are beginning to open up in the gene therapy of disease. An exciting aspect of gene therapy of disease is that it appears these new approaches will make available a great number of new and potentially invaluable diagnostic studies in nuclear medicine.

M. D. Blaufox, MD, PhD

Uptake of 201Tl Into Primary Cell Cultures From Human Thyroid Tissue Is Multiplied by TSH
Mruck S, Pfahlberg A, Papadopoulos T, et al (Friedrich-Alexander-Universität Erlangen-Nürnberg, Germany)
J Nucl Med 43:145-152, 2002   5–12

Background.—Thyroglobulin (Tg) is an accurate marker of tumor in the clinical follow-up of patients who have undergone thyroidectomy with differentiated carcinoma of the thyroid. The elevation of the Tg concentration in patients' sera is a sensitive and specific reflection of the progression of differentiated thyroid cancer. When the Tg level indicates the onset of recurrence, it is of vital importance to identify the site of Tg production. Wholebody scintigraphy after iodine 131 administration is the procedure of first choice; however, a loss of the ability of metastases to concentrate iodine is a frequently observed complication in progressive thyroid carcinoma. This inability of metastases to concentrate iodine makes the recurrence undetectable and also untreatable with radioiodine. In such cases, several alternative radiopharmaceuticals are used, including thallium 201. The effect of thyroid-stimulating hormone (TSH) on thyroid 201Tl uptake in vitro was evaluated.

Methods.—Adherent monolayers of human thyroid tissue obtained from patients undergoing surgical treatment of nodular goiter were cultured after mechanical disintegration and enzymatic digestion by neutral protease. The studies were performed exclusively on paranodular tissue components. Tg accumulation was calculated after repetitive measurements of Tg concentrations by radioimmunoassay. The statistical significance of differences in Tg release and 201Tl uptake was corroborated in a generalized estimating equations analysis, taking into account the variability of unbalanced replicate measurements.

Results.—There was a 2-fold greater release of Tg and 3-fold greater uptake of ^{201}Tl in cells cultured in the presence of TSH.

Conclusions.—The uptake of ^{201}Tl in human thyroid cells is significantly increased by TSH. These data suggest that withdrawal of thyroid hormone substitution can improve the sensitivity of ^{201}Tl scintigraphy for the detection of thyroid remnants or cancer recurrences. These findings deserve further investigation in patients and in cell cultures from thyroid carcinomas.

▶ This rather surprising study demonstrates a responsiveness of ^{201}Tl uptake in human thyroid cells to TSH stimulation. It has generally been presumed that the agents substituted for ^{131}I in evaluating metastatic thyroid disease, such as ^{201}Tl, technetium 99m sestamibi, and fluorine 18 FDG, are not TSH dependent but rather are taken up through some mechanism specific to tumor activity rather than thyroidal function. This in vitro study causes some concern, because if thallium uptake by thyroid tumor cells depends on TSH, then perhaps uptake of other agents may also be influenced by this factor. It is very likely that any dependence noted here on TSH is simply a function of cell growth and metabolic activity. However, as the authors point out, some recent studies have suggested a dependence of FDG on TSH as well. If these in vitro studies are verified in human beings, they can have a very significant effect on our approach to identifying metastatic thyroid disease in patients who have negative whole body scans.

M. D. Blaufox, MD, PhD

Antithyroid Drugs as a Factor Influencing the Outcome of Radioiodine Therapy in Graves' Disease and Toxic Nodular Goitre?
Körber C, Schneider P, Körber-Hafner N, et al (Univ of Würzburg, Germany)
Eur J Nucl Med 28:1360-1364, 2001   5–13

Introduction.—Factors that affect the outcome of radioiodine therapy for benign thyroid diseases are under question. Antithyroid medication negatively impacts the effectiveness of radioiodine in patients with Graves' disease (GD). Factors that significantly influence the therapeutic outcome of GD and to what degree these factors are involved were examined in a longitudinal investigation.

Methods.—Patients with GD and toxic nodular goiter (TNG) referred for therapeutic dosimetry were evaluated to determine the influence of gender, age, antithyroid drugs, target radiation dose, target mass, applied activity, delivered dose, interval between last meal and application, and TSH, FT_3, and FT_4 levels on the outcome of radioiodine therapy. Follow-up was 8 months in 144 patients with GD (111 female, 33 male) and in 563 patients with TNG (434 female, 129 male). Treatment was considered successful when the TSH level was normal or increased.

Results.—Treatment was successful in 98 patients with GD and 418 with TNG. Forward stepwise multiple regression analysis models showed that only the target mass in GD and the applied activity in TNG were significantly correlated with therapy outcome. The predictive value of all evaluated variables was extremely low for both disease groups. Concomitant antithyroid medication had no impact on GD and adversely affected radioiodine therapy in TNG.

Conclusion.—No evaluated factor was significantly correlated with the general outcome of radioiodine therapy. In patients with TNG, antithyroid medication tended to decrease the therapeutic efficacy of radioiodine therapy. Because the TSH levels during radioiodine therapy were higher in the TNG group receiving antithyroid drugs, this effect may be due to the "steal phenomenon."

▶ The treatment of hyperthyroidism with radioiodine is certainly a remarkable achievement for nuclear medicine. However, despite repeated investigations, the exact treatment approach in many aspects of thyroid disease remains controversial and appears to reflect an art more than a science. It is particularly difficult to determine how best to treat a patient who is receiving antithyroid therapy and who is a candidate for radioiodine treatment. While treatment in patients who have not received antithyroid drugs is relatively straightforward, many questions arise in those individuals who have received some type of thyroid suppression. This article helps to provide some perspective, both for patients with Graves' disease and for those with toxic nodular goiter, in anticipating the possible effects of prior antithyroid therapy. In Graves' disease, the success rate for patients who received antithyroid drugs was the same as those who did not, but it was significantly lower in those with toxic nodular goiter. This is surprising because among the patients with toxic nodular goiter who received antithyroid drugs, the thyroid radiation dose was actually higher. Unfortunately, the authors' attempts to sort out the specific factors that contributed to their results were unsuccessful. It certainly would be of great clinical value to determine if there are differences between effects of specific antithyroid drugs on the resulting success rate for treatment at any given dose.

M. D. Blaufox, MD, PhD

I-123 Diagnostic Thyroid Tumor Whole-Body Scanning With Imaging at 6, 24, and 48 Hours
Gerard SK, Cavalieri RR (San Francisco VA Med Ctr; Univ of California, San Francisco)
Clin Nucl Med 27:1-8, 2002   5–14

Introduction.—The use of iodine-123 (^{123}I) instead of iodine-131 (^{131}I) for diagnostic whole-body thyroid tumor scanning (DxRaI) for patients with differentiated thyroid cancer eliminates the risk of stunning and provides significantly superior image quality. Because of the shorter half-life (13 hours) of ^{123}I, images have been acquired primarily 6 or 24 hours after injection, potentially reducing the sensitivity for identifying weakly avid thyroid tumor or remnant. The effectiveness of ^{123}I for DxRaI was compared with that of ^{131}I for the same purpose. Also investigated was whether increased doses of ^{123}I would improve detection of weakly avid tumors.

Methods.—Thirteen diagnostic studies were performed in 10 patients referred for diagnostic imaging and ^{131}I treatment of differentiated thyroid cancer, either follicular or papillary. Nine additional studies were performed after thyroidectomy, and 4 were performed after ^{131}I ablation. Anterior and posterior whole-body scanning with [123]I (111-185 MBq [3-5 mCi]) was performed using low-energy, high-resolution collimators under withdrawal conditions, imaging at 6, 24, and in most patients, 48 hours and compared with post-^{131}I treatment scans acquired early (2-3 days) and late (7-10 days) in all except 1 patient.

Results.—Of 37 sites or tumors detected in posttreatment scans, 26 were identified in the DxRaI ^{123}I scan (sensitivity, 70%). In the 11 sites missed by ^{123}I, 7 were observed only in the late posttreatment scans, thereby indicating the sensitivity of ^{123}I imaging versus the early post-^{131}I treatment scans to be 26/30 or 86.7%. In 10 cases, 48-hour ^{123}I imaging was attempted and produced images of acceptable quality in 8 cases. Lesion detection was improved on the 48-hour images; in 1 case, this allowed detection of a site of tumor recurrence that was verified as positive on the ^{131}I posttreatment scan.

Conclusion.—The use of ^{123}I doses of 111 to 185 MBq for DxRaI offers acceptable levels of sensitivity overall and may allow 48-hour imaging for improved identification of weakly avid tumor or remnant without any risk of stunning.

▶ The debate over the use of ^{123}I versus ^{131}I for whole-body scanning in patients with thyroid cancer seems to be heating up. On the one hand, you have suggestions that stunning may be caused by ^{131}I and on the other, that shorter imaging times for ^{123}I may lead to lesions being missed. A key word in this article is that ^{123}I provides acceptable levels of sensitivity. If the article is reviewed carefully, it is apparent that ^{131}I appears to have performed significantly better. Although the image quality with ^{123}I is reported to have been equal or better than ^{131}I, this is not the critical issue. In scanning patients with suspected metastatic disease, one needs to identify the lesions. The critical number is which agent identifies more lesions, regardless of the observers' qualitative evaluation of the quality of the scan. Although the authors come out in favor of ^{123}I, their data seem to support [131]I.

M. D. Blaufox, MD, PhD

Clinical Comparison of Whole-Body Radioiodine Scan and Serum Thyroglobulin After Stimulation With Recombinant Human Thyrotropin

Haugen BR, Ridgway EC, McLaughlin BA, et al (Univ of Colorado, Denver)
Thyroid 12:37-43, 2002
5–15

Introduction.—Recombinant human thyrotropin (rhTSH) has been created to promote sensitive monitoring for thyroid cancer recurrence without the morbidity of hypothyroidism associated with hormone withdrawal. The sensitive monitoring for thyroid cancer recurrence or persistence includes whole-body radioiodine scanning (WBS) and determination of serum thyroglobulin (Tg) after endogenous or exogenous thyrotropin (TSH) stimula-

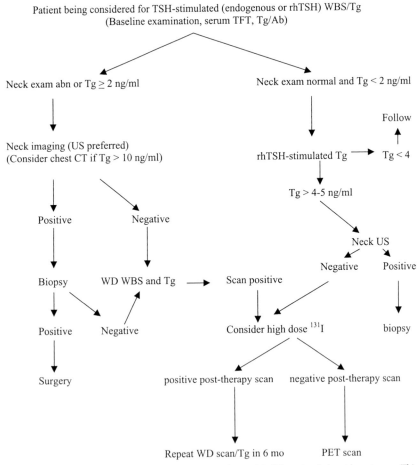

FIGURE 3.—Proposed algorithm for monitoring patients with differentiated thyroid carcinoma. This algorithm is based on the results of this study, review of the literature, and experience of the authors. (Courtesy of Haugen BR, Ridgway EC, McLaughlin BA, et al: Clinical significance of whole-body radioiodine scan and serum thyroglobulin after stimulation with recombinant human thyrotropin. *Thyroid* 12:37-43, 2002.)

tion. The experience with rhTSH was reviewed in 83 patients to compare the clinical relevance of a positive WBS and/or serum Tg.

Methods.—Between February 1999 and August 2000, 107 WBS and/or serum Tg measurements were performed in 102 patients after they underwent stimulation with rhTSH. All patients had undergone a near-total thyroidectomy for differentiated thyroid cancer.

Results.—Ten patients had a positive WBS. Of these, 8 had activity limited to the thyroid bed. The rhTSH-stimulated Tg was 2 ng/mL or more in 25 patients and 5 ng/mL or more in 13 patients. For patients with a negative WBS, 11 of 20 with a Tg of 2 ng/mL or more and 7 of 9 with a Tg of 5 ng/mL or more received therapy or further assessment on the basis of a positive WBS alone. Three patients who did not receive therapy or further assessment had a subsequent negative WBS 10 to 12 months later, indicating a lack of clinically significant disease. Twenty patients had a negative WBS and a serum Tg of 2 ng/mL or more. Of 20 patients, 11 had a Tg less than 5 ng/mL; 4 of these patients underwent neck US. One patient had a biopsy-confirmed recurrence (rhTSH-stimulated Tg of 4 ng/mL). Subsequent assessments at 6 months or later, were negative in 8 patients. Of the 9 patients with a Tg of 5 ng/mL or more and a negative WBS, 7 underwent further assessment, and 6 of these 7 had identified disease. An algorithm for monitoring patients with undifferentiated thyroid carcinoma was developed (Fig 3).

Conclusion.—The rhTSH-stimulated WBS and Tg levels are complementary, and Tg is a more sensitive indicator of disease recurrence or persistence. An rhTSH-stimulated Tg greater than 4 to 5 ng/mL frequently resulted in further assessment; a Tg less than 4 ng/mL rarely resulted in further immediate assessment.

▶ Recombinant human thyrotropin is becoming more widely used and promises to have a significant effect on how we follow up our patients with thyroid cancer. The use of this agent coupled with the ready availability of serum thyroglobulin measurements is significantly changing our approach to the thyroid. There is a possibility after 50 years of controversy that we may be moving toward a uniform protocol for treatment and diagnosis of thyroid cancer.

M. D. Blaufox, MD, PhD

Decreased Thyroid Uptake of Tc-99m Pertechnetate in Patients With Advanced-Stage Sjögren Syndrome: Evaluation Using Salivary Gland Scintigraphy
Taura S-I, Murata Y, Aung W, et al (Tokyo Med and Dental Univ)
Clin Nucl Med 27:265-269, 2002   5–16

Introduction.—Recent reports indicate a high prevalence of thyroid disease in patients with Sjögren syndrome, an autoimmune disease often diagnosed by using salivary gland scintigraphy. To clarify the relation between Sjögren syndrome and thyroid dysfunction, the correlation between thyroid uptake of Tc-99m pertechnetate and the histopathologic grade of labial biopsy specimens or stage of Sjögren syndrome was investigated.

Methods.—Seventy-three patients with Sjögren syndrome underwent salivary gland scintigraphy and a labial biopsy. On the basis of biopsy findings, 32 patients were considered to have early-stage disease (histopathologic grade 1 or 2) and 41 to have advanced-stage disease (histopathologic grade 3 or 4). Dynamic salivary gland scintigraphy was performed after administration of 370 MBq (10 mCi) Tc-99m pertechnetate. The thyroid gland was included in the imaging area. A control group used for comparison of the thyroid uptake ratio consisted of 25 healthy persons.

Results.—Control and patient groups were similar in mean age (50.4 and 50.8 years, respectively). Patients with advanced-stage disease, however, were significantly older than those with early-stage disease. All control subjects and all patients but 1 were women. The thyroid uptake ratio of the early-stage Sjögren group did not differ significantly from that of the control group, but the advanced-stage patient group had a significantly lower ratio. There were no significant correlations between thyroid uptake ratio and any of the salivary gland parameters.

Conclusion.—Because the thyroid and salivary glands share developmental, functional, and pathologic similarities, the possibility exists for a relationship between thyroid disease and Sjögren syndrome. Patients with advanced Sjögren syndrome had significantly less thyroid uptake of Tc-99m pertechnetate than either healthy control subjects or early-stage patients. No relationship was found, however, between thyroid uptake and parotid or submandibular gland function.

▶ This is a remarkably large study of patients with Sjögren syndrome. It is interesting that in a subgroup of the patients, the investigators were able to show some apparent reduction in thyroid uptake of Tc-99m pertechnetate. There remains a need to measure the actual thyroid uptake in these patients with the use of standard uptake measurements and to add a perspective on the significance of this observation. The range of normal uptake of iodine and pertechnetate by the thyroid is really quite large, and any retrospective division of patients to separate out high- and low-uptake groups is subject to many potential confounding errors. The authors should pursue these observations to determine the clinical significance of their findings.

M. D. Blaufox, MD, PhD

High Dose [131]I Therapy for the Treatment of Hyperthyroidism Caused by Graves' Disease
Alexander EK, Larsen PR (Brigham and Women's Hosp, Boston)
J Clin Endocrinol Metab 87:1073-1077, 2002   5–17

Background.—In the United States, radioactive iodine (^{131}I) is the most widely used therapy for patients with hyperthyroidism caused by Graves' disease. There have been a number of dosing regimens proposed, from those based on high-precision dosimetry and US-guided volume determination to large, fixed doses of ^{131}I intended to cause hypothyroidism soon after treatment. Regardless of the protocol, most patients ultimately have hypothyroidism develop after ^{131}I treatment. The results of a high-dose ^{131}I therapy protocol based on the measurement of 24-hour thyroid ^{131}I uptake designed to deliver 8 mCi to the thyroid gland 24 hours after ^{131}I administration were presented. The clinical experience with this protocol over a 7-year period was reviewed.

Methods.—A total of 261 patients (219 women and 42 men) with hyperparathyroidism caused by Graves' disease were treated with a mean dose of 14.6 mCi of ^{131}I between 1993 and 1999. Before ^{131}I treatment, 207 (79%) patients had received an antithyroid drug (propylthiouracil or methimazole). The thyroid status of these patients was determined 1 year after treatment in relation to age, pretreatment with an antithyroid drug, pretreatment thyroid size, and dose of ^{131}I retained in the thyroid 24 hours after treatment.

Results.—Eighty-six percent of the patients were euthyroid or hypothyroid 1 year after treatment, and 14% of patients had persistent hyperthyroidism requiring a second treatment. Patients with persistent hyperthyroidism were younger, had larger thyroid glands, higher pretreatment thyroid ^{131}I uptake values, and higher serum T4 concentrations. These patients were more likely to have been treated with antithyroid medication before the administration of [131]I. Transient hypothyroidism followed by thyrotoxicosis developed in 5 of these patients. There was an asymptotic, inverse relation between the retained dose of ^{131}I at 24 hours and persistent hyperthyroidism, which revealed a failure rate of 5% to 10%.

Conclusions.—A dose of ^{131}I that results in accumulation of 8 mCi in the thyroid 24 hours after administration is effective for the treatment of hyperthyroidism in patients with Graves' disease. However, younger patients with larger thyroid glands, higher serum T4 concentrations, and higher 24-hour thyroid ^{123}I uptake values are at a higher risk for treatment failure, as are patients pretreated with antithyroid medication for more than 4 months. In these patients, a higher dose of ^{131}I may be advisable.

▶ The balance between the dose of ^{131}I therapy for Graves' disease that will cause remission of disease and the dose that will cause hypothyroidism has always been a perplexing problem in endocrinology. This issue is further compounded by the effects of medical treatment before ^{131}I therapy on the potential for a cure. This report addresses this issue by grouping patients who are hypothyroid and euthyroid at 1 year under successful treatment. Clearly, given that definition, the success of treatment is directly related to the dose of ^{131}I per gram of thyroid tissue and to the pre-^{131}I treatment regimen. Even given this high-dose approach to the treatment of Graves' disease, there still remain a significant number of patients who will not respond to treatment. There is a need for some scientific and clearly rational estimation of ^{131}I dose in this disease, and it appears that we have more work to do before this will be achieved.

M. D. Blaufox, MD, PhD

Determination of the Optimal Minimum Radioiodine Dose in Patients With Graves' Disease: A Clinical Outcome Study

Howarth D, Epstein M, Lan L, et al (Pacific Med Imaging, Newcastle, NSW, Australia; John Hunter Hosp, Newcastle, NSW, Australia; St George Hosp, Sydney, NSW, Australia)

Eur J Nucl Med 28:1489-1495, 2001   5–18

Background.—In the past few decades, most patients with Graves' disease have been treated with 1 or more of 3 modalities: medical therapy, total thyroidectomy, and radioiodine therapy. In Australia, a widely accepted initial treatment regimen for these patients is to use an antithyroid medication with biochemical thyroid function tests to monitor the patient's response. Patients are referred for thyroidectomy or radioiodine therapy only if relapse or treatment failure occurs after 6 to 18 months of tolerated therapy or the patient experiences an adverse reaction to treatment. There is a reluctance to refer patients for radioiodine therapy, largely because of the belief that it has not been proved safe and effective. Recently, however, data have been published that establish both the safety and the efficacy of radioiodine therapy in the treatment of Graves' disease. The determination of the optimal minimum therapeutic dose of iodine-131 (^{131}I) for the treatment of Graves' disease was investigated in a single-blinded randomized prospective study.

Methods.—The study included 58 patients (50 women and 8 men), aged from 17 to 75 years, who were analyzed by clinical, biochemical, and immunologic assessment, thyroid US, technetium-99m thyroid scintigraphy, and 24-hour thyroid ^{131}I uptake. The patients were then randomized to receive either 60 Gy or 90 Gy thyroid tissue-absorbed dose of radioiodine. The primary outcomes were clinical and biochemical response to treatment. The median follow-up was 37.5 months.

Results.—All but 1 patient completed final follow-up. A euthyroid state was obtained in 26 (46%) of 57 patients, while 27 (47%) of 57 patients were rendered hypothyroid, and 4 (7%) remained hyperthyroid. A total of 34 (60%) patients continued to be hyperthyroid at 6 months after the initial radioiodine dose, and 21 patients required additional radioiodine therapy. Of the 29 patients who received a dose of 90 Gy, 17 (59%) patients remained hyperthyroid at 6-month follow up. Of the 28 patients who received a dose of 60 Gy, 17 (61%) remained hyperthyroid at 6-month follow up. Thus, no significant difference was noted in treatment response. Five patients in the 90-Gy group and 2 patients in the 60-Gy group were hypothyroid at 6-month follow up. Nonresponders to low-dose therapy had a significantly larger thyroid gland mass and significantly higher levels of serum thyroglobulin at 6 months.

Conclusions.—For patients in whom low-dose radioiodine treatment for Graves' disease is considered, a 39% response rate can be obtained at 6 months with a dose of 60 Gy, which minimizes early hypothyroidism. These findings demonstrate that no significant advantage can be gained in response rate obtained with a dose of 90 Gy. Doses in excess of 120 Gy may be required for more rapid therapeutic effect at the expense of an increased rate of hypothyroidism. Patients who could be less responsive to low-dose therapy may be identified with the use of US determination of thyroid mass and measurement of serum thyroglobulin levels.

▶ What is the best dose of radioiodine to use in treating Graves' disease? I do not know. The authors are not sure they know. Do you know?

M. D. Blaufox, MD, PhD

Dose Selection for Radioiodine Therapy of Borderline Hyperthyroid Patients With Multifocal and Disseminated Autonomy on the Basis of ^{99m}Tc-Pertechnetate Thyroid Uptake

Reinhardt MJ, Joe A, von Mallek D, et al (Univ Hosp Bonn, Germany; Univ Hosp Freiburg, Germany; Inselspital Bern, Switzerland)
Eur J Nucl Med 29:480-485, 2002

5–19

Background.—Although radioiodine therapy (RIT) has been used for almost 60 years in the treatment of hyperthyroidism, there is little consensus among the experts regarding the best method of dose determination. Marinelli's formula has been developed to provide a consistent framework for absorbed dose calculations using universally accepted units and measurements. The formula requires determination of the effective half-life and the maximum uptake of radioiodine, usually derived from a radioiodine uptake test prior to RIT, and the target volume. It is easy to determine the target volume in the case of single hyperfunctioning thyroid nodule, but it is almost impossible to determine the target volume when there is a multifocal and disseminated pattern of functional autonomous cells. A "dosimetric compromise" has been suggested to overcome this problem. The results of use of a modified dosimetric approach in which RIT is performed using pretreatment technetium-99m pertechnetate thyroid uptake under thyrotropin suppression ($TcTU_s$)–adapted dose selection in more than 400 patients with goiters and multifocal and disseminated thyroid autonomy were described.

Methods.—The mean age of the patients in this study was 70 ± 9 years, and the mean thyroid volume was 54 ± 26 ml. More than half the patients (261) had at least 1 documented previous episode of overt hyperthyroidism. Tissue absorbed doses were adapted to the pretreatment $TcTU_s$. Normalization of $TcTU_s$ and thyrotropin (TSH), thyroid volume reduction, and frequency of hypothyroidism and recurrent hyperthyroidism were evaluated 1 year after a single radioiodine therapy.

Results.—The presented dose strategy resulted in normalization of $TcTU_s$ in 96% of patients and an increase in TSH to the normal range in 92% of patients. Only 5 patients demonstrated recurrent hyperthyroidism. Thyroid volume decreased from 54 ± 26 ml before treatment to 34 ± 20 ml after treatment, a mean reduction of 37%. The frequency of hypothyroidism was only 0.9%.

Conclusions.—Dose selection adapted to pretreatment $TcTU_s$ is recommended for elimination of functional autonomous tissue with a single radioiodine therapy in elderly patients with enlarged thyroid glands and relevant autonomous masses who are at risk of developing iodine-induced hyperthyroidism.

▶ I have commented many times on the problems in choosing the appropriate dose of radioiodine for treatment of hyperthyroidism. This study uses the interesting approach of relating the dose to 99mTc-pertechnetate. The results in this large series of patients appear to be very satisfactory, and it appears to present a reasonable alternative approach.

M. D. Blaufox, MD, PhD

Scintigraphic Evaluation of Primary Congenital Hypothyroidism: Results of the Greek Screening Program
Panoutsopoulos G, Mengreli C, Ilias I, et al (Sotiria Hosp, Athens, Greece; Inst of Child Health, Athens, Greece)
Eur J Nucl Med 28:529-533, 2001   5–20

Introduction.—Screening for primary congenital hypothyroidism (CH) has been conducted in Greece since 1979. By early 2000, heel prick measurement of thyrotropin had been performed in 1,976,719 newborns, leading to a diagnosis of CH in 584 children. These children received L-thyroxine (L-T_4) replacement therapy and were studied with different scintigraphic modalities between 2 and 3 years of age. The scintigraphic findings were presented, and the various methods of scanning were compared.

Methods.—Among the children identified as having CH, 413 were examined after withdrawal of L-T_4 for 3 weeks. Scintigraphic studies were used to further evaluate and classify the children as having either an aplastic (AT) or an ectopic thyroid gland (ET) or as showing thyroidal dyshormonogenesis (DN, with a nomotopic gland). Ninety-six children (group A) were studied with technetium-99m pertechnetate and a rectilinear scanner, 73 (group B) with technetium-99m pertechnetate and a gamma camera equipped with a pinhole collimator, and 220 (group C) with iodine-123 sodium iodide and the same gamma camera. Thyroglobulin (Tg) was measured in 191 children from group C, and US was performed in 49.

Results.—In group A, 61.5% of children had AT, 26.0% had ET, and 12.5% had DN; 28.8% of group B children had AT, 52.0% had ET, and 19.2% had DN; 23.2% of group C children had AT, 63.2% had ET, and 13.6% had DN. For both AT and ET, there were statistically significant differences between group A and groups B and C. The imaging quality of iodine-123 sodium iodide was superior to that of technetium-99m pertechnetate, with notably less background activity. Scintigraphy was more concordant with Tg measurements than with US.

Conclusion.—Newer scintigraphic modalities, especially with iodine-123 sodium iodide, indicate that ET is the most common finding in CH. Despite its higher cost, scintigraphy with iodine-123 sodium iodide is the most appropriate nuclear medicine method for reevaluation and classification of children with CH. Neck US and TG measurements have limited value.

▶ This extraordinarily large study provides some very valuable information about the value of screening for CH and the follow-up of these children. In this study, scintigraphy played a vital role in the follow-up. A side benefit of the report is the demonstration of the very clear advantage of using ^{123}I-Na for thyroid imaging over pertechnetate while still maintaining an acceptable radiation dose. Ultrasound, as probably would be expected, did not provide as much valuable information when compared against thyroid function studies.

M. D. Blaufox, MD, PhD

Immunohistochemical Analysis of Sodium Iodide Symporter Expression in Metastatic Differentiated Thyroid Cancer: Correlation With Radioiodine Uptake
Castro MR, Bergert ER, Goellner JR, et al (Mayo Clinic and Mayo Found, Rochester, Minn)
J Clin Endocrinol Metab 86:5627-5632, 2001   5–21

Introduction.—The ability of thyroid cancers to concentrate radioiodine (RAI) partially depends upon the expression and functional integrity of the sodium iodide symporter (NIS). Some differentiated thyroid carcinomas (DTCs) and most undifferentiated thyroid carcinomas do not have the ability to concentrate iodide and are thus insensitive to ^{131}I therapy. Variation of NIS protein expression may be important in this behavior and was therefore examined. The NIS expression in primary DTC tumors was examined to ascertain if it correlates with the subsequent RAI uptake by metastatic lesions in the same patients.

Methods.—Paraffin-embedded tissue specimens were reviewed from 60 patients with metastatic thyroid cancer who had undergone total or near-total thyroidectomy for DTC and had known presence or absence of RAI uptake in their tumor deposits determined by total body scanning after thyroid hormone withdrawal. Tissue sections from the primary intrathyroidal tumors were immunostained using a monoclonal antibody against human NIS. Two independent reviewers assessed slides for specific immunostain (IS). Whole-body scan (WBS) uptake was recorded for each patient. The relationship between the results of IS and WBS was examined.

Results.—In 43 patients with positive WBS, 37 also had positive IS of their tumors. For 6 patients with negative IS, a positive WBS was observed; in 3, TSH at the time of surgery was <0.3 mIU/L. Ten of the 17 patients with negative WBS also had negative IS. Positive IS accurately predicted a positive scan result in 84% of patients. The ability of the IS to identify all cases with a positive scan result was 86%; it increased to 90% when patients who were receiving thyroid hormone therapy at the time of surgery were excluded.

Conclusion.—Sodium iodide symporter IS of the thyroidal primary tumor in patients with papillary and follicular thyroid cancers can predict the behavior of subsequent deposits of metastatic and recurrent cancer in terms of iodine trapping and concentration.

▶ The sodium iodide symporter has been attracting increasing attention in recent years. If these results are confirmed, this technique could potentially be helpful in deciding which patients with thyroid cancer are best observed with an iodine scan and which ones might be better suited to observation with FDG imaging on PET. Some recent studies suggest that certain breast cancers express the iodide symporter, raising the possibility of imaging these individuals with radioiodine.

M. D. Blaufox, MD, PhD

Comparison of ^{123}I and ^{131}I for Whole-Body Imaging in Thyroid Cancer
Sarkar SD, Kalapparambath TP, Palestro CJ (Long Island Jewish Med Ctr, New Hyde Park, NY)
J Nucl Med 43:632-634, 2002   5–22

Background.—A number of medical centers are now using ^{123}I for evaluation of thyroid cancer, partly out of a concern about stunning of thyroid tissue by [131]I. However, the efficacy of ^{123}I for the identification of thyroid cancer metastases has not been clearly elucidated, particularly for distant metastases from the neck. This study compared ^{123}I and ^{131}I whole-body imaging in patients with and without metastases.

Methods.—The study group comprised patients with differentiated thyroid cancer who were referred for pretherapy radioiodine imaging. Twelve patients underwent 13 sets of ^{123}I and ^{131}I studies. All patients had previously undergone thyroidectomy; 3 of the patients had prior ^{131}I treatment, and at the time of imaging, the endogenous serum thyroid-stimulating hormone levels were generally μU/ml or greater. All but 1 patient received ^{131}I treatment, which was administered within 1 week after imaging. After thyroid hormone withdrawal, whole-body imaging was performed at about 24 and 72 to 96 hours after administration of 74 to 185 MBq (2 to 5 mCi) [123]I and 111 to 185 MBq (3-5 mCi) [131]I, respectively. The images were compared by 2 independent readers for ease of lesion detection. Findings were confirmed by posttherapy imaging, CT, ^{18}F-FDG PET, or follow-up or previous radionuclide imaging, when available.

Results.—Both ^{123}I and ^{131}I demonstrated residual thyroid tissue in 9 patients. [131]I detected metastases in 5 studies of 4 patients. In 4 of 5 studies, ^{123}I missed metastases shown by ^{131}I in 8 body regions, including the neck, mediastinum, lungs, and bone and only retrospectively detected 3 other sites of metastasis (Fig 2). No lesion was better visualized with ^{123}I than with [131]I.

Conclusions.—While ^{123}I appears to be adequate for imaging residual thyroid tissue, it appears that it is less sensitive than ^{131}I for imaging thyroid cancer metastases.

▶ There has been an ongoing debate about the relative value of ^{123}I versus ^{131}I studies for thyroid metastases. At our institution, we had been pretty well convinced that ^{123}I could be conveniently substituted for [131]I. The findings of this study, although in a small group of patients, suggest that we should rethink this position. Dr Sarkar, who is the lead author on this article, recently joined my department and has extended his series. He is convinced that equivalent doses of ^{131}I and ^{123}I result in greater sensitivity for [131]I.

M. D. Blaufox, MD, PhD

FIGURE 2

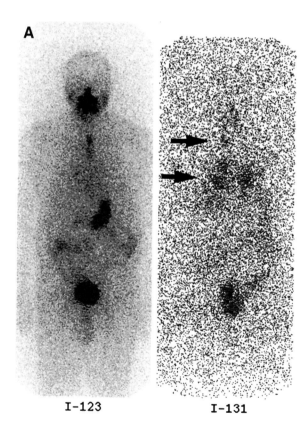

I-123   I-131

(Continued)

FIGURE 2 (cont.)

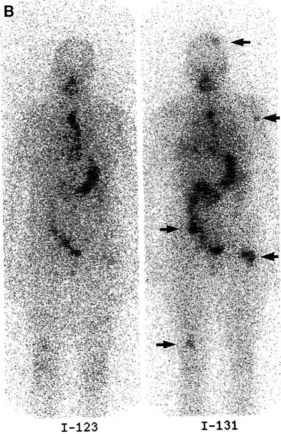

I-123   I-131

FIGURE 2.—**A,** A 63-year-old man with Hürthle cell thyroid cancer had distant metastases and persistent disease despite 2 prior treatments with [131]I. Anterior whole-body ^{123}I image (*left*) is negative for metastases. Midline chest activity is in esophagus. Corresponding ^{131}I image (*right*) shows diffuse pulmonary and right cervical nodal metastases (*arrows*). This patient received a larger amount of [123]I (185 MBq) than of [131]I (148 MBq). **B,** A 53-year-old woman with follicular thyroid cancer and distant metastases received 4 prior ^{131}I treatments for persistent disease. Anterior whole-body ^{123}I image (*left*) shows metastases in left hip, right femur, and left proximal humerus. These foci are better seen on ^{131}I image (*right*), which additionally shows diffuse uptake in lungs and focal lesions in skull and right iliac bone (*arrows*). Midline chest activity is in esophagus. (Reprinted by permission of the Society of Nuclear Medicine, courtesy of Sarkar SD, Kalapparambath TP, Palestro CJ: Comparison of ^{123}I and ^{131}I for whole-body imaging in thyroid cancer. *J Nucl Med* 43:632-634, 2002.)

Better Yield of ¹⁸Fluorodeoxyglucose-Positron Emission Tomography in Patients With Metastatic Differentiated Thyroid Carcinoma During Thyrotropin Stimulation
van Tol KM, Jager PL, Piers A, et al (Univ Hosp Groningen, The Netherlands)
Thyroid 12:381-387, 2002   5–23

Background.—The use of FDG PET for glucose metabolism is a promising means for the detection of many types of tumors because of the high glycolytic demand of these tumors. There have been several published reports regarding the relevance of FDG-PET scanning in patients with differentiated thyroid carcinoma; in this form of cancer, the uptake of FDG seems to be associated with poor differentiation of low iodine uptake on diagnostic ¹³¹I scanning. The clinical significance of this phenomenon is not fully understood, but in practice FDG-PET scanning is now the method of choice for the detection of ¹³¹I-negative metastases of differentiated thyroid carcinoma. The withdrawal of thyroid hormones is thought not to be necessary for FDG-PET scanning, but only a few reports have described the possible influence of the serum thyrotropin (TSH) level on FDG uptake in thyroid carcinoma tissue, and these studies have provided conflicting results. The effects of serum TSH on FDG-PET uptake patterns in patients with suspected recurrent or metastatic differentiated thyroid cancer were determined.

Methods.—This prospective study evaluated 8 patients. After the second FDG-PET scan, a therapeutic ¹³¹I dose was administered, and posttherapy scans were obtained 10 days later. The FDG-PET scans were compared with each other and with the ¹³¹I posttherapy whole body scans by 2 independent observers. The findings on FDG-PET scans were verified using other imaging modalities or biopsies.

Results.—Median TSH was 0.04 mU/L during TSH suppression and 64 mU/L during TSH stimulation. The FDG-PET scans during TSH suppression revealed abnormalities in 4 patients, while the FDG-PET scans during TSH stimulation showed abnormalities in 5 patients (Fig 2). One patient was only positive during TSH stimulation. In 2 other patients, the FDG-PET scan during stimulation of TSH clearly demonstrated more lesions, and in all positive patients lesion contrast was better during TSH stimulation. In 2 patients, a change in clinical management resulted from FDG-PET findings during TSH stimulation.

Conclusions.—In this study, the performance of FDG PET during TSH stimulation was either superior to or equal to performance of FDG PET during TSH suppression, but never inferior. For detection of metastatic or recurrent differentiated thyroid carcinoma, FDG PET should be performed during hypothyroidism, which leads to TSH stimulation.

▶ The role of PET in the evaluation of patients with metastatic thyroid cancer is gradually being clarified and assuming a place in clinical medicine. One of the questions that has yet to be answered definitively is whether or not FDG PET in thyroid cancer can be performed during thyrotropin suppression. This study suggests that, in fact, thyrotropic stimulation does enhance the findings on

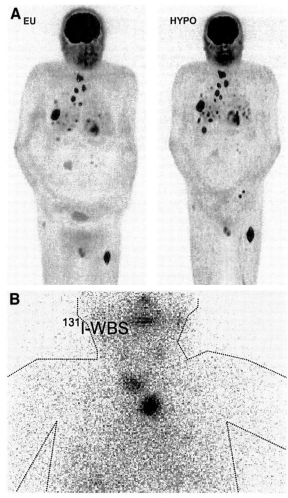

FIGURE 2.—Widespread metastatic papillary thyroid carcinoma in a 60-year-old male (patient 3). **A,** Compared to the FDG-PET scan during TSH suppression (*EU*), the FDG-PET scan during TSH stimulation (*HYPO*) is showing many more lesions in both lungs. Other metastatic lesions are also better visualized during TSH stimulation. **B,** On the posttherapy ^{131}I whole-body scan (^{131}I-WBS), only uptake in the mediastinal area is seen. (Courtesy of van Tol KM, Jager PL, Piers DA, et al: Better yield of [18]fluorodeoxyglucose-positron emission tomography in patients with metastatic differentiated thyroid carcinoma during thyrotropin stimulation. *Thyroid* 12:381-387, 2002.)

FDG PET. Further studies are needed to determine if this is just a random occurrence or if the overall yield would be significantly improved if patients in whom a PET scan is being performed for thyroid cancer were subjected to thyroid TSH stimulation.

M. D. Blaufox, MD, PhD

Clinical Impact of ¹⁸F-FDG PET in Thyroid Carcinoma Patients With Elevated Thyroglobulin Levels and Negative ¹³¹I Scanning Results After Therapy
Helal BO, Merlet P, Toubert M-E, et al (Hôpital Antoine Béclère, Clamart, France; Service Hospitalier Frédéric Joliot, CEA, Orsay, France; Hôpital Saint-Louis, Paris; et al)
J Nucl Med 42:1464-1469, 2001   5–24

Introduction.—The use of ¹⁸F-FDG with PET allows detection of differentiated thyroid carcinoma (DTC) metastases with impaired iodine-trapping ability. The potential contribution of FDG PET in the follow-up of 37 patients with DTC, increased thyroglobulin (Tg) levels, and negative whole-body scan results obtained after high doses of ¹³¹I were prospectively examined.

Methods.—The ability of FDG PET to detect metastases was examined in the aforementioned cohort. Patients underwent additional conventional imaging procedures to identify residual disease. Patients were placed in 2 groups: group 1, positive conventional imaging findings; group 2, patients with negative conventional imaging findings (10 and 27 patients, respectively).

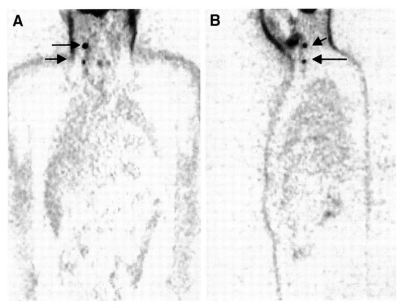

FIGURE 2.—A 28-year-old man with papillary thyroid cancer who had previously required 2 cervical lymph node dissections. Neck sonography was negative, but FDG depicted on the coronal (A) and sagittal (B) slices 2 right cervical lymph nodes that were confirmed pathologically to be metastases (patient 27, group 2). (Reprinted by permission of the Society of Nuclear Medicine from Helal BO, Merlet P, Toubert M-E, et al: Clinical impact of ¹⁸F-FDG PET in thyroid carcinoma patients with elevated thyroglobulin levels and negative ¹³¹I scanning results after therapy. *J Nucl Med* 42:1464-1469, 2001.)

Results.—Twenty-eight patients had positive FDG-PET findings. Tumor sites were accurately localized in 89% of patients. In group 1, FDG PET verified 17 of 18 previously known tumor sites and identified 11 additional sites. In group 2, FDG-PET findings were positive in 19 of 27 patients who had not previously identified metastases (Fig 2). The PET imaging was effective for both low- and high-stage tumors. As a result of FDG data, there was a change in the clinical treatment of 29 of 37 patients and further surgical resection in 23 patients, 4 of whom achieved disease-free status, and external radiation therapy in 4 patients.

Conclusion.—Metastases not detected by ^{131}I posttherapy whole-body scanning in patients with increased Tg levels can be identified using FDG PET. It should be used as a first-line investigation in patients with persistent disease and negative findings on ^{131}I whole-body scans after treatment.

▶ A recent review by Medicare approved reimbursement for PET imaging of head and neck tumors with the specific exclusion of thyroid disease. Increasing evidence is accumulating to suggest that this may not have been a wise decision. It is apparent that a significant number of metastatic deposits of thyroid cancer that are missed with ^{131}I imaging are detected with FDG PET. If the study by Castro et al[1] is confirmed, there could conceivably be a rational basis on which to choose those patients who should be sent directly for ^{131}I imaging (the majority) and those who would benefit more from PET scans.

M. D. Blaufox, MD, PhD

Reference

1. Castro MR, Bergert ER, Goellner JR, et al: Immunohistochemical analysis of sodium iodide symporter expression in metastatic differentiated thyroid cancer: Correlation with radioiodine uptake. *J Clin Endocrinol Metab* 86(11):5627-5632, 2001.

Risk of Malignancy in Thyroid Incidentalomas Identified by Fluorodeoxy-glucose-Positron Emission Tomography
Cohen MS, Arslan N, Dehdashti F, et al (Washington Univ, St Louis)
Surgery 130:941-946, 2001   5–25

Background.—The incidence of thyroid malignancy in the general population is about 40 to 1000 cases per million per year, compared with a prevalence of 4% to 7% for benign nodules. In some cases, thyroid nodules are identified incidentally during imaging evaluation for benign or malignant disease processes. FDG PET will often reveal enhanced glucose uptake, which is evidence of increased metabolic activity in thyroid tumors. The incidence of new thyroid lesions found on routine FDG PET was investigated in a retrospective review.

Methods.—Data for all patients who underwent FDG-PET imaging at 1 institution from June 1996 through March 2001 were evaluated. Patients with a newly diagnosed thyroid lesion were identified. Thyroid incidentaloma was defined as a thyroid lesion that was seen initially on FDG-PET imaging in a patient who had no history of thyroid disease. Follow-up data were documented where available.

Results.—Of 4525 FDG-PET examinations, 102 (2.3%) demonstrated thyroid incidentalomas. Of these 102 patients, 87 (85.3%) had no thyroid histology resulting from other malignancies. Fifteen patients underwent thyroid biopsy: 7 (47%) patients with thyroid cancer, 6 (40%) patients with nodular hyperplasia, 1 patient with thyroiditis, and 1 patient with atypical cells of indeterminate origin. Malignant lesions had higher average standardized uptake values than benign lesions.

Conclusions.—The incidence of thyroid incidentaloma identified by FDG-PET was 2.3%. Of the thyroid incidentalomas that underwent biopsy, 47% were malignant. In light of the risk of malignancy, patients with new lesions identified on PET scan should have a tissue diagnosis when such a diagnosis will influence the patient's outcome and management. Discriminating benign from malignant tissue may be aided by standardized uptake values.

▶ Occasional visualization of the thyroid on an FDG-PET scan is pretty well established, and this study has identified the incidence at about 2.3% on the basis of 4525 PET scans. Some of these patients may have thyroid carcinoma. However, the authors' estimate of 47% is potentially erroneous since only 15 of 102 of the patients identified had thyroid histology performed. Given the fact that the vast majority of patients with visualization of the thyroid on the PET scan were not biopsied, it is impossible to determine what the true prevalence is. However, even if we assume that none of those patients had a thyroid malignancy, the prevalence of thyroid cancer would approximate 7%, which is well above the prevalence of thyroid malignancy in the general population. Given the fact that the patients who were not biopsied had known malignancies, their risk of a second malignancy would be greater from the general population, suggesting that the true prevalence may be significantly higher than the 7% lower limit. The moral clearly is that visualization of the thyroid on PET scans should not be dismissed as an incidental finding.

M. D. Blaufox, MD, PhD

False-Positive Findings on ¹³¹I Whole-Body Scans Because of Posttraumatic Superficial Scabs
Regalbuto C, Buscema M, Arena S, et al (Univ of Catania, Italy)
J Nucl Med 43:207-209, 2002   5–26

Background.—The 2 main investigations used to detect residual thyroid tissue and local or distant metastases after thyroidectomy for differentiated thyroid cancer are whole-body scanning (WBS) with iodine 131 and serum thyroglobulin measurement (Tg). WBS and Tg are usually concordant, but in some patients there may be discordance between the 2 studies. A negative WBS result in the presence of a positive Tg result is usually interpreted as a false-negative result because of an insufficient ^{131}I concentration in malignant tissue. WBS is frequently performed after therapeutic administration of radioiodine (3700 to 5500 MBq) to increase sensitivity; this allows the detection of even small foci of ^{131}I accumulation. There have been several reports of a variety of tissues or pathologic processes associated with nonspecific ^{131}I uptake. Posttraumatic superficial scabs, a newly identified cause of false-positive WBS findings, are reported.

Methods.—The study group was composed of 4 women aged 34 to 59 years who had undergone thyroidectomy for differentiated thyroid cancer. All patients were clearly hypothyroid at the time of the study. WBS was conducted after therapeutic administration of 3700 MBq [131]I.

Results.—WBS showed an area of uptake in the lower limbs at a site that corresponded to a slight abrasion of the skin that had occurred from a few hours before to 24 hours after radioiodine administration (Fig 1). In 2 patients, a radioiodine concentration in the scab was demonstrated by the disappearance of the radioactivity in the leg after the scab was removed and by detection of radioactivity in the collected material.

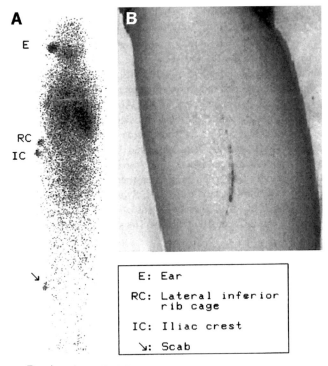

Posterior scan

FIGURE 1.—**A,** Posterior scan after 3700 MBq ^{131}I were administered to patient 1 shows focus of uptake (*arrow*) in lower third of left leg on lateral side. **B,** Photograph shows lateral view of cutaneous lesion in same area. (Courtesy of Regalbuto V, Buscema M, Arena S, et al: False-positive findings on ^{131}I whole-body scans because of posttraumatic superficial scabs. *J Nucl Med* 43:207-209, 2002. Reprinted by permission of the Society of Nuclear Medicine.)

Conclusions.—Posttraumatic superficial scabs may be a source of false-positive findings on WBS. Although high doses of ^{131}I may provide increased sensitivity, such doses may also increase the number of false-positive results.

▶ Nonspecific uptake of radiopharmaceuticals has always been both a strength and a weakness of nuclear medicine. In many situations, nonspecific uptake can lead to very valuable diagnostic studies. In others, nonspecific uptake is a source of difficulty in interpretation of studies and the cause of false-positive results. This small case report demonstrates a rather unexpected source of false-positive results in ^{131}I WBS. Posttraumatic superficial scabs are a relatively common condition. They are also a condition that many of us do not think of immediately as a cause of false-positive results. This should be added to the list and should serve as a reminder that evaluation of ^{131}I uptake on a WBS should be performed with care and with a full knowledge of its normal distribution and potential confounding factors.

M. D. Blaufox, MD, PhD

6   Renal

Introduction

Although work in the renal area has been relatively slow the last couple of years, we are beginning to see some renewed interest. Most importantly, people are now beginning again to look at the role of PET in renal disease and the possible role in patients with urologic tumors. Another important question that has been studied this year is the relative role of ACE inhibition versus angiotensin receptor blockade in evaluating renovascular hypertension.

An area that has always concerned me is how best to do a diuretic renogram in children and especially in neonates. Data are now emerging that I believe are on a more secure ground than the old "well tempered renogram." It now appears that even at a relatively early age it is possible to assess obstructive uropathy reliably in the neonate, and perhaps the approach of injecting the diuretic with the radionuclide is the simplest and most reliable.

Most of the articles reviewed here are addressed in the specific comments, but I would like to highlight the appearance of a new study of exercise renography from Italy. I cannot understand why more attention has not been paid to this potentially very valuable modality. There clearly exists in all disease, a period in which the patient functions adequately, but when stressed will reveal subclinical disease. Exercise renography promises to provide this information and also to separate a variety of pathologies in diseases such as essential hypertension. Once again, I put forth for any investigators looking to find a worthwhile project, the potential to investigate the exercise renogram and its useful role in clinical renal disease.

What is still lacking is a good, solid immunologic approach to kidney disease. The potential exists but we see virtually no articles appearing in this area. Since a significant number of renal diseases are immunologic in basis, this really deserves further study. So, too, does the problem of renal disease in diabetes.

M. Donald Blaufox, MD, PhD

Uptake of Cis-4-[18F]Fluoro-L-Proline in Urologic Tumors

Langen K-J, Börner AR, Müller-Mattheis V, et al (Insts of Medicine and Nuclear Chemistry, Jülich, Germany; Heinrich-Heine-Univ, Düsseldorf, Germany)
J Nucl Med 42:752-754, 2001   6-1

Background.—18F-FDG PET is of limited value in the diagnosis of renal malignancies. However, radiolabeled amino acids may help overcome some of the diagnostic limitations of FDG. Unfortunately, most of the interesting amino acids proposed for PET can only be labeled with the short-lived positron emitter 11C (with a 20-minute half-life), whose use is restricted to a few PET centers with a cyclotron and a radiochemistry laboratory on site. Recently the diastereoisomers cis-4-[18F]fluoro-L-proline (cis-FPro) and trans-4-[18F]fluoro-L-proline (trans-FPro) labeled with fluorine 18, which has a half-life of 110 minutes, have been presented. Animal experiments have shown that more cis-FPro than trans-FPro accumulates in osteosarcomas, and tissue homogenates showed protein incorporation of only cis-FPro. The potential of cis-FPro for tumor imaging in human beings was investigated.

Methods.—The study group included 6 men and 2 women ranging in age from 37 to 81 years. Three of the patients had primary renal cell carcinomas, 1 had a local recurrence of renal cell carcinomas, 1 had squamous renal cell carcinoma, 1 had an adrenal hemangioma, 1 had inguinal metastases of penile squamous carcinoma, and 1 had suspected metastatic disease from pros-

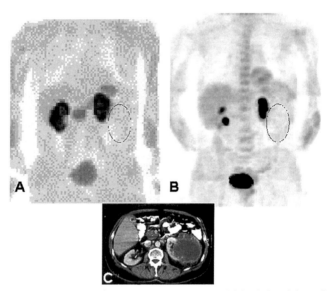

FIGURE 1.—PET and CT scans of 72-year-old man (patient 2) with left-sided renal clear-cell carcinoma. A, Reprojected whole-body scan with cis-FPro shows negative findings (*dotted oval*). Note uptake in renal cortex and pancreas. B, Reprojected whole-body scan with FDG shows negative findings (*dotted oval*). C, Transaxial CT scan at tumor level shows large, hypodense mass in left kidney. (Courtesy of Langen K-J, Börner AR, Müller-Mattheis V, et al: Uptake of Cis-4-[18F]fluoro-L-proline in urologic tumors. *J Nucl Med* 42:752-754, 2001. Reprinted by permission of the Society of Nuclear Medicine.)

tate cancer. PET scans of the trunk were acquired 1 hour and 3 to 5 hours after IV injection of cis-FPro. Findings were compared with findings from ^{18}F-FDG-PET scans and CT.

Results.—There was no significant uptake of cis-FPro in any of the tumors or metastases, whereas FDG uptake was seen in 1 of the 3 primary renal cell carcinomas, in the local recurrence of renal cell carcinoma, in the squamous renal cell carcinoma, and in the metastases of penile cancer (Fig 1).

Conclusions.—These findings suggest that cis-FPro is not a promising PET tracer in oncology.

▶ Although it has not been clearly explained, the diagnostic value of ^{18}F-FDG PET in the evaluation of renal malignancies has not been very successful. It certainly makes a lot of sense to look for a radiopharmaceutical that would have a more reliable uptake by renal tumors. It is not unreasonable to approach this problem with labeled amino acids. However, as the investigators point out, there are limitations on the use of these agents because of the short half-life of ^{11}C. It is unfortunate that the ^{18}F-labeled analogue that was used in this study has proven to be unsuccessful. Perhaps a similar approach will lead to a PET tracer that will have a useful role in the genitourinary tract or perhaps supplement FDG in general oncologic imaging.

M. D. Blaufox, MD, PhD

Mapping of Local Renal Blood Flow With PET and H$_2$^{15}O
Alpert NM, Rabito CA, Correia DJA, et al (Massachusetts Gen Hosp, Boston; Pfizer Global Research and Development, Groton, Conn; Harvard Med School, Boston; et al)
J Nucl Med 43:470-475, 2002   6–2

Background.—Total renal blood flow (RBF) can be reduced by a variety of clinical disorders, including renovascular hypertension and renal failure and drug treatment. However, less is known about the effects of other events, such as trauma, on local RBF. Currently there is not a completely satisfactory method for measuring RBF. Several methods for measuring local RBF in animals have been described, but these methods are highly invasive and so are unsuitable for human investigation. PET can provide a quantitative, low-risk, minimally invasive assessment of local RBF. A noninvasive method for the mapping of regional RBF in humans using PET and H$_2$^{15}O was described.

Methods.—The study group comprised 15 subjects, of whom 5 had normal renal function and 10 had renal disease. The procedure involved a whole-body PET scanner, IV bolus injection of 1110 to 1859 MBq H$_2$^{15}O and sequential imaging at 3 seconds per frame. ^{131}I-Iodohippuran was used for independent assessment of effective renal plasma flow in each subject. Hippuran clearance and RBF were measured twice, before and after treatment with probenecid, to verify that RBF was not affected. Flow maps were analyzed by regions of interest (largely excluding the medulla and collecting system) for each kidney on each slice and pooled to yield mean RBF.

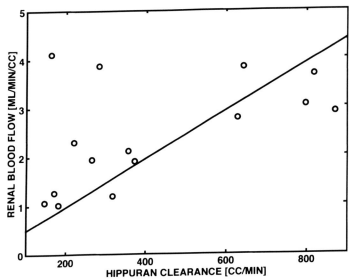

FIGURE 2.—Comparison of hippuran clearance rates (mL/min) and mean RBF (mL/min/cm³) in control state. Solid line is linear regression. RBF = constant · hippuran clearance rate. (Reprinted by permission of the Society of Nuclear Medicine, courtesy of Alpert NM, Rabito CA, Correia DJA, et al: Mapping of local renal blood flow with PET and $H_2^{15}O$. *J Nucl Med* 43:470-475, 2002.)

Results.—Mean RBF in the 5 healthy subjects was 3.4 ± 0.4 mL/min/g, and there was no difference in flow between kidneys. Before treatment with probenecid, RBF was linearly related to hippuran clearance. Probenecid treatment significantly reduced hippuran clearance, but RBF was unchanged (Fig 2). In comparison with healthy control subjects, RBF was significantly decreased in patients with renal disease. The flow maps for all subjects were of good quality and exhibited characteristic patterns, with higher values in all subjects.

Conclusions.—Parametric mapping of RBF with PET and $H_2^{15}O$ provides a straightforward, noninvasive method for quantitative mapping of RBF that may be useful not only in research but also in the management of patients whose therapy alters renal tubular transport.

▶ As I have noted many times in my commentaries, the application of PET to renal problems has been very limited. Dr Szabo, working at Johns Hopkins, has been 1 of the few people who have seriously approached this application in this area. It is gratifying to see that another group has shown some interest, and even more important, they suggest that their approach may provide clinically useful information. The only qualifying factor is the fact that, in order to do these studies using ¹⁵O, it is necessary to have ready availability of a cyclotron production facility. It would be nice if someone could come up with a method using a positron agent with a longer half-life which would allow more general application of the technique. It also is a little frustrating that although a technique measuring renal blood flow was described in 1971 by

Mike Ter-Pogossian,[1] we really have not made a great deal of progress toward its clinical application.

M. D. Blaufox, MD, PhD

Reference

1. Peters PE, Ter-Pogossian MM, Rockoff ML, et al: Measurement of renal blood flow by means of radioactive water labeled with oxzygen-15, in Blaufox MD, Funck-Brentano JL (eds): *Radionuclides in Nephrourology*. Grune & Stratton, 1971, pp 27-36.

ACE Inhibition Is Superior to Angiotensin Receptor Blockade for Renography in Renal Artery Stenosis

Karanikas G, Becherer A, Wiesner K, et al (Univ of Vienna)
Eur J Nucl Med 29:312-318, 2002   6–3

Introduction.—Angiotensin-converting enzyme (ACE) inhibitors are used in combination with renography to diagnose renovascular hypertension (RVH). The more recently developed angiotensin II receptor subtype 1 (AT1) antagonists also prevent the vasoconstrictive effect of angiotensin II on the efferent renal vessels, an effect considered essential for the demonstration of RVH by captopril renography. Renographic changes induced by captopril and the AT1 receptor antagonist valsartan were compared in patients with a high probability for RVH.

Methods.—Patients were 13 women and 12 men ranging in age from 33 to 83 years. Renal artery stenosis, verified by angiography in all patients, was unilateral in 17 and bilateral in 8. Stenosis was moderate (50%-70%) in 6 vessels and severe (>70%) in 27 vessels. Captopril, valsartan, and baseline renography were performed within 48 hours with technetium-99m mercaptoacetyltriglycine. Patients were hydrated with 10 mL of fluid per kilogram of body weight 45 minutes before renography. Changes in renographic curves after intervention were evaluated by means of the Santa Fe consensus on ACE inhibitor renography.

Results.—The studies were well tolerated, and no patients experienced side effects. Captopril renography was positive for RVH in 25 of 33 stenosed vessels, but valsartan renography was positive in only 10. Blood pressure during the studies, reduction in blood pressure after the studies, and plasma renin concentration were comparable for captopril and valsartan. Although urinary flow was higher after valsartan than after captopril, this difference did not account for the greater sensitivity of captopril in demonstrating renal artery stenosis.

Conclusion.—Captopril renography proved much more sensitive than valsartan renography in identifying a clinically significant renal artery stenosis. Because there was no positive valsartan result with a negative captopril finding, combining the tests would not increase sensitivity.

▶ This is truly a very interesting study with very surprising results. I would have predicted that a receptor antagonist for angiotensin would perform as well as a converting enzyme inhibitor, if not better. The authors' technique of analyzing the studies tended to minimize the potential effect of pelvic retention. Given this technique, I would have expected the 2 methods to behave similarly. The only explanation the authors suggest is that of an increased urinary flow rate in the receptor antagonist patients; however, I do not think, nor do they truly think, that this explains why an ACE inhibitor appeared to perform so much better than a receptor antagonist. The 1 potentially confounding factor that the authors do not discuss is that of prior medication. It would be nice to know the medication history in the patients in whom the receptor antagonist caused a false-negative result in order to determine whether any drug interaction may have occurred. In the discussion, the issue was raised of the difference in the effect on the bradykinin system of the 2 drugs. It is precisely this difference that would have led me to think that you would have fewer false-positives with a receptor blocker and an equal number of true positives. The reason for this is that the bradykinin system also affects the urinary outflow tract and can cause urinary stasis, with resultant changes in the renographic pattern. However, its effect on renal blood flow also should be considered and perhaps has a more important role. Regardless of the cause, further study of this subject is needed. It certainly would be attractive to be able to use a receptor antagonist to differentiate renovascular hypertension from renal artery stenosis, and if the medications are a confounding factor, this would be important to know also.

One other comment worth making is that in the cases shown, it appears that the duration of action of valsartan is shorter than that of captopril. The false-negatives that the authors show certainly have some significant change in the pattern of the renogram of the involved kidney, although not nearly so dramatic as that of the captopril. Another consideration is that perhaps one cannot apply the same criteria for valsartan as for captopril in determining true positives and false positives. Perhaps 1 other chore the authors should undertake is to go back and determine whether different criteria for the 2 agents would lead to similar sensitivities and specificities.

M. D. Blaufox, MD, PhD

Interobserver Agreement on Captopril Renography for Assessing Renal Vascular Disease

Krijnen P, Oei H-Y, Claessens RAMJ, et al (Erasmus Univ, Rotterdam, The Netherlands; Univ Hosp Rotterdam-Dijkzigt, The Netherlands; Bosch Medicentrum, Hertogenbosch, The Netherlands; et al)
J Nucl Med 43:330-337, 2002   6–4

Background.—Captopril-stimulated renography is widely used to screen selected groups of patients with hypertension for the presence of renal vascular disease. In patients with renovascular hypertension, captopril causes changes in the scintigraphic images of the kidney distal to stenosis by demonstrating decreased uptake or delayed excretion with cortical retention, or both. However, evaluation of this noninvasive test is a complex task, and the lack of interobserver agreement on the assessment and interpretation of renographic parameters may contribute to differences in sensitivity and specificity between studies. The interobserver agreement on the assessment of renographic parameters was assessed in a series of captopril renography examinations as well as the agreement on the judgment regarding the presence of hemodynamically significant renal artery stenosis.

Methods.—A total of 658 renograms from 503 hypertensive patients suspected of having renal vascular disease were evaluated by 3 experienced nuclear medicine physicians. The patients for this study were obtained from a large Dutch multicenter study, the Dutch Renal Artery Stenosis Intervention Cooperative (DRASTIC) study. Interobserver agreement on several renographic parameters was assessed by the κ statistic and the intraclass correlation coefficient (ICC).

Results.—There was high interobserver agreement on the time to excretion, with a pooled ICC of 0.90. The pooled κ was 0.65 or higher for the pattern of the time-activity curves, the visual aspect of the scintigraphic images, and the judgment on the presence of renal artery stenosis. In contrast, there was low interobserver agreement on cortical retention ($\kappa = 0.46$) and pelvic retention ($\kappa = 0.52$). Pelvic retention complicated the interpretation of renographic findings.

Conclusions.—This assessment of interobserver agreement in captopril renography for the assessment of renal vascular disease found satisfactory interobserver agreement on most of the renographic parameters, but the assessment of cortical retention was more difficult, particularly in the presence of pelvic retention. Caution is advised in the interpretation of captopril renography if pelvic retention is suspected. Interobserver variability is 1 possible explanation for the differences in diagnostic test performance observed between studies.

▶ It is interesting that the lay public generally believes that a test has an all-or-none result. No matter how difficult or how complex the examination, most laypeople think that the physician simply looks at the results and has an answer that is 100%. Nothing could be further from the truth, as this study of interobserver agreement on captopril renography once again reveals. The concept of clinical skills, which are learned by practicing physicians and reflect both education and experience, has yet to be replaced. It would be very nice if we could teach all physicians to interpret all studies with 100% accuracy, but this does not just seem possible. An encouraging note of this report is the fact that interobserver agreement on most renographic parameters was considered to be satisfactory. Relative kidney uptake, the pattern of the time-activity curves, and the time to excretion had good interobserver agreement, and these are, of course, important parameters. However, the presence of pelvic retention, which can be a very important cause of false-positive results, appears to be more difficult and results in poorer interobserver agreement. This problem should be potentially approachable by automated region of interest, which can be used to generate time-activity curves or some form of factor analysis. However, a truly practical program is still needed.

M. D. Blaufox, MD, PhD

Effect of Percutaneous Nephrolithotomy on Differential Renal Function as Measured by Mercaptoacetyl Triglycine Nuclear Renography
Chatham JR, Dykes TE, Kennon WG, et al (Tripler Army Med Ctr, Honolulu, Hawaii; North Texas Ctr for Laparoscopy and Stone Disease, Fort Worth)
Urology 59:522-526, 2002   6–5

Background.—Percutaneous nephrolithotomy is the preferred method of approaching complex renal calculi. Traditionally, complex calculi were treated with open procedures, including anatrophic nephrolithotomy, pyelolithotomy, or radial nephrolithotomy. It is well recognized in the western world that a percutaneous approach is preferable to an open surgical approach for the treatment of most cases of complex renal calculi. The effects of minimally invasive techniques on renal function are thought to be negligible, but this presumption has not been evaluated with the latest renography agents. The effects on differential renal function of percutaneous nephrolithotomy for the treatment of complex renal calculi were evaluated.

Methods.—A total of 45 patients underwent percutaneous nephrolithotomy from July 1999 to December 2000. Of these 45 patients, 19 consented to participate in this study. All patients completed a quantitative assessment of differential renal function preoperatively and postoperatively with technetium 99m mercaptoacetyl triglycine nuclear renography and serum creatinine measurements.

Results.—The 13 female and 6 male patients ranged in age from 11 to 75 years, with a median age of 49 years. The mean stone burden was 1432 mm^2 (range, 156 to 5220 mm^2), and the mean surgical time was 2.57 hours (range, 1.17 to 5.08 hours). The median duration of hospital stay was 2 days, with a range of 1 to 19 days. Of these patients, 13 (68%) were stone free after 1 procedure. Four patients underwent ureteroscopy with stone extraction for residual fragments, and 1 patient underwent secondary extracorporeal shock wave lithotripsy. One patient underwent nephrectomy for poor renal function. For the entire group, there was an increase in renal function from 36.8% preoperatively to 38.5% postoperatively. Renal function was preserved in 16 (84%) of the patients, and function improved in 7 (37%) patients. There was no change in serum creatinine levels.

Conclusions.—Percutaneous nephrolithotomy for the treatment of complex renal calculi does not cause a loss of renal function as measured by nuclear scintigraphy. In this study, operative and hospitalization times were decreased with percutaneous nephrolithotomy, and stone clearance was similar when compared with historical open nephrolithotomy.

▶ Radionuclides are seriously underused in nephrourology. This study shows one more example of how radionuclides can play a valuable role in assisting the nephrologist or urologist to evaluate a group of patients. The results here are quite reassuring because the major concern of nephrolithotomy is, of course, loss of renal function after the surgery. The renal nuclear medicine technique here provides the urologist with a simple, noninvasive means of assessing various approaches to this disease.

M. D. Blaufox, MD, PhD

End-Stage Renal Disease After Treatment With ^{90}Y-DOTATOC
Cybulla M, Weiner SM, Otte A (Univ Hosp Freiburg, Germany; Obere Lachen, Freiburg, Germany)
Eur J Nucl Med 28:1552-1554, 2001   6–6

Background.—DOTA-D-Phe¹-tyr³-octreotide (DOTATOC) is a newly developed somatostatin analogue that can be stably labeled with the β-emitter yttrium-90 (^{90}Y) and used for receptor-mediated internal therapy. A number of studies have documented the benefits of ^{90}Y-DOTATOC therapy for patients with somatostatin receptor-positive tumors; however, only short-term efficacy and safety data were available when these studies and cases were published. The dose-limiting factor in ^{90}Y-DOTATOC therapy is renal toxicity, so long-term renal safety data are essential for the validation and possible modification and optimization of this promising anticancer therapy. This case report on long-term outcome of DOTATOC therapy suggests that it may not be possible to stipulate a clear-cut cumulative DOTATOC dose limit for the avoidance of renal toxicity.

Case Report.—Woman, 78, suffering from a carcinoid of the small intestine with multiple metastases in the liver and metastases in the mesenteric and supraclavicular lymph nodes was treated with ^{90}Y-DOTATOC therapy after poor response to other chemotherapy options. She was administered 4 single doses of ^{90}Y-DOTATOC at 6-week intervals, for a cumulative dose of 9620 MBq. Restaging showed stable metastatic disease. Before and during DOTATOC therapy, the patient's serum creatinine and urea nitrogen levels were within the reference range; however, a progressive deterioration of renal function occurred 15 months after the end of DOTATOC therapy, resulting in end-stage renal disease. Urinalysis showed a slight degree of proteinuria of 700 mg/day without hematuria, leukocyturia, or casts. With the exception of DOTATOC therapy, no obvious risk factor was apparent for the chronic renal insufficiency. For this patient, however, kidney biopsy was not a feasible option to prove the presence of radiation-induced nephritis. Intermittent hemodialysis was initiated as the creatinine clearance decreased to less than 10 mL/min. The patient died of intracerebral bleeding 4 months after the initiation of hemodialysis.

Conclusions.—This is a case of delayed renal insufficiency after a relatively low cumulative dose of ^{90}Y-DOTATOC. This report demonstrates the need for additional studies to determine the optimal dose of ^{90}Y-DOTATOC, under which renal protection regimen that will balance risks and benefits to provide optimal management.

▶ An ongoing concern of radioimmunotherapy and radio-receptor mediated therapy is the potential for damage to the kidney, which is the main excretory organ of most of these agents. It is certainly of concern that at a relatively modest radiation dose, this patient developed end-stage renal disease. This would appear to be strong justification for a continued search for some type of adjuvant therapy that would enhance renal excretion and reduce the risk. The use of Hartmann-Hepa 8% solution, Proteinsteril Hepa 8% and Mg 5-Sulfat Amp 10% (30 mL) in this case was not successful. The problem to be solved is to find some agent that will enhance renal excretion of a radiotherapeutic compound and reduce renal toxicity while not significantly impairing its therapeutic efficacy.

M. D. Blaufox, MD, PhD

F + 0 Renography in Neonates and Infants Younger Than 6 Months: An Accurate Method to Diagnose Severe Obstructive Uropathy
Boubaker A, Prior J, Antonescu C, et al (Centre Hospitalier Universitaire Vaudois, Lausanne, Switzerland)
J Nucl Med 42:1780-1788, 2001   6–7

Introduction.—The proper management of unilateral ureteropelvic junction obstruction (UJO) in infants is controversial. Early surgery is recommended by some, whereas others prefer conservative management and close follow-up. Function of the affected kidney (AK), as determined by renography, is considered, but only 1 previous study has dealt with absolute renal function in unilateral UJO in children by using ^{99m}Tc-dimercaptosuccinic acid (DMSA). In 9 infants with proven unilateral UJO, the response to F+0 renography and the relative and absolute kidney function were studied before and after surgery.

FIGURE 2

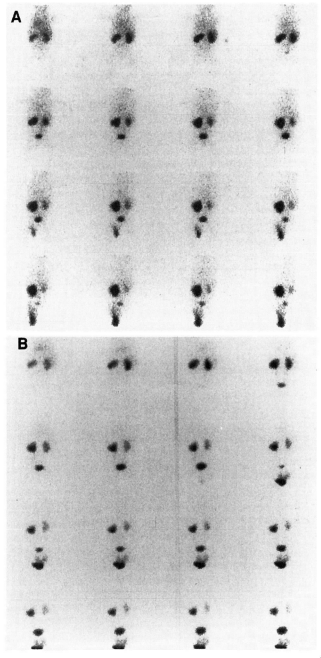

(Continued)

FIGURE 2 (cont.)

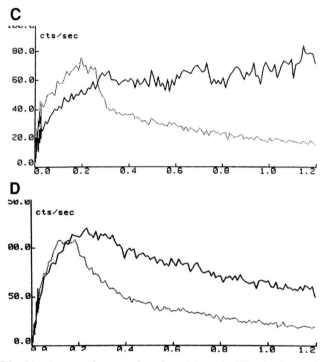

FIGURE 2.—Diuretic renography was performed on a 2.5-month-old boy in whom grade 2 hydrone-phrosis on left side was diagnosed during pregnancy and confirmed at birth. A, One-minute posterior views at diagnosis show parenchymal thinning of the left kidney and no response to furosemide, whereas right kidney appears normal. B, Same views obtained at follow-up show persistent left parenchymal thinning and improvement in left urinary flow under furosemide. C, Background-corrected renal curves (left kidney, *dark line*; right kidney, *dotted line*) at diagnosis show decreased tracer uptake by left kidney (AI, 6.50 % ID) and typical obstructive curve pattern (EI, 0.66). Contralateral kidney was normal (AI, 8.94 %ID; EI, 4.35). D, After surgery, left kidney improved in function and drainage (AI, 9.43 %ID; EI, 2.15) and right kidney remained normal (AI 9.40 %ID; EI, 6.43). *Abbreviations: AI*, Accumulation index; *EI*, elimination index; *%ID*, percentage of injected activity. (Reprinted by permission of the Society of Nuclear Medicine, from Boubaker A, Prior J, Antonescu C, et al: F+0 renography in neonates and infants younger than 6 months: An accurate method to diagnose severe obstructive uropathy. *J Nucl Med* 42:1780-1788, 2001.)

Methods.—The mean age of the infants (8 boys and 1 girl) was 2.4 months. Results obtained at diagnosis and after pyeloplasty were evaluated and compared with a control group of 10 infants with symmetric renal function and an initially dilated but not obstructed renal pelvis. Renography was performed for 20 minutes after injection of ^{123}I-hippuran (OIH) (0.5-1.0 MBq/kg) immediately followed by furosemide (1 mg/kg). Response to furosemide was quantified by an elimination index (EI); an EI of 3 or greater was considered definitely normal, and an EI of 1 or less was considered definitely abnormal.

Results.—At diagnosis of UJO, all AKs had definitely abnormal EIs and were significantly lower than the EIs of the normal kidneys (NKs) and of the 20 control kidneys. Pyeloplasty resulted in significant improvement in the

EIs of the AKs (from a mean of 0.56 to a mean of 2.81). The accumulation index of the AKs increased at follow-up, but remained lower than that of the NKs (Fig 2).

Conclusion.—The use of ^{123}I-OIH renography with early furosemide injection (F+0) allows AKs to be reliably diagnosed in neonates and infants younger than 6 months. This method can also determine whether parenchymal function is normal or impaired and whether surgery is successful.

▶ Two things about Lasix renography are becoming apparent in the literature and beginning to change our concept of how to use this diagnostic test. As first proposed by George Sfakianakis and advocated by Monica Rossleigh from Australia, the use of F renography in neonates and infants has shown that the test is reliable in this age group. Previously we had been taught that Lasix renography in infants is unreliable and that the test should be delayed for as long as possible. We now have an article from Dr Delaloye's group that further supports the use of this test. Several other small confirmatory reports have appeared in the literature. It appears now that in neonates, there is good reason to consider doing F diuretic renography if obstruction is considered, and there is every reason to perform this test early to aid in diagnostic management.

M. D. Blaufox, MD, PhD

Renal Fibrosis: Prediction From Acute Pyelonephritis Focus Volume Measured at [99m]Tc Dimercaptosuccinic Acid SPECT
Chiou Y-Y, Wang S-T, Tang M-J, et al (Natl Cheng Kung Univ, Tainan, Taiwan, Republic of China)
Radiology 221:366-370, 2001   6–8

Introduction.—In children with febrile urinary tract infection (UTI), routine clinical and laboratory parameters are not good indicators for differentiating acute pyelonephritis (APN) from UTI without parenchymal involvement. The value of the volume of an APN lesion derived from dimercaptosuccinic acid (DMSA) renal SPECT imaging as a predictor for the development of subsequent renal fibrosis was assessed in children with APN.

Methods.—The study included 44 children with APN who underwent technetium-99m (^{99m}Tc) DMSA renal SPECT during acute infection and at follow-up 6 to 10 months later. By quantitative analysis, the volume of photopenic lesions and the ratio of radioactivity in the photopenic lesion to that in normal renal tissue were determined. Sensitivity, specificity, and positive and negative predictive values were ascertained.

Results.—In the 44 children, 69 APN foci were evaluated. Thirty-seven (54%) lesions were normal on follow-up renal scans and 32 (46%) developed scars. Significant differences in the photopenic lesion volume were identified between the 2 groups ($P < .01$) (Fig 2). When photopenic lesion volume showed a positive diagnosis lesion volume (≥ 4.6 cm^3), sensitivity,

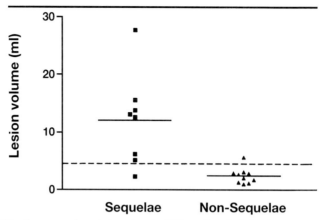

FIGURE 2.—Scattergram shows lesion volume in children with multiple foci that progressed to different outcomes; sequelae and nonsequelae groups. The volume of lesions that progressed to sequelae (12.1 cm^3 ± 2.8) was significantly larger ($P = .001$) from that of lesions that resolved without sequelae (2.4 cm^3 ± 0.4). The *dotted line* represents a lesion volume of 4.6 cm^3. (Courtesy of Chiou Y-Y, Wang S-T, Tang J-J, et al: Renal fibrosis: Prediction from acute pyelonephritis focus volume measured at ^{99m}Tc dimercaptosuccinic acid SPECT. *Radiology* 221:366-370, 2001. Radiological Society of North America.)

specificity, positive and negative predictive values were 96.7%, 92.3%, 90.6%, and 97.3%, respectively.

Conclusion.—Quantitative analysis of acute DMSA renal SPECT findings is useful in predicting renal fibrosis in patients with APN. The volume of an acute pyelonephritis lesion can be helpful in predicting the development of fibrosis.

▶ One of the major concerns in a child with a UTI is, of course, the risk of permanent sequelae. This has a significant effect on the aggressiveness of the antibiotic therapy and the intensity of the follow-up. Unfortunately, the criteria for gathering prognostic information have not been uniform, and they involve a considerable amount of subjective interpretation. This study provides an interesting approach by measuring the actual size of the involved area in children with infection undergoing DMSA imaging. Many of the parameters studied had considerable overlap, but the lesion volume appeared to correlate very well with the development with sequelae. It is interesting that the volume of the lesions was the only predictor of scarring since one would suspect that multiple lesions would present a greater risk than solitary lesions as an indication of the extent of the disease and the risk of permanent tissue injury.

M. D. Blaufox, MD, PhD

The Incidence of Left Iliac Fossa Uptake of ^{99m}Tc-DTPA in Renal Scanning

Roman MR, Gruenewald SM, Saunders CA (Westmead Hosp, Sydney, Australia)

Eur J Nucl Med 28:1842-1844, 2001

6–9

Introduction.—Several cases of extrarenal uptake of technetium-99m DTPA (^{99m}Tc-DTPA) have been reported, usually in cases of tumor, abscess, or a "phantom kidney." A relatively common observation has been increased uptake in the left iliac fossa (LIF). The incidence of this phenomenon was examined in a retrospective analysis.

Methods.—The departmental database was searched for all patients who underwent renal DTPA scan between January 1, 1996 and December 31, 1997. The presence and grade of increased iliac fossa activity were ascertained by consensus of 3 observers. Patients with increased uptake were cross-referenced against the New South Wales (Australian) Cancer Council database to exclude the possibility of a neoplastic lesion.

Results.—Increased LIF uptake was observed in 41 (18%) of the 231 consecutive patients (18 men, 23 women; mean age, 43 years). In the 41 patients with increase LIF uptake, 2 patients (5%) had severe uptake, 12 (29%) had moderate uptake, and 27 (66%) had mild uptake. No increased uptake in the right iliac fossa was observed. One patient with increased uptake had a malignant lesion and was excluded. No other patients had developed malignancy at a mean follow-up of 4.1 years.

Conclusion.—Increased LIF uptake is a common, benign finding most likely the result of activity within the descending colon. It occurs in about 18% of the population and is important to recognize to avoid misdiagnosis.

▶ The uptake or apparent uptake of some renal agents in the abdomen has often been a source of confusion. It has usually been attributed to gastrointestinal (GI) activity. This can be especially difficult in patients studied with MAG3, which is excreted by the liver. These investigators report a relatively high incidence of uptake in patients studied with DTPA renography. It is very likely that some of this may be due to our use of larger doses of radioactivity than are absolutely necessary for imaging purposes. The authors here use 600 MBq, which may be sufficient activity to make areas of uptake that might otherwise be minimal or hardly noticed apparent on reviewing the scans. It is interesting that all of the uptake noted was in the left iliac fossa, and the authors' suggestions that this is most likely due to the GI tract certainly would appear to be reasonable. I would be curious to know if this phenomenon is noticeable in patients receiving doses of less than 100 MBq. At our institution where smaller doses are used, this has not presented a problem in interpretation of the scans.

M. D. Blaufox, MD, PhD

Exercise Renal Scintigraphy Shows Renal Ischemia in a Transplanted Kidney

Fanti S, Mirelli M, Curti T, et al (S Orsola-Malpighi Hosp, Bologna, Italy)
Clin Nucl Med 27:483-485, 2002   6–10

Background.—Renal scintigraphy has been used for years in the evaluation of transplanted kidneys. Renographic studies have also been used to study vascular occlusion, obstruction, urine leakage, and hematomas. Radionuclide imaging has also been used in the differential diagnosis of acute tubular necrosis, acute rejection, and cyclosporine toxicity. Captopril renal scintigraphy has been used for the identification of a transplanted kidney as a cause of hypertension. Stenosis of a renal artery supplying a transplanted kidney is not rare, occurring in about 3% of patients. However, renal artery stenosis may not be the only cause of ischemia in a transplanted kidney, and hypertension may not necessarily be a consequence of unilateral renal ischemia. A patient with an unusual arterial supply to a transplanted kidney whose hemodynamic situation could be evaluated properly only by an unusual scintigraphic approach was described.

Case Report.—A 52-year-old man was referred for evaluation of a possible "steal phenomenon" involving a transplanted kidney. The patient had a history of chronic renal failure and required peritoneal dialysis since January 1997. At that time, a 55-mm abdominal aortic aneurysm was also discovered. In June 1998, the aneurysm was repaired in an endovascular approach in which a bifurcated stent graft replaced the aneurysm. Although the procedure had a good initial outcome, progressive worsening of renal function was noted during follow-up. As a result, the patient received a left pelvic renal transplant in January 2000, at which time the transplanted renal artery was connected to the left external iliac artery. The patient did well until February 2001, when a thrombotic occlusion of the left femoral artery occurred. A femoro-femoral bypass was performed to ensure renal perfusion through reversed flow via the external iliac artery. A few months later, the patient noticed reduced urine production after walking and also had oliguric episodes after prolonged walking, which resolved at rest. Blood pressure was always within normal limits. A steal phenomenon of the kidney was considered likely. Exercise renography was performed, which showed parenchymal trapping of radiotracer as a result of exercise, indicating ischemia of the transplanted kidney. The patient underwent surgery for removal of the stent, and an aortoiliac bypass was performed.

Conclusions.—Exercise renography has been used as a research tool for the investigation of the pathophysiologic nature of hypertension. This appears to be the first reported use of exercise renography to demonstrate renal ischemia and the first exercise renographic study performed in a patient with an organ transplant.

▶ I have long been an advocate of exercise renography and have felt that the use of this tool in renal nuclear medicine has been severely limited. Although this is only a report of a single case, the report here helps to confirm the potential role of exercise renography in patients with transplanted kidneys in whom this also would appear to be an ideal application.

M. D. Blaufox, MD, PhD

Kidney Allografts and Remaining Contralateral Donor Kidneys Before and After Transplantation: Assessment by Quantitative ^{99m}Tc-DMSA SPECT

Even-Sapir E, Gutman M, Lerman H, et al (Tel-Aviv Univ, Israel)
J Nucl Med 43:584-588, 2002   6–11

Background.—The renal cortical agent dimercaptosuccinic acid (DMSA) labeled with ^{99m}Tc detects the functioning proximal tubular mass. Its uptake correlates with effective renal plasma flow, glomerular filtration rate, and creatinine clearance. The quantitative measurement of ^{99m}Tc-DMSA is therefore a good index for renal function. Previous studies have shown that ^{99m}Tc-DMSA uptake differentiates between normal and diseased kidneys. Accurate determination of renal mass and function is critical both before transplantation for kidney donor selection and after transplantation for follow-up. The potential role of quantitative ^{99m}Tc-DMSA SPECT (QDMSA) in the clinical setting of renal transplantation was assessed. The remaining donor kidney and the donated kidney were evaluated before and after transplantation.

Methods.—A baseline QDMSA study was performed in 19 kidney donors before nephrectomy. The kidneys remaining in 16 donors were studied at 1 to 2 months and at 6 to 15 months after harvesting. The parameters obtained in each SPECT study included functional volume, concentration of ^{99m}Tc-DMSA per cubic centimeter of renal tissue, and total kidney uptake. Clinical evaluation and determination of serum creatinine levels took place at the same time as SPECT.

Results.—Clinical examination showed that 14 grafts had normal function and 5 were impaired. The mean ±SD of kidney uptake values expressed as percentage of baseline values were 131% ± 30% in normal grafts versus 57% ± 5% in impaired grafts at 1 week; 173% ± 57% versus 65% ± 10% at 1 to 2 months; and 190% ± 50% versus 69% ± 14% at 6 to 15 months after transplantation (Fig 1). Uptake values in the donors' remaining kidneys were 159% ± 27% of baseline values at 1 to 2 months and 164% ± 30% at 6 to 15 months after nephrectomy. Allografts and remaining kidneys demonstrated a similar increase in total kidney uptake as a result of an increase in functional volume as well as concentration.

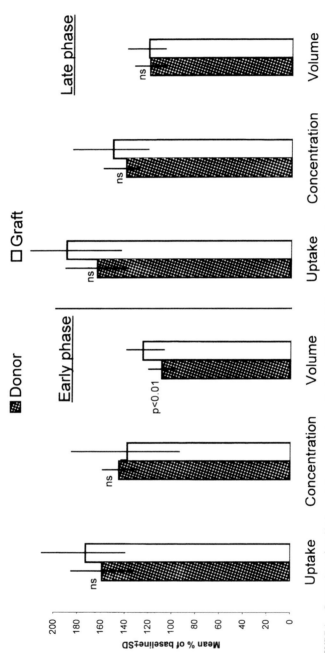

FIGURE 1.—Comparison of total kidney uptake, concentration, and volume of ^{99m}Tc-DMSA in normal allografts and in donors' remaining kidneys early (1-2 months) and late (6-15 months) after transplantation. *Abbreviation: ns,* Not statistically significant. (Reprinted by permission of the Society of Nuclear Medicine, courtesy of Even-Sapir E, Gutman M, Lerman H, et al: Kidney allografts and remaining contralateral donor kidneys before and after transplantation: Assessment by quantitative ^{99m}Tc-DMSA SPECT. *J Nucl Med* 43:584-588, 2002.)

Conclusions.—Quantitative ^{99m}Tc-DMSA SPECT has the potential to provide a noninvasive assessment tool in kidney transplantation from living donors.

▶ This article provides an approach to measuring renal allograft function. I am not really sure why one would prefer to use Tc-DMSA over either Tc-DTPA, which would give you the GFR or Tc-MAG$_3$, which would give you some estimate of renal tubular function. However, it is a potentially useful alternative approach. Once again, I am faced with the specter that I encountered in last year's YEAR BOOK OF NUCLEAR MEDICINE of work that I personally had done more than 30 years ago apparently being overlooked. Back in the time when I was a renal transplant fellow at Peter Bent Brigham Hospital, I studied a series of patients who had received kidney transplants from living related donors. Studies carried out using para amino hippuric acid and inulin, compared the function in the transplant donor and the recipient. Although radioactive materials were not used, the studies described definitively what level of renal function one could reasonably expect in a successful renal transplant and how that would compare to the function in the donor.[1]

M. D. Blaufox, MD, PhD

Reference

1. Blaufox MD, Lewis EJ, Jagger P, et al: Physiologic responses of the transplanted human kidney, sodium regulation and renin secretion. *N Engl J Med* 280: 62-66, 1969.

Segmental Infarction With Graft Dysfunction: An Emerging Syndrome in Renal Transplantation?
Kanchanabat B, Siddins M, Coates T, et al (Queen Elizabeth Hosp, Woodville, South Australia)
Nephrol Dial Transplant 17:123-128, 2002   6–12

Background.—Unlike total graft thrombosis, segmental infarction is not commonly recognized. There are only a few previous studies of focal perfusion defects after renal transplantation, and the incidence in these studies has ranged from 4% to 42%. This variation in incidence of segmental infarction reflects the heterogeneity of the patient populations and the small numbers of patients in these studies. Segmental allograft infarction has been reported in association with rejection, prolonged ischemia, and multiple renal arteries; the condition is at present poorly defined. The clinical manifestations, risk factors, prognosis, and natural history of segmental allograft infarction were characterized.

Methods.—A retrospective study reviewed the renal scans obtained from all renal transplant recipients at 1 institution over a 3-year period (1997 to 2000). Segmental infarction was diagnosed on the basis of a significant elevation in lactate dehydrogenase and a photopenic perfusion defect. The graft characteristics, operative details, clinical course, and long-term outcomes were evaluated in these patients.

Results.—Segmental infarction was identified in 13 (4.7%) of 277 consecutive renal transplant recipients. The onset of infarction occurred within 24 hours after transplantation in 9 patients. All these patients received marginal grafts, and in 5 patients the transplant operation was complicated by major blood loss. Eight of the patients with segmental infarction exhibited primary nonfunction or had renal failure develop after the onset of infarction. In 4 patients, infarction occurred after 24 hours but within 35 hours to 10 days of transplantation. One patient demonstrated primary nonfunction, and renal function deteriorated after the onset of infarction in the remaining 3 patients. Long-term graft function was impaired in these patients, and 6 patients had nadir creatine clearances below 60 mL/min.

Conclusions.—Segmental infarction appears to have a multifactorial pathogenesis, which reflects the combination of an initiating anatomic lesion and potentiating thrombogenic milieu. Segmental infarction usually occurs in the early postoperative period, and a prompt diagnosis can be difficult. Prophylactic heparin may therefore be warranted in persons at highest risk. In this study, there was no correlation between the infarct area and the graft function, and the long-term function of the graft is compromised out of proportion to the extent of parenchymal loss. This finding underscores the role of predisposing factors, particularly marginal graft quality, in determining the functional outcome of the graft.

▶ The occurrence of segmental infarction in a renal graft is certainly not surprising considering the multiple risk factors involved. This study shows the significance of that complication. However, from the nuclear medicine point of view, it also very nicely shows the great value of renal scanning in transplant recipients. Although it is likely over the next several years that in vitro tests for the detection of renal transplant rejection will evolve, these tests will not totally replace the use of radionuclides for evaluating renal transplantations. This study shows the value of radionuclide imaging in segmental infarction as one of the applications that is best served with nuclear medicine techniques.

M. D. Blaufox, MD, PhD

7 Gastrointestinal

Introduction

This chapter starts with articles on antibody white cell labeling to detect inflammatory bowel problems. Several articles on interesting applications of hepatobiliary scintigraphy follow. The chapter then moves on to gastrointestinal bleeding studies and protein losing enteropathy. The chapter ends with cases using colloid and heat-treated red blood cells.

Alexander Gottschalk, MD

---

^{99m}Tc Anti-CD 15 Monoclonal Antibody (LeuTech) Imaging Improves Diagnostic Accuracy and Clinical Management in Patients With Equivocal Presentation of Appendicitis

Rypins EB, Kipper SL, Weiland F, et al (Tri-City Med Ctr, Oceanside, Calif; Sutter Roseville Med Ctr, Calif; Mem Med Ctr, Springfield, Ill; et al)
Ann Surg 235:232-239, 2002   7–1

Background.—Appendicitis is the most common cause of acute abdominal pain requiring surgery. Appendicitis often has an atypical presentation, which can result in misdiagnosis or a delay in diagnosis, particularly in early cases in which the patients may be discharged from an emergency department only to return with perforated appendicitis. The standard of care for patients with equivocal presentation of appendicitis is hospital admission for observation or early operation. In this equivocal population, adjunctive imaging tests have been used with mixed results. A promising novel monoclonal antibody, technetium 99m-labeled anti-CD 15, which specifically targets neutrophils and may be used for imaging appendicitis in patients with an equivocal presentation, was evaluated.

Methods.—This prospective, multicenter, open-label study enrolled 200 patients (121 women, 79 men) with a mean age of 30.5 ± 16.5 years (range, 5 to 86 years) (Table 1). A management plan was developed for each patient before imaging and evaluated after imaging with ^{99m}Tc-labeled anti-CD 15 (LeuTech) to determine the effects of imaging on patient management. Imaging was performed with a standard gamma camera for 30 to 90 minutes.

Results.—A histopathologic diagnosis of acute appendicitis was established in 59 patients. LeuTech identified 53 of these patients (90% sensitivity) and was negative in 122 of 141 patients without appendicitis (87%

TABLE 1.—Enrollment Criteria for Equivocal Presentation of
Acute Appendicitis

1. Equivocal presentation included one or more of the following:
2. Atypical history/symptoms
   - Absence of periumbilical pain migrating to RLQ
   - No gradual onset of pain
   - No increasing intensity of pain over time
   - Pain not aggravated by movement and coughing
3. Atypical physical examination
   - Absence of Mcburney's point tenderness
   - Absence of referred tenderness to RLQ with palpation in other quadrants
   - Absence of abdominal muscular spasm with RLQ tenderness
4. Fever <101°F
5. White blood cell count <10,500/mm^3

Abbreviation: RLQ, Right lower quadrant.
(Courtesy of Rypins EB, Kipper SL, Weiland F, et al: ^{99m}Tc anti-CD 15 monoclonal antibody (LeuTech) imaging improves diagnostic accuracy and clinical management in patients with equivocal presentation of appendicitis. *Ann Surg* 235(2):232-239, 2002.)

specificity). The accuracy, positive predictive value, and negative predictive value were 88%, 74%, and 95%, respectively. The diagnostic efficacy was unchanged in a subgroup of 48 pediatric patients. Diagnostic images for appendicitis were achieved within 8 minutes after injection in 50% of patients and within 47 minutes in 90% of patients. Significant shifts in patient management decisions were manifest after LeuTech results. LeuTech was well tolerated, and there were no serious adverse events reported.

Conclusions.—LeuTech is a convenient, safe, and rapid imaging test for the diagnosis of appendicitis in adult and pediatric patients with equivocal signs and symptoms.

▶ When a tracer is easy to use and works, it is likely to go far. The fact that this article is in a surgery journal is also encouraging. But if the competition is spiral CT and the CT technologist is always at the hospital and the nuclear medicine technologist has to be called in or is not present in the evenings, which technique do you think the ER doctor will use? If you want to use LeuTech, be ready to use it 24 hours a day. How about cross-training the on-call x-ray technologist? We do not need major imaging skill here—no SPECT, etc. Just turn on the camera and aim at the right lower quadrant. (Also, please make skin contact.)

A. Gottschalk, MD

Scintigraphic Head-to-Head Comparison Between ^{99m}Tc-WBCs and ^{99m}Tc-LeukoScan in the Evaluation of Inflammatory Bowel Disease: A Pilot Study
Stokkel MPM, Reigman HIE, Pauwels EKJ (Leiden Univ, The Netherlands)
Eur J Nucl Med 29:251-254, 2002   7–2

Background.—To assess the extent of inflammatory changes in the gastrointestinal tract in patients with inflammatory bowel diseases (IBDs) such as ulcerative colitis or Crohn's disease, scintigraphy with technetium (Tc) 99m-labeled white blood cells (WBCs) is generally used. Among its disadvantages are the length of tracer preparation time required, the need to handle blood, and the inability to detect stenosis, fistulae, and malignancies. A relatively new agent, LeukoScan, has been used to detect soft tissue and bone infections, with results for ^{99m}Tc-LeukoScan comparable with those reported for ^{99m}Tc-WBC scintigraphy. A one-on-one comparison of the 2 methods was undertaken to see whether ^{99m}Tc-LeukoScan proved useful in the evaluation of IBD.

Methods.—The 6 patients (4 males and 2 females; mean age, 35) all had histologically proven IBD and increased uptake on ^{99m}Tc-WBC images. The 2 scans were taken 2 to 7 days apart, and active IBD was then confirmed endoscopically.

Results.—All 6 patients' ^{99m}Tc-WBC images showed significantly increased uptake in at least 2 bowel segments, denoting inflammation, whereas only 3 of the ^{99m}Tc-LeukoScan images showed uptake and it was slight. Because no inflammation could be confirmed at these sites, it was assumed that the increased uptake resulted from liver excretion. In the other 3 patients, no increased uptake was found.

Conclusions.—LeukoScan proved to be of no value in assessing IBD when compared with the effectiveness of ^{99m}Tc-WBC images.

▶ A bummer.

A. Gottschalk, MD

The Usefulness of Hepatobiliary Scintigraphy in the Diagnosis of Complications After Adult-to-Adult Living Donor Liver Transplantation
Kim JS, Moon DH, Lee SG, et al (Univ of Ulsan, Seoul, Korea)
Eur J Nucl Med 29:473-479, 2002   7–3

Introduction.—It is well known that hepatobiliary scintigraphy (HBS) is useful in evaluating postoperative complications after various types of biliary surgery or cadaveric whole liver transplantation; its use after adult living donor liver transplantation (LDLT) has not been described. Since adult LDLT necessitates different surgical approaches and involves a different postoperative anatomy than does whole liver transplantation, the pattern of postoperative complications may differ. The scintigraphic findings of the postoperative complications after adult-to-adult LDLT were examined, as well as the usefulness of HBS in diagnosing complications.

Methods.—Eighty-two HBS studies performed with technetium-99m DISIDA were evaluated in 60 adult patients who received a living donor's hepatic lobe (right lobe, 32; left lobe, 28). Indications for HBS included abnormal symptoms, abnormal liver function tests, or both (n = 54), or suspected bile leak or biloma (n = 28). The median number of days between transplantation and scintigraphy was 69. Classifications of scintigraphic findings were hepatic parenchymal dysfunction, total biliary obstruction, segmental biliary obstruction, bile leak, and normal graft.

Results.—Scintigraphic findings were verified on liver biopsy in 17 patients and by radiologic and clinical follow-up in 65 patients. There were 29 events associated with biliary complications (6 total biliary obstructions, 8 segmental biliary obstructions, and 15 bile leaks) and 19 linked to nonbiliary complications (15 rejections, 2 infections, and 2 vascular compromises) in 38 patients. HBS yielded the correct diagnosis in all 8 segmental, 5 of 6 total biliary obstructions, and all 15 cases of bile leaks. Of the 19 nonbiliary complications, 16 demonstrated parenchymal dysfunction regardless of etiology and 3 revealed total biliary obstruction on scintigraphy. All except 3 of 34 normally functioning grafts were normal on scintigraphy. The diagnostic sensitivity and specificity of scintigraphy for biliary obstruction in 54 patients who had abnormal symptoms or liver function studies were 93% (100% for segmental, 83% for total) and 88% (35/40), respectively. The sensitivity and specificity for bile leak were each 100% (15/15, 13/13) in the 28 patients with suspected bile leak or biloma.

Conclusion.—HBS is diagnostically accurate in the assessment of biliary complications in patients who have undergone adult-to-adult LDLT. This approach is limited as a means of differential diagnosis of nonbiliary complications.

▶ If you have biliary complications, a test that evaluates the biliary tree should find them. If the complication does not involve the biliary tree, the test will not do as well. This makes sense to me.

A. Gottschalk, MD

Scintigraphy of the Small Intestine: A Simplified Standard for Study of Transit With Reference to Normal Values
Grybäck P, Jacobsson H, Blomquist L, et al (Karolinska Hosp, Stockholm)
Eur J Nucl Med 29:39-45, 2002   7–4

Introduction.—Noninvasive approaches are preferred in the evaluation of small intestine transit; scintigraphic methods are considered standard. Assessment of the small-bowel transit is complex because of its anatomical position. To avoid any influence of the gastric emptying rate on scintigraphic results, ^{99m}Tc-HIDA was used to assess small-bowel transit, because it is a tracer that is excreted in bile and, therefore, delivered directly into the duodenum.

Methods.—Thirty healthy research subjects underwent administration of 120 MBq of ^{99m}Tc-HIDA. Dynamic 1-minute image acquisitions were obtained. The duodenum and cecum were easily detected on the digitized images. Small-bowel transit time was determined from the difference in the arrival time of the radiopharmaceutical in the proximal duodenum and cecum, as determined by assessment of the count rate against background activity (Scint 1) and by the visual appearance of activity (Scint 2). A hydrogen breath test was performed simultaneously to assess scintigraphic transit. Scintigraphic transit tests were also performed in 23 patients who had motility disorders and had undergone manometry of the small bowel.

Results.—In healthy research subjects, the transit time of ^{99m}Tc-HIDA was 77.9 minutes (Scint 1) or 79.3 minutes (Scint 2), and the lactulose transit time was 100.1 minutes. Seventeen of the 23 patients with motility disorders, 17 (73.9%) had a dysmotility pattern that was confirmed by manometry; in 14 patients, ^{99m}Tc-HIDA transit was prolonged.

Conclusion.—For identification of transit abnormalities, scintigraphy with ^{99m}Tc-HIDA to assess small-bowel transit is a readily available technique in the clinical setting. This approach is clinically feasible. The transit time of ^{99m}Tc-HIDA had good correlation with the results of the hydrogen breath test (lactulose transit time) in healthy research subjects.

▶ Using Tc-99m HIDA as a tracer for these studies is a clever idea, allowing the stomach to be bypassed. But, just as the authors point out that gastric emptying rate is a variable that complicates the study if an oral tracer is used, I have to worry if the "biliary" emptying rate in any way affects these data— especially worrisome because normal limits ranged between 21 and 153 minutes.

A. Gottschalk, MD

Cholecystokinin-Stimulated Mebrofenin (^{99m}Tc-Choletec) Hepatobiliary Scintigraphy in Asymptomatic Postcholecystectomy Individuals: Assessment of Specificity, Interobserver Reliability, and Reproducibility
Pineau BC, Knapple WL, Spicer KM, et al (Wake Forest Univ, Winston-Salem, NC; Med Univ of South Carolina, Charleston)
Am J Gastroenterol 96:3106-3109, 2001   7–5

Purpose.—In patients who have undergone cholecystectomy, sphincter of Oddi dysfunction (SOD) can lead to recurrent, biliary-type pain. Previous reports have suggested that cholecystokinin-stimulated hepatobiliary scintigraphy (CCK-HBS) is a highly accurate noninvasive test for diagnosis of SOD. The specificity, interobserver reliability, and reproducibility of CCK-HBS were evaluated in symptom-free postcholecystectomy patients.

Methods.—The study included 20 postcholecystectomy patients with no symptoms and a normal liver screening profile. All underwent 2 CCK-HBS studies on separate occasions, an average of 24 weeks apart. The first scan was performed on average of 43 months after cholecystectomy. The studies were read by 3 nuclear medicine physicians in blinded fashion.

Results.—Interobserver agreement was good for both scans, with κ values of 0.554 and 0.507, respectively. However, intraobserver agreement was poor, with κ values of 0.062 to 0.385 for first and second scans read by the same nuclear medicine specialist. In this population, the CCK-HBS scans had an overall specificity of 77.5%. However, when 2 negative CCK-HBS scans were used as the definition of true-negative, specificity dropped to 60%.

Conclusions.—Cholecystokinin-stimulated hepatobiliary scintigraphy shows low specificity in symptom-free postcholecystectomy patients. The findings question the value of CCK-HBS in evaluation of patients with suspected SOD. Interobserver agreement is good, but reliability is low when the test is repeated in the same patient over time.

▶ Studies like this are often hard to do, and we need more of them. You might argue that the time of cholecystokinin infusion and the tracer used are important variables, but then you should do a study like this to show it. So often the group used to "prove" the efficiency of any test is loaded with the disease in question, which makes the test look great. Alternatively, patients with the disease are analyzed to find the "unique characteristics." When subsequently used in a random group of patients only suspected of having the disease, the test works poorly. My favorite example of this is the use of the plain chest radiograph to diagnose pulmonary embolism (PE). You doubtless know that there are many radiographic signs of PE on the chest film—all with peer-reviewed articles to support their use. My old chief, Dick Greenspan, took chest films from PIOPED and asked a group of chest radiologists to read each case and state whether or not the patient had PE. You will recall that all PIOPED patients were suspected of having PE, but only about one third did (angiogram proven). Dick made it a point to get real professionals to read the chest films and noted that some had even described some of the signs of PE noted here. I was not asked to participate, but had I been asked, and had I chosen to flip a coin and never look at the films, my diagnostic skill would have been right up there with the best of them.

A. Gottschalk, MD

Comparison of Sphincter of Oddi Manometry, Fatty Meal Sonography, and Hepatobiliary Scintigraphy in the Diagnosis of Sphincter of Oddi Dysfunction

Rosenblatt ML, Catalano MF, Alcocer E, et al (St Luke's Med Ctr, Milwaukee, Wis)
Gastrointest Endosc 54:697-704, 2001   7–6

Background.—The sphincter of Oddi is a complex structure comprising smooth muscle fibers surrounding the distal common bile duct, pancreatic duct, and major duodenal papilla. Sphincter of Oddi dysfunction (SOD) affects about 1% to 5% of patients after a cholecystectomy. Sphincter of Oddi manometry (SOM) is the diagnostic standard for SOD. However, SOM is an invasive, technically difficult technique that is frequently complicated by pancreatitis. Thus, a need exists for a sensitive and accurate noninvasive imaging modality for the diagnosis of SOD. Two tests that are used for this purpose are quantitative hepatobiliary scintigraphy (HBS) and fatty meal sonography (FMS); however, results of these tests vary. The accuracy of SOM, HBS, and FMS in the diagnosis of SOD were compared in a large cohort of patients.

TABLE 3.—Comparison of SOM with HBS in the Diagnosis
of SOD (n = 304)

| | | SOM | | |
		Normal	Abnormal	Total
	Abnormal	50	36	86
HBS	Normal	181	37	218
	Total	231	73	304

Abbreviations: SOM, Sphincter of Oddi manometry; *HBS*, hepatobiliary scintigraphy; *SOD*, sphincter of Oddi dysfunction.
(Courtesy of Rosenblatt ML, Catalano MF, Alcocer E, et al: Comparison of sphincter of Oddi manometry, fatty meal sonography, and hepatobiliary scintigraphy in the diagnosis of sphincter of Oddi dysfunction. *Gastrointest Endosc* 54:697-704, 2001.)

Methods.—A total of 304 consecutive patients with suspected SOD were evaluated by SOM, FMS, and HBS after cholecystectomy. Findings on SOM were judged abnormal if basal pressure was increased (>40 mm Hg); phasic activity was increased (amplitude >350 mm Hg); the frequency of contractions was greater than 8 per minute; more than 50% of propagation sequences were retrograde; or the response to cholecystokinin was paradoxical. Findings on FMS were considered abnormal if ductal dilation was greater than 2 mm at 45 minutes after fatty meal ingestion. Quantitative HBS was performed with sequential images obtained every 5 minutes for 90 minutes to monitor excretion of the radionuclide. The time-to-peak, half-time, and downslope were calculated on the basis of predetermined ranges.

Results.—SOD was diagnosed in 73 of 304 patients (24%), and SOM was used as the reference standard. HBS findings were abnormal in 86 patients, and FMS findings were abnormal in 22 patients (Table 3). A true-positive result was obtained in 15 patients by FMS and in 36 patients by HBS. False-positive results were obtained by FMS in 7 patients and by HBS in 50 patients. The sensitivity was 21% for FMS and 49% for HBS, whereas specificities were 97% and 78%, respectively. FMS, HBS, or findings from both were abnormal in 90% of patients with Geenen-Hogan type I SOD, in 50% of patients with type II SOD, and in 44% of patients with type III SOD (Table 5). Sphincterotomy was performed in 73 patients, and 40 of these patients

TABLE 5.—Accuracy of FMS and HBS in the Diagnosis of SOD*

Study	Sensitivity	Specificity	PPV	NPV
FMS	21%	97%	68%	79%
HBS	49%	78%	42%	83%
Both†	53%	77%	42%	84%

*SOM is used as the reference standard.
†Refers to either FMS or HBS findings being abnormal.
Abbreviations: SOM, Sphincter of Oddi manometry; *HBS*, hepatobiliary scintigraphy; *SOD*, sphincter of Oddi dysfunction; *PPV*, positive predictive value; *NPV*, negative predictive value.
(Courtesy of Rosenblatt ML, Catalano MF, Alcocer E, et al: Comparison of sphincter of Oddi manometry, fatty meal sonography, and hepatobiliary scintigraphy in the diagnosis of sphincter of Oddi dysfunction. *Gastrointest Endosc* 54:697-704, 2001.)

had a long-term response. Of patients with SOD, 11 of 13 patients (85%) with abnormal HBS and FMS findings had a good long-term response. *Conclusions.*—This is the largest trial reported to date comparing SOM, FMS, and HBS in the diagnosis of SOD. In this series, FMS and HBS correlated poorly with SOM in the diagnosis of SOD. A slight increase in sensitivity can be obtained when FMS and HBS are used together. The accuracy of both FMS and HBS decreases across the spectrum of SOD from type I to type III; however, FMS and HBS may help to predict a long-term response to endoscopic sphincterotomy in patients with elevated sphincter of Oddi basal pressure.

▶ I was hoping to write a "little girl" type comment here. You know, "when she is good she is very very good, but when she is bad she is horrid." However, unfortunately, when HBS is good (specificity, 78%) she is only fair, and when she is bad (sensitivity, 49%), she is lousy. The authors end by suggesting that someone try adding an associated morphine provocative test to the HBS study. It seems that the data could only get better. I hope someone takes them up on this suggestion.

A. Gottschalk, MD

Tc-99m DISIDA Scan Findings in Two Large Choledochal Cysts in the Same Patient
Hwang K-H, Park CH, Kim OH, et al (Ajou Univ, Suwon, Korea)
Clin Nucl Med 26:1047-1048, 2001   7–7

Purpose.—Choledochal cysts may be detected by prenatal US. An infant with 2 large choledochal cysts is described, and the results of Tc-99m DISIDA scanning are presented.

   Case Report.—Girl, 5 days, underwent Tc-99m DISIDA hepatobiliary scintigraphy to evaluate 2 cystic masses of the liver and right abdomen. The lesions had been detected on prenatal ultrasonography and confirmed by abdominal CT at the age of 3 days (Figs 1 and 2). Both cysts showed delayed filling with bile, consistent with choledochal cysts. Excision of the lower cyst confirmed the diagnosis of choledochal cyst. The hepatic cyst was left untreated.

Discussion.—An unusual case of 2 choledochal cysts in a newborn is described, including the Tc-99m DISIDA scan and surgical findings.

▶ An unusual variant of an entity that most of us thought we knew all about. This case is a new wrinkle for me.

A. Gottschalk, MD

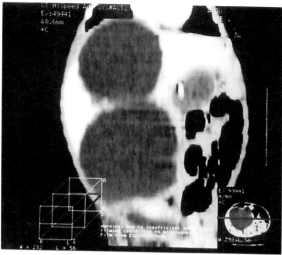

FIGURE 1.—A 3-day-old female neonate had a CT scan of the abdomen for 2 large cystic masses, 1 in the liver and the other in the right abdomen, that were detected by prenatal US. A 2-dimensional coronal reconstruction image of the abdominal CT showed 2 large cysts, 1 in the liver and the other in the right abdomen. (Courtesy of Hwang K-H, Park CH, Kim OH, et al: Tc-99m DISIDA scan findings in two large choledochal cysts in the same patient. *Clin Nucl Med* 26(12):1047-1048, 2001.)

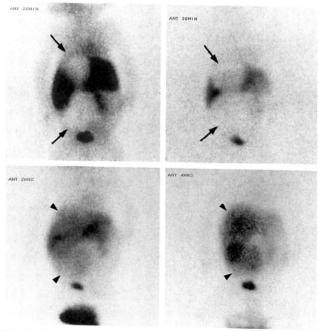

FIGURE 2.—On the fifth day after birth, Tc-99m DISIDA hepatobiliary scintigraphy was performed. Two large photon-deficient cystic structures were seen on early images (*arrows*). These areas filled with bile on 2-hour and 4-hour late images (*arrowheads*). These findings show the classic appearance of a choledochal cyst. The patient was treated by excision of the lower choledochal cyst, cholecystectomy, and choledochojejunostomy. Histologic analysis verified a large choledochal cyst. The hepatic choledochal cyst was left alone, with no surgical intervention. (Courtesy of Hwang K-H, Park CH, Kim OH, et al: Tc-99m DISIDA scan findings in two large choledochal cysts in the same patient. *Clin Nucl Med* 26(12):1047-1048, 2001.)

Repeated Bleeding Scintigraphy May Reveal That Stationary Foci of Activity Represent Sites of Active Hemorrhage
Krynyckyi BR, Zuckier LS, Tatlidil R, et al (Yeshiva Univ, Bronx, NY; New York Univ; Sifa Hosp, Izmir, Turkey)
Clin Nucl Med 27:25-29, 2002   7–8

Introduction.—Radionuclide bleeding scintigraphy is of value in localizing the source of gastrointestinal (GI) bleeding. Tracer activity is generally visualized extravasating from the blood pool into the lumen, then moving in sequential images. When the focus of activity does not move, it is thought to represent a fixed structure—such as collection in the urinary tract or blood vessels—rather than extravasation into the bowel. Three cases in which stationary foci of activity did represent GI bleeding are described and illustrated.

Patients.—The patients were 2 women and 1 man with an age range of 47 to 85 years. All underwent Tc-99m–labeled red blood cell (Tc-RBC) bleeding scans for assessment of GI bleeding episodes. The scans showed stationary foci of increased activity in various locations. One patient with a static focus in the right lower quadrant of the abdomen was eventually found to have a vascular ectasia of the cecum. In the second patient, a persistent focus of increased uptake was noted above the urinary bladder on 2 consecutive bleeding scans. This patient had extensive sigmoid diverticulosis, detected on colonoscopy, and the bleeding resolved spontaneously. No specific bleeding site was identified (Fig 2).

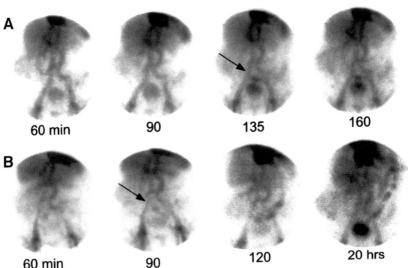

FIGURE 2.—A, A focus of activity just superior to the urinary bladder (*arrow*) appeared late in the study but did not improve with time. B, A repeated study shows a similar focus, which appeared by 90 minutes but progressed retrograde into the sigmoid and descending colon. Colonoscopy showed extensive sigmoid diverticulosis, but the specific bleeding site could not be identified. (Courtesy of Krynyckyi BR, Zuckier LS, Tatlidil R, et al: Repeated bleeding scintigraphy may reveal that stationary foci of activity represent sites of active hemorrhage. *Clin Nucl Med* 27(1):25-29, 2002.)

FIGURE 3

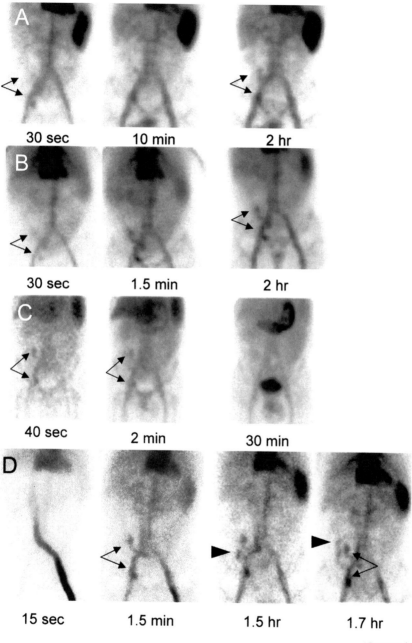

30 sec   10 min   2 hr

30 sec   1.5 min   2 hr

40 sec   2 min   30 min

15 sec   1.5 min   1.5 hr   1.7 hr

(*Continued*)

FIGURE 3 (cont.)

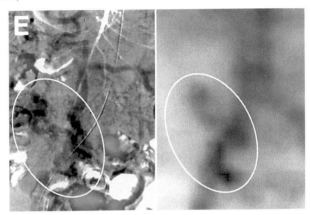

FIGURE 3.—A, B, A stationary serpiginous region of activity (*arrows*) overlying the right iliac vessels was present on the initial frames and throughout studies performed on 2 different days, with no evidence of motion within the bowel. C, A Meckel's scan of same patient shows a similar region of activity (*arrows*) on initial frames and fading with time with clearance of activity from the blood pool. No accumulation of pertechnetate is evident. D, An additional Tc-RBC study again shows the stationary focus of activity (*arrows*) seen on earlier studies. However, at approximately 1.5 hours, extravasated activity accumulated and moved adjacent to the fixed region (*bold arrowheads*). E (*left*), An angiogram shows mesenteric venous diverticula (within the oval), with no evidence of active bleeding, closely corresponding to that stationary focus of activity visualized on the scintigraphic studies (E, *right panel*). (Courtesy of Krynyckyi BR, Zuckier LS, Tatlidil R, et al: Repeated bleeding scintigraphy may reveal that stationary foci of activity represent sites of active hemorrhage. *Clin Nucl Med* 27(1):25-29, 2002.)

In the third patient, a fixed region of increased uptake was found over the right iliac vessels. This patient proved to have portal vein thrombosis with diffuse mesenteric varices (Fig 3).

Discussion.—In some patients with GI bleeding who are undergoing bleeding scintigraphy, fixed foci of activity may prove to represent areas of bleeding. In 2 of the patients reported here, the fixed foci did actually correspond to extravasated blood; it is unclear why the blood did not subsequently move in these cases. The third case of fixed activity was associated with extensive varices, which led to the bleeding. These possible explanations should be considered in the management of patients with stationary foci of activity, leading to further evaluations to localize the bleeding site.

▶ I think the authors' approach of repeating the red-cell study, continuing it for a longer time, or directing an angiogram to the area makes sense. I also suspect that most of us have seen a case or 2 like this from time to time. I think it is likely that only those cases presenting an unusual diagnosis that does not represent GI bleeding get written up. I applaud these authors for bucking this trend.

A. Gottschalk, MD

Protein-Losing Enteropathy Detected on Tc-99m HSA and Tc-99m MDP Scintigraphy

Seok JW, Kim SJ, Lee SH, et al (Pusan Natl Univ, Korea)
Clin Nucl Med 27:431-433, 2002   7–9

Background.—The excessive loss of gastrointestinal protein is associated with various disorders. Identifying the site of enteric protein loss may require the use of technetium (Tc) 99m human serum albumin (HSA) scintigraphy or Tc-99m methylene diphosphonate (MDP) scintigraphy. A protein-losing enteropathy was detected in a hospitalized patient with the use of Tc-99m HSA scintigraphy, with confirmation using Tc-99m MDP scintigraphy.

Case Report.—Man, 34, was hospitalized for left ankle edema, pain and tenderness in the left calf, and fever. Right leg pain and swelling, fever, and fatigue had been present for a year before admission, and pitting edema of both legs was found along with left calf pain on physical examination. Hypoproteinemia, hypoalbuminemia, hypocalcemia, increased levels of C-reactive protein, and increased lactate dehydrogenase concentrations were detected; whereas renal and liver function tests were normal. Antibiotics relieved the fever, bilateral leg edema, and left calf pain, but hypoalbuminemia and hypoproteinemia persisted. Liver disease and endogenous degradation of plasma protein were ruled out. Four hours after injecting Tc-99m HSA, the right middle abdomen revealed definite intestinal activity (Fig 1). Whole-body images were obtained 3 hours after injecting Tc-99m MDP, and scintigraphy showed increased uptake in the right middle abdomen, which confirmed the findings of Tc-99m HSA (Fig 2). A diagnosis of protein-losing enteropathy was made and a low-fat diet advised for the patient on discharge.

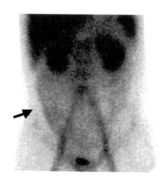 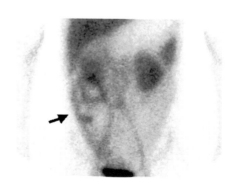

A   4 HRS   **B   8 HRS**

FIGURE 1.—With Tc-99m HSA scintigraphy, **A**, the 4-hour and, **B**, 8-hour anterior abdominal images showed definite intestinal activity in the right middle abdomen conforming to the ascending colon. (Courtesy of Seok JW, Kim SJ, Lee SH, et al: Protein-losing enteropathy detected on Tc-99m HSA and Tc-99m MDP scintigraphy. *Clin Nucl Med* 27(6):431-433, 2002.)

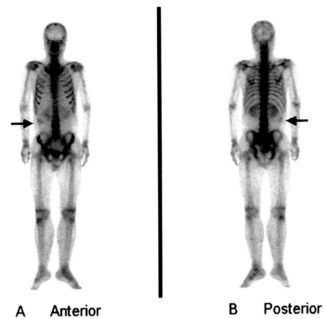

A   Anterior   B   Posterior

FIGURE 2.—Tc-99m MDP scintigraphy was performed 3 hours after radionuclide administration. A, Anterior and, B, posterior whole-body images show increased accumulation in the right middle abdomen corresponding to the involvement seen in the region identified by Tc-99m HSA scintigraphy. (Courtesy of Seok JW, Kim SJ, Lee SH, et al: Protein-losing enteropathy detected on Tc-99m HSA and Tc-99m MDP scintigraphy. *Clin Nucl Med* 27(6):431-433, 2002.)

Conclusions.—The right middle abdomen of this patient, which corresponded to the ascending colon, showed definite intestinal activity that led to the diagnosis of protein-losing enteropathy. Both the diagnosing study and the confirmatory investigation can generally be performed within 24 hours, allowing rapid identification of leakage and enabling treatment planning.

▶ I believe my standard red-cell bleeding study comment belongs here, too. It goes like this, "Once you remove the patient from underneath the camera, you cannot be certain the bleeding site you find is the site the blood initially came from." A corollary to this is the thought that pee, pus, water, and blood run downhill, and that anything in the small gut may get to the ileum in a hurry. If you don't believe me, read on.

A. Gottschalk, MD

Tc-99m Sulfur Colloid and Tc-99m Tagged Red Blood Cell Methods Are Comparable for Detecting Lower Gastrointestinal Bleeding in Clinical Practice

Ponzo F, Zhuang H, Liu FM, et al (Univ of Pennsylvania, Philadelphia)
Clin Nucl Med 27:405-409, 2002   7–10

Background.—To successfully treat patients who have acute lower gastrointestinal tract bleeding, it is essential to identify the source of the bleeding accurately. The greatest sensitivity is achieved with nuclear medicine studies, specifically, scintigraphic techniques. It has been noted that the use of technetium (Tc) 99m red blood cell (RBC) images may provide misleading data because of the delayed images; optimal patient treatment does not result when the gastrointestinal bleeding is detected only with interrupted delayed imaging. The effectiveness of Tc-99m RBC scintigraphy was compared with Tc-99m sulfur colloid (SC) scintigraphy for their abilities to detect and locate sites of lower gastrointestinal bleeding.

Methods.—A retrospective review of 359 consecutive cases of gastrointestinal bleeding yielded the data for analysis. In all, 193 Tc-99m SC scans lasting 30 minutes per scan and 138 Tc-99m RBC scans lasting 1 hour per scan were performed, along with 28 Tc-99m SC images, followed immediately by Tc-99m RBC images over a period of several hours. Results of the 2 techniques were compared.

Results.—Forty-seven of the 193 Tc-99m SC images (24.4%) showed the bleeding site compared with 38 of the 138 Tc-99m RBC images (27.5%). This difference was not significant. When the 2 scans were used consecutively, only 4 (14.8%) showed positive bleeding sites after an extended time, and only 1 of these was noted on Tc-99m SC within the first hour of the evaluation. More sites would be expected to be identified over the longer period required for the Tc-99m RBC technique, which proved to be the case. The rate of positive results in studies performed during regular working hours was 30.7%, whereas that for studies performed in off hours was 14.1%, a significant difference. Focusing just on those studies performed during working hours, Tc-99m SC studies did have a slightly greater sensitivity than Tc-99m RBC studies (34.7% vs 31.5%). Sensitivity for the off-hour Tc-99m SC studies was 14.3%, whereas that for off-hour Tc-99m RBC studies was 13.3% (Table 1).

TABLE 1.—Localization Rate of Gastrointestinal Scintigraphic Methods

	Sulfur Colloid			Red Blood Cell		
	Working Hours	Off Hours	Total	Working Hours	Off Hours	Total
Patients, n	95.0	98.0	193.0	108.0	30.0	138.0
Positive studies, n	33.0	14.0	47.0	34.0	4.0	38.0
Bleeding localization rate, %	34.7	14.3	24.4	31.5	13.3	27.5

(Courtesy of Ponzo F, Zhuang H, Liu FM, et al: Tc-99m sulfur colloid and Tc-99m tagged red blood cell methods are comparable for detecting lower gastrointestinal bleeding in clinical practice. *Clin Nucl Med* 27(6):405-409, 2002.)

Conclusions.—Equal sensitivity was shown for Tc-99m SC and Tc-99m RBC in locating the site of lower gastrointestinal tract bleeding.

▶ To me it makes sense to do emergency "middle of the night studies" with colloid. These authors make the point that delayed studies are nothing more than an expensive stool guaiac test once the patient's time under the camera is interrupted. About 2 decades ago, the group at Colorado studied a patient with intermittent bleeding that was evading diagnosis with labeled red-cells. He was imaged after hours and an off-duty registered nurse was hired to stay with him while he was sedated and under the camera/computer combo taking continuous 1-minute images for 3 hours or so. In those days, this was a technologic feat. At about 2½ hours, the patient bled from the terminal ileum and this was easily seen when the whole series was played back as a closed loop movie. With current equipment, this could be peformed anywhere. Think of the cost savings in the workup from just decreased hospitalization and useless (nonbleeding) abdominal angiograms alone if this were implemented.

A. Gottschalk, MD

Concurrent Occurrence of Chylothorax, Chylous Ascites, and Protein-Losing Enteropathy in Systemic Lupus Erythematosus

Lee C-K, Han JM, Lee KN, et al (Univ of Ulsan, Seoul, Korea)
J Rheumatol 29:1330-1333, 2002   7–11

Background.—Systemic lupus erythematosus (SLE) is a chronic inflammatory disease affecting the skin, joints, kidneys, lungs, nervous system, serous membranes, and other organs. Chylothorax or chylous ascites are characterized by chyle in the pleural or peritoneal fluid and result from damage or blockage of the lymphatics. Protein-losing enteropathy is characterized by leakage of protein that results in hypoproteinemia and generalized edema. Although protein-losing enteropathy is associated with a wide variety of disorders, it is not usually associated with SLE. The concurrent occurrence of chylothorax, chylous ascites, and protein-losing enteropathy have never been reported in a patient with SLE. Two patients with SLE whose initial manifestations of the disease were chylous effusion and protein-losing enteropathy were described.

Case 1.—A 47-year-old Korean woman with a 9-month history of progressive abdominal distension, generalized weakness, urinary frequency, and edema was admitted for evaluation. She had no history of any previous disease. Physical examination showed diminished sounds of breathing over the bilateral fields and a malar rash. Abdominal distension with shifting dullness and pitting edema on the bilateral lower extremities were noted. The patient was diagnosed with SLE associated with protein-losing enteropathy, cystitis, and chylous effusion on the basis of a positive ANA, a positive Rho

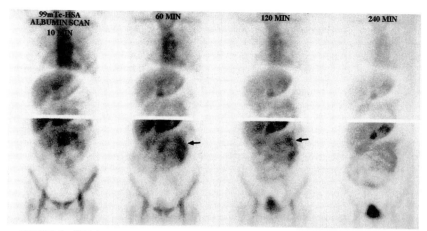

FIGURE 1.—^{99m}Tc-human serum albumin scintigraphy shows protein loss from small bowel (jejunum). Serum albumin was shown to leak into jejunum (*arrow*). (Courtesy of Lee C-K, Han JM, Lee KN, et al: Concurrent occurrence of chylothorax, chylous ascites, and protein-losing enteropathy in systemic lupus erythematosus. *J Rheumatol* 29:1330-1333, 2002.)

antibody, leukopenia, serositis, a malar rash, and low complement (Fig 1).

Case 2.—A 68-year-old Korean man presented with a 7-month history of generalized weakness, increased abdominal girth, weight loss, and edema. On initial examination, decreased sounds of breathing in the bilateral lower lung field, abdominal distension with shifting dullness, and pitting edema on the bilateral lower extremities were noted. Needle biopsy of the kidney showed findings compatible with a lupus nephritis, and it was believed that this presentation was most compatible with a lupus-induced protein-losing enteropathy and chylous effusion. He eventually died from acute respiratory failure. *Klebsiella pneumoniae* was cultured in the blood and bronchoalveolar lavage fluid. *Strongyloides stercoralis* larvae were found in the ascites and stool in cultures performed just before the patient died.

Conclusions.—Chylothorax and chylous ascites are manifestations of many types of disease rather than diseases themselves, so the prognosis depends on the treatment of the underlying disease. However, supportive measures are often needed to relieve the symptoms of chylothorax or chylous ascites along with treatment of the primary disease. These patients were started on low-fat diets with medium-chain triglyceride supplementation to decrease lymphatic flow. The patient in case 1 failed to respond to corticosteroid therapy, but was successfully treated with monthly IV cyclophosphamide therapy for 3 months. The patient in case 2 responded initially to corticosteroid therapy but later died of infectious complications. It is suggested that SLE should be included as a cause of chylothorax and chylous ascites.

▶ I suspect this concurrence has been around for awhile, but these authors were the first to look for it. Since we all see SLE from time to time, remember the possibility; you may make the diagnosis and be labeled a diagnostic guru by your colleagues.

A. Gottschalk, MD

Scintigraphic Follow-up of the Effects of Therapy With Hydroxyurea on Splenic Function in Patients With Sickle Cell Disease
Santos A, Pinheiro V, Anjos AC, et al (Campinas State Univ, Brazil; Centro Infantil Domingos A Boldrini, Campinas, Brazil; Cidade Universitária Zeferino Vaz, Campinas, SP, Brazil)
Eur J Nucl Med 29:536-541, 2002   7–12

Introduction.—In patients with sickle cell disease (SCD), functional asplenia may develop as a chronic complication secondary to repeated episodes of polymerization of hemoglobin S. Increased plasma concentrations of fetal hemoglobin (HbF) decrease the polymerization of hemoglobin S. Hydroxyurea is a chemotherapeutic agent that can increase HbF levels in red blood cells. It may be useful in the treatment of SCD. The effect of long-term hydroxyurea therapy on the recovery of splenic function was examined in 21 patients with SCD.

Methods.—Patients ranged in age from 3 to 22 years; 14 patients had SS hemoglobinopathy and 7 had $S\beta^0$ hemoglobinopathy. Patients underwent liver/spleen scintigraphy before and after 6 and 12 months of therapy. All studies were submitted to visual inspection and semiquantitative analyses by using spleen/liver ratios.

Results.—Imaging before therapy revealed functional asplenia in 9 patients with SS and 1 patient with $S\beta^0$, and impaired splenic function in 5 patients with SS and 6 with $S\beta^0$. After therapy, splenic function improved in 10 patients, was unchanged in 8, and worsened in 3.

Conclusion.—Liver/spleen imaging revealed that splenic function can be improved with hydroxyurea therapy in some patients with SCD. Improvement was not always possible and frequently did not produce normal splenic function, even after 1 year of treatment.

▶ If you see SCD patients with any frequency, this approach could at least partially revitalize your colloid liver/spleen scan business. These authors used abdominal shielding in some of their cases. I never can understand this. You cannot shield the left lobe of the liver, which overlies the splenic bed and is often relatively large when the spleen gets small. Also, if you use a parallel hole collimator, what do you gain with a shield?

A. Gottschalk, MD

Multiple Hepatic Adenomas: Tc-99m RBC Liver SPECT Findings With Pathologic Correlation

Lim ST, Sohn M-H, Kwak J-Y, et al (Chonbuk Natl Univ, Chonju, Korea)
Clin Nucl Med 27:270-274, 2002   7–13

Introduction.—It is not unusual to detect a lesion in the liver incidentally on US or CT of the abdomen. When found, the origin of such a mass should be determined noninvasively. Tc-99m red blood cell (RBC) scintigraphic findings of multiple hepatic adenomas incidentally seen on US examination in a man with rheumatoid arthritis (RA) after 3 years of steroid therapy were described.

Case Report.—Man, 24, was hospitalized for evaluation of multiple hepatic masses found incidentally on US. The patient had been taking prednisolone for 3 years for treatment of RA. He had no other remarkable personal or family history. Physical examination and liver function studies were normal. Results of tests for α-fetoprotein, carcinoembyronic antigen, carbohydrate antigens 19-9 and 125, and hepatitis B surface antigen and antibody were negative. US showed multiple ovoid and hyperechoic masses in both hepatic lobes; diameters ranged from 1.5 to 3.5 cm (right lobe, 3 nodules; left lobe, 1 nodule). Liver SPECT showed 2 areas of increased blood pooling in the right lobe of the liver. The 2 other masses demonstrated no blood pooling and the same activity as normal liver (Fig 2). CT scan of the liver revealed marked, relatively homogeneous enhancement of the masses, except for small areas within the 2 large masses in both he-

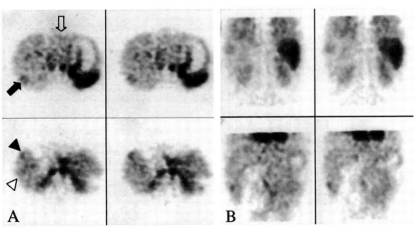

FIGURE 2.—Selected (**A**) transaxial and (**B**) coronal images of Tc-99m RBC liver SPECT through the hepatic masses show 2 areas of blood pooling in the right lobe of the liver (*black arrow* and *arrowhead*). The other 2 masses show no blood pooling and the same activity as normal liver (*open arrow* and *open arrowhead*). (Courtesy of Lim ST, Sohn M-H, Kwak J-Y, et al: Multiple hepatic adenomas: Tc-99m RBC liver SPECT findings with pathologic correlation. *Clin Nucl Med* 27(4):270-274, 2002.)

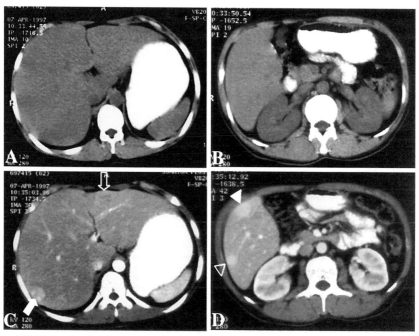

FIGURE 3.—**A** and **B,** A nonenhanced CT scan through the middle and lower portion of the liver shows no visible mass with isodensity in the liver. **C** and **D,** The contrast-enhanced CT scan through the same level as shown in **panels A** and **B** shows relatively homogenous contrast enhancement of the masses except for focal low-density areas within the 2 large tumors. Peripheral rims with low density, indicating capsules, are also evident around the 2 large tumors (*arrows*). (Courtesy of Lim ST, Sohn M-H, Kwak J-Y, et al: Multiple hepatic adenomas: Tc-99m RBC liver SPECT findings with pathologic correlation. *Clin Nucl Med* 27(4):270-274, 2002.)

patic lobes. They seemed to be surrounded by low-density rims (Fig 3). Gadolinium-enhanced MR images demonstrated homogeneous enhancement of the masses. Peripheral rims with low-signal intensities were identified around the 2 large tumors (Fig 4). Selective angiography revealed 3 hypervascular masses in the right lobe and a hypovascular mass in the left lobe of the liver. The patient underwent surgical excision of the 2 large tumors in both lobes of the liver. Histologic examination revealed hepatic adenomas with capsules. The surgically resected hepatic adenoma on the right lobe had many dilated sinusoids made up of thin-walled capillaries. The hepatic adenoma of the left lobe had fatty changes without dilated sinusoids. No malignant degeneration was observed.

Conclusion.—This case is an example of how false-positive findings can be mistaken for hemangioma.

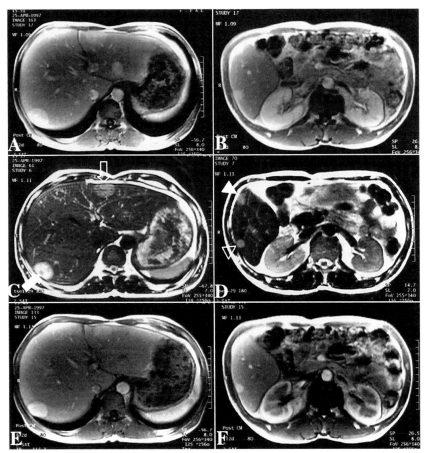

FIGURE 4.—An axial magnetic resonance image of the liver shows multiple well-defined masses of different sizes with high-signal intensities on (**A** and **B**) T1 weighted and (**C** and **D**) T2 weighted scan. E and F, A gadolinium-enhanced image shows homogenous enhancement of the masses with peripheral rims around the two large masses. (Courtesy of Lim ST, Sohn M-H, Kwak J-Y, et al: Multiple hepatic adenomas: Tc-99m RBC liver SPECT findings with pathologic correlation. *Clin Nucl Med* 27(4):270-274, 2002.)

▶ It is good to remember that nothing is perfect, and red-cell scanning of hepatic hemangioma comes as close as we usually get. Remember the use of steroids in this patient—if you can find that out before you read a red-cell study. You may be able to suggest adenoma as a possible diagnosis.

A. Gottschalk, MD

Intrathoracic Splenosis: Superiority of Technetium Tc 99m Heat-Damaged RBC Imaging

Hagman TF, Winer-Muram HT, Meyer CA, et al (Indiana Univ, Indianapolis; Richard L Roudebush VA Med Ctr, Indianapolis, Ind)

Chest 120:2097-2098, 2001   7–14

Background.—Intrathoracic splenosis is a rare diagnosis usually made after an invasive procedure. The radiographic and CT findings in intrathoracic splenosis are nonspecific, but when combined with a history of splenic injury they should suggest the possibility of this diagnosis. A patient is described with intrathoracic splenosis diagnosed on the basis of technetium Tc 99m heat-damaged red blood cell scan after false-negative results on ^{99m}Tc sulfur colloid scan.

Case Report.—An HIV-positive man, 52, underwent emergency splenectomy after being involved in a motor vehicle accident in 1983. In 1997, a routine peripheral blood smear showed the presence of a few Howell-Jolly bodies. Chest radiographs obtained in January 1999 showed healed left rib fractures and several nodular opacities in the lower left hemithorax. Chest CT showed multiple pleural-based nodules, up to 2 cm in diameter, at the posterolateral base of the left hemithorax and on the left hemidiaphragm (Fig 1). At this time, residual splenic tissue was also noted in the left upper quadrant of the abdomen. There was no change in the appearance of the nodules on a follow-up CT in October 1999. However, the patient's history prompted a concern for the possibility of intrathoracic splenosis, and a ^{99m}Tc sulfur colloid scan was performed. Although residual splenic tissue was seen in the thorax, there was no splenic

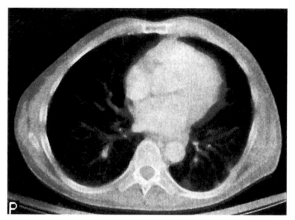

FIGURE 1.—Chest CT scan image demonstrates multiple ill-defined nodules at left posterolateral hemithorax. These resemble pulmonary nodules but are in pleura. (Courtesy of Hagman TF, Winer-Muram HT, Meyer CA, et al: Intrathoracic splenosis: Superiority of technetium Tc 99m heat-damaged RBC imaging. *Chest* 120:2097-2098, 2001.)

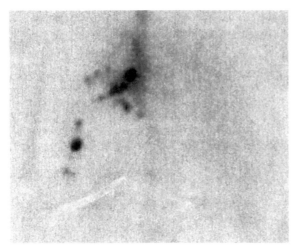

FIGURE 2.—^{99m}Tc heat-damaged red blood cell scan, posterior view, shows multiple areas of increased activity at left lower hemithorax, indicating intrathoracic splenic tissue. (Courtesy of Hagman TF, Winer-Muram HT, Meyer CA, Jennings SG, et al: Intrathoracic splenosis: Superiority of technetium Tc 99m heat-damaged RBC imaging. *Chest* 120:2097-2098, 2001.)

tissue present. These negative results and the presence of Howell-Jolly bodies in the peripheral blood smear made the diagnosis of intrathoracic splenosis appear unlikely. However, serial radiographs and CT scans in the following year showed no growth or alteration of the pleural-based nodules, and the possibility of intrathoracic splenosis was again entertained. A ^{99m}Tc heat-damaged red blood cell scan was performed and showed multiple areas of increased activity in the left lower hemithorax, which confirmed the diagnosis of intrathoracic splenosis (Fig 2).

Conclusions.—The diagnosis of intrathoracic splenosis is rare but should be considered in any patient with pleural-based nodules in the left hemithorax with a history of thoracoabdominal trauma and splenectomy or splenic injury. Noninvasive confirmation of the diagnosis with ^{99m}Tc heat-damaged red blood cell scintigraphy can spare patients additional invasive procedures or additional follow-up imaging.

▶ An easy diagnosis to make if you think of the possibility and remember heat-damaged red blood cells as the tracer. The technique is simple—my colleagues and I described it years ago.[1]

A. Gottschalk, MD

Reference

1. Armas R, Thakur ML, Gottschalk A: A simple method of spleen imaging with Tc-99m-labeled erythrocytes. *Radiology* 132:215-216, 1979.

8 Vascular

Introduction

It is very likely that with improving techniques for preventing disease, we will be encountering an increased number of vascular problems in the aging population. Although significant progress has been made in noninvasive evaluation of blood flow using magnetic resonance, there still clearly is a role for nuclear medicine. The lead article in this chapter takes advantage of the fact that thallium can be used to assess lower limb vascularity in diabetic patients. This is a logical and potentially very valuable method of assessing clinical or subclinical peripheral vascular disease in a group of patients who are at very high risk. The association between coronary artery disease and generalized peripheral vascular disease is well known. It makes clear sense that we should be using more tests to gain as much information as we can from a single injection of radionuclide. Other articles included in this section are a description of the role of labeled leukocytes in aortic prosthetic reconstruction. Here, too, is another potential valuable use also related to an aging population, an increasing prevalence of vascular disease, and the complications of its treatment. I believe that over the next several years we will see increasing applications of the technology in this particular area.

Isotope lymphography also continues to be a useful vascular application of radionuclides. We see articles coming out on a sporadic basis. Fortunately, this is a situation in which, although nuclear medicine has a valuable role, the number of cases is relatively limited.

Another important vascular application is in cases such as frostbite or electrocution where tissue injury can be massive; it is important to gain an early recognition of potentially viable tissue versus nonviable tissue.

Nuclear medicine has been and remains an important application in vascular disease and tissue injury in which blood flow may be disturbed or interrupted. In order for us to see greater application of these techniques, it is important that the vascular surgeons and other professionals who deal with these types of problems be made aware of this potential. A great deal of attention is devoted to magnetic resonance and invasive radiographic techniques. However, the noninvasive safe nuclear medicine techniques remain out there for our application and have had a role in these areas since the introduction of nuclear medicine. They will undoubtedly continue to have a

183

significant role in the future. Hopefully, we can develop more specific labels to follow these problems of this type.

M. Donald Blaufox, MD, PhD

Lower-Limb Vascularization in Diabetic Patients: Assessment by Thallium-201 Scanning Coupled With Exercise Myocardial Scintigraphy
Cosson E, Ramadan A, Paycha F, et al (Paris-Nord Univ; Louis Mourier Hosp, Colombes, France; Sainte Catherine les Arras, France)
Diabetes Care 24:870-874, 2001   8–1

Background.—Nearly 4 decades of follow-up for the Framingham Heart Study have demonstrated that the risk of development of intermittent claudication was increased by associated coronary heart disease and diabetes. The prevalence of coronary artery disease and peripheral vascular disease (PVD) is high in the population with diabetes. More than half of patients with diabetes die from cardiovascular disease, and the morbidity resulting from PVD is very high. Claudication is a strong predictor of subsequent cardiovascular events. Myocardial scintigraphy is suggestive of silent myocardial ischemia (SMI) in 20% to 30% of diabetic patients with other risk factors. It is common for these patients to exhibit angiographically normal coronary arteries and endothelial dysfunction while myocardial microvascular changes are occurring. Thallium 201 (^{201}Tl) scanning was used to evaluate the circulation in the muscles of the lower limb in patients with diabetes who do not have clinical peripheral vascular disease but do have a high cardiovascular risk profile.

Methods.—The study group included 80 patients with diabetes; almost all of them had type 2 diabetes, with more than 1 additional cardiovascular risk factor but no claudication. Stress testing was performed, followed by administration of 1.5 MBq/kg ^{201}Tl and myocardial single-photon emission CT followed by scanning of the lower limb. Blood flow was considered abnormal if the asymmetry in uptake of ^{201}Tl between the 2 buttocks or thighs or calves was greater than 10% (Fig 1).

Results.—Muscle perfusion defects were observed in 42% of patients, primarily in the calves, and these defects were correlated with the presence of retinopathy and with the HbA_{1c} level. Patients with defects in the buttock and/or thigh had a higher prevalence of nephropathy and retinopathy than patients who had isolated defects in the calf.

Conclusions.—These findings suggest that scanning of the lower limb, coupled with myocardial scintigraphy, is a practical method for the investigation of peripheral muscle circulation. In diabetic patients without clinical arterial disease, proximal perfusion defects are associated with increased prevalence of retinopathy and nephropathy, and thus, may be the result of microvascular disease in the muscles of the lower limb. Distal defects may be indicative of silent macrovascular disease of the lower limb.

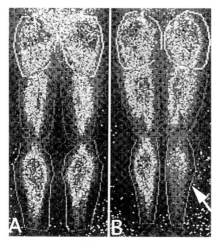

FIGURE 1.—Examples of lower limb (LL) ^{201}Tl scintigraphy. **A:** Patient with a normal result of LL ^{201}Tl scanning (posterior view). The right-to-left ratios for buttocks, thighs, and calves were 0.99, 0.98, and 0.97, respectively. **B:** Patient with an abnormal result of LL [201]T1 scanning. The right-to-left ratios for buttocks, thighs, and calves were 0.96, 0.92, and 0.63, respectively. The test showed a defect of perfusion in the right calf *(arrow)*. (Courtesy of Cosson E, Ramadan A, Paycha F, et al: Lower-limb vascularization in diabetic patients: Assessment by thallium-201 scanning coupled with exercise myocardial scintigraphy. *Diabetes Care* 24:870-874. Copyright 2001 American Diabetes Association. Reprinted with permission from The American Diabetes Association.)

▶ A few studies have sporadically appeared which have combined thallium imaging of the heart with an evaluation of other parts of the body. This particular study may have been successful because it selected a high-risk group for this combined procedure. Diabetics are at significant risk of having peripheral vascular disease and those with suspected coronary artery disease would certainly be at great risk. It is noteworthy that the presence of abnormalities of muscle perfusion correlated with the hemoglobin A_{1c} level. This appears to be further evidence that tight control of blood glucose concentrations reduces cardiovascular risk in diabetics. This is an attractive, noninvasive method to study it, and we should see more studies of this type in the future.

M. D. Blaufox, MD, PhD

The Role of Preoperative Tc-99m HMPAO-Labeled Leukocyte Total-Body Scans in Aortic Prosthetic Reconstruction
Liberatore M, Fiore V, Iurilli AP, et al (Univ of Rome "La Sapienza")
Clin Nucl Med 26:1024-1027, 2001   8–2

Background.—Infection of an aortofemoral vascular graft is a serious and life-threatening complication of reconstructive vascular surgery. Although the incidence of vascular graft infection ranges from less than 1% to 6%, mortality and morbidity rates are high, ranging from 20% to 75% and 24% to 31%, respectively. Vascular graft infection can result from direct intraoperative contamination, bacteremia, the proximity of bacterial infection in the bowel, or from remote septic foci. The utility of Tc-99m exametazime

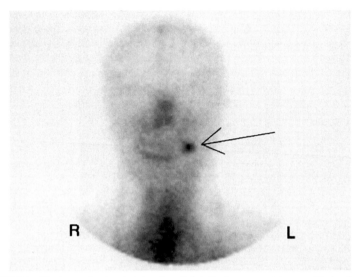

FIGURE 4.—Two hours after the administration of labeled leukocytes, static images of the head and neck were acquired in the anterior view. Focal uptake of the labeled cells in the left superior dental arch is seen clearly (*arrow*). The final diagnosis was dental abscess. (Courtesy of Liberatore M, Fiore V, Iurilli AP, et al: The role of preoperative Tc-99m HMPAO-labeled leukocyte total-body scans in aortic prosthetic reconstruction. *Clin Nucl Med* 26(12):1024-1027, 2001.)

(HMPAO)-labeled total-body leukocyte scanning (TBLS) for the detection of remote septic foci before operation for patients undergoing aortofemoral vascular surgery was investigated.

Methods.—A consecutive series of 58 patients (51 men and 7 women), aged from 50 to 79 years, were screened before surgery for inflammatory or infectious disease. A clinical score was assigned to each patient. TBLS was then performed for each patient, and the relation between the clinical score and the TBLS result was determined. Patients with positive results on TBLS were examined, and the causes of the findings were treated before these patients underwent surgery.

Results.—A positive finding on TBLS was obtained in 10 (17%) of 58 patients. Of the 31 patients with a clinical score of 0, 3 patients had positive findings of TBLS. No positive TBLS findings were noted among the 13 patients with a clinical score of 1. For patients with clinical scores of 2, 3, or 4, TBLS findings were positive in 7 (50%) of 14 patients (Fig 4). No signs of prosthetic vascular graft infection were observed in any of the patients during postoperative follow-up.

Conclusions.—TBLS is useful for identifying relevant infective foci that could result in vascular graft infection for patients about to undergo aortofemoral surgery provided they have high clinical scores for inflammatory or infectious disease.

► Infection of vascular grafts is a very significant and life-threatening problem. Once infection occurs, treatment can be very difficult. I once had as a patient an individual who had been placed on ampicillin because of an infected aortic graft. He was seen again at a time when I was a resident and after his being on antibiotics several years. Since he had been asymptomatic and afebrile during this time, the attending physician stopped the antibiotic. The patient subsequently died of septicemia. This certainly made this problem vivid in my mind. This study presents an interesting approach to evaluating this potential problem and perhaps charting a therapeutic course to prevent it.

M. D. Blaufox, MD, PhD

Value of Isotope Lymphography in the Diagnosis of Lymphoedema of the Leg
Burnand KG, McGuinness CL, Lagattolla NRF, et al (St Thomas' Hosp, London; Sal Manyia Med Centre, Manama, Bahrain)
Br J Surg 89:74-78, 2002   8–3

Introduction.—Isotope lymphography has been reported to have good sensitivity and specificity in diagnosing lymphedema of the leg and has nearly replaced lymphography in the diagnosis of lymphedema. Its accuracy has only been evaluated in small trials. It is not known whether isotope lymphography can identify patients with a proximal lymphatic obstruction who may be appropriate candidates for lymphatic bypass surgery. The accuracy of isotope lymphography in diagnosing lymphedema and the presence and level of proximal lymphatic obstruction in the leg were determined.

Methods.—The study included 395 patients with suspected lymphedema who underwent isotope lymphography between 1985 and 1995. Contrast lymphography was also performed in 29 patients in this cohort when the isotope results were thought to be misleading or were due to lymphatic bypass surgery.

Results.—For the 29 patients who underwent both investigations, isotope lymphography identified 20 (83.3%) of 24 abnormal lymphatic systems. Four legs with obstructed groin lymphatics were reported as normal by isotope lymphography. Two legs with normal contrast lymphograms were incorrectly diagnosed as having lymphedema. Detectable groin nodes on the scintigrams were suggestive of either normal lymphatics or proximal lymphatic obstruction. An increase in isotope uptake during 30 to 60 minutes of less than 50%, or a total absence of isotope within groin nodes, was a sensitive indicator that lymphatic bypass surgery was not appropriate.

Conclusion.—Isotope lymphography is moderately sensitive in the assessment of lymphedema; that is, it will mistakenly classify some normal legs as lymphedematous. This method, however, usually identifies correctly those patients who are suitable for undergoing lymphatic bypass surgery.

▶ This is a remarkably large series of patients, and most importantly, the first author is from a department of surgery, which would put him in a position to critically evaluate the results and their impact on his practice. It is interesting that they conclude that in some cases, contrast lymphography may still be needed. Isotope lymphography is certainly a simpler less-traumatic procedure for the patient, but apparently, it does not obviate the occasional need for contrast lymphography. Most importantly, they suggest further studies when the results do not agree with the clinical picture. One of the long-standing requirements of the American Board of Nuclear Medicine is a close correlation between the patients' clinical presentation and the nuclear medicine studies performed. All patients are expected to be interviewed and examined. This study certainly supports that approach to the use of nuclear medicine and confirms its value.

M. D. Blaufox, MD, PhD

Imaging of Frostbite Injury by Technetium-99m-Sestamibi Scintigraphy: A Case Report
Aygit AC, Sarikaya A (Trakya Univ, Edirne, Turkey)
Foot Ankle Int 23:56-59, 2002   8–4

Introduction.—For patients with severe frostbite injury requiring an amputation, the early diagnosis and treatment of frozen tissue decreases length of hospital stay and allows for maximum amputation stump length preservation. A patient with frostbite injury for whom technetium-99m (^{99m}Tc)-sestamibi was used to assess skeletal muscle perfusion and to direct early surgical intervention is discussed.

Case Report.—Man, 34, was taken to the emergency department on the fourth day postinjury with frostbite involving both lower extremities. He had diffuse edema, numbness, and dense cyanosis distal to the proximal part of the first metatarsophalangeal joint on the dorsal and medial aspects of the first ray. He underwent ^{99m}Tc sestamibi scintigraphy and MRI. At 30 minutes after 15 mCi IV of ^{99m}Tc sestamibi, 5-minute static images of his plantar feet and posterior calf were obtained, using a large-field-of-view gamma camera (Philips digital). Scintigraphic images revealed diffusely decreased uptake in the soft tissue of both calves and feet, possibly resulting from viable, yet ischemic tissue. He underwent T1- and T2-weighted spin-echo, gradient-echo, and short-time inversion recovery MRI in the sagittal and axial planes of both legs below the knees and the feet. The MRI showed only increased signal intensity of muscular structures that probably corresponded with ischemia. Both Rheomacrodex and aspirin were used as platelet aggregation inhibitors. Five days after therapy, ^{99m}Tc sestamibi scan revealed prominently increased uptake in both calves and feet and partial skin necrosis was observed. The patient underwent debridement of the necrotic skin and subcutaneous tissue. No bone was exposed and split-thickness skin grafting was used for coverage of the skin defect. Healing was good at 15 days postgrafting.

Conclusion.—For patients with frostbite injury, evaluation and treatment of soft-tissue perfusion can be performed using ^{99m}Tc sestamibi.

▶ A significant problem in dealing with patients with frostbite is to determine the definition of irreparable damage to minimize loss of tissue. Determination of viability is an essential component of proper treatment. This is an example of nuclear medicine doing what it does best. The uptake of sestamibi by skeletal muscle is an indication of function and viability. It is indirectly a measurement of perfusion since it requires blood flow to reach the involved sites. This study suggests that this may be a simpler method and a reliable one for studying patients with this problem.

M. D. Blaufox, MD, PhD

9 Central Nervous System

Introduction

I had great enthusiasm for this chapter this year, and placed half of my choices for this volume of the YEAR BOOK here. I begin with selections on epilepsy. These are followed by many articles on the dementing diseases, which begin with β-CIT imaging to characterize Parkinson's and move onto some FDG work on Parkinson's. Next, I selected articles on Alzheimer's, starting with PET and ending with SPECT. Then you will find articles on ischemic disease, with several discussing SPECT to evaluate thrombolytic therapy. A heterogeneous group on some unusual diseases follows, and the chapter ends with articles discussing brain databases.

Alexander Gottschalk, MD

Interictal 99ᵐTc-HMPAO SPECT in Temporal Lobe Epilepsy: Relation to Clinical Variables

Avery RA, Zubal IG, Studholme C, et al (Yale Univ, New Haven, Conn)
Epilepsia 42:869-874, 2001
9–1

Background.—No systematic study has been done on the factors affecting blood flow observed by interictal SPECT images in patients with temporal lobe epilepsy. In this study, interictal SPECT results were evaluated with respect to a number of clinical variables in a large population of patients with temporal lobe epilepsy. All patients had undergone temporal lobectomy.

Methods.—Interictal 99ᵐTc-hexamethylpropyleneamineoxime (HMPAO) SPECT scans were obtained from 61 patients with temporal lobe epilepsy before an anterior temporal lobectomy. SPECT was analyzed with use of a region-of-interest analysis in the cerebellum, anterior temporal lobe, lateral temporal lobe, mesial temporal lobe, whole temporal lobe, and inferior frontal lobe. Asymmetry indices (AIs) were also calculated, and a correlative analysis of AIs and clinical variables was performed.

Results.—A significant difference was found in the AIs calculated for patients with temporal lobe epilepsy compared with those of control patients in the anterior, lateral, and whole temporal regions. No consistent overall correlation was found between the AIs and the clinical variables. In patients with right temporal lobe epilepsy only, AIs in the lateral and whole temporal lobe were positively correlated with age of onset. Also in patients with right temporal lobe epilepsy only, the duration of epilepsy was negatively correlated with the anterior and mesial temporal lobe AI. No correlations were identified between clinical variables and AIs in patients with left temporal lobe epilepsy.

Conclusions.—The significant correlation of age at onset and duration of epilepsy with asymmetry indices in patients with right temporal lobe epilepsy but not in patients with left temporal lobe epilepsy suggests that physiologic processes may be determined to some degree by the laterality of temporal lobe epilepsy.

▶ I join the authors in having no clue why the left side does not show decreased blood flow while the right side does. I recently selected an article from the Pennsylvania group[1] showing that patients without epilepsy have decreased left temporal blood flow, and I wonder if this could in anyway affect these data.

A. Gottschalk, MD

Reference

1. Ivancevic V, Alavi A, Souder E, et al: Regional cerebral glucose metabolism in healthy volunteers determined by FDG-PET: Appearance and variance in the transaxial, coronal, and sagittal planes. *Clin Nucl Med* 25:596-602, 2000. (2001 YEAR BOOK OF NUCLEAR MEDICINE, pp 216-217.)

The Usefulness of Subtraction Ictal SPECT Coregistered to MRI in Single- and Dual-Headed SPECT Cameras in Partial Epilepsy
Kaiboriboon K, Lowe VJ, Chantarujikapong SI, et al (Saint Louis Univ)
Epilepsia 43:408-414, 2002   9–2

Background.—There are several useful electrophysiologic and imaging tests for localization of the area of seizure onset (epileptogenic zone) in patients with refractory partial epilepsy. The traditional standard for localization in the epileptogenic zone has been scalp and invasive EEG. However, new neuroimaging tests have shown clinical utility in seizure localization. Ictal SPECT is a useful test for localizing regional blood flow changes in the epileptogenic zone in patients with partial epilepsy. However, interictal SPECT is of limited value in sensitivity and specificity for localization in the epileptogenic zone. Comparison of ictal and interictal studies is often helpful in determining the region of ictal blood-flow changes; however, the visual comparison between ictal and interictal SPECT studies is particularly difficult. Subtraction ictal SPECT coregistered to MRI (SISCOM) has been shown to produce an accurate SPECT-to-SPECT coregistration and normalization, allowing valid ictal subtraction images. The clinical utility of SISCOM was evaluated and SISCOM images derived from single- and dual-headed SPECT cameras for localization of partial epileptic seizures were compared.

Methods.—This retrospective study evaluated 38 partial epilepsy patients using SISCOM. A single-headed camera was used to obtain SPECT images in the first 15 patients, and a dual-headed camera was used for SPECT images in the next 23 patients. Side-by-side ictal-interictal SPECT evaluation and SISCOM images were blindly reviewed and classified as either localizing to 1 of 16 sites or nonlocalizing. Results were compared with seizure localization by any of 3 traditional techniques, including surgical outcome and invasive and noninvasive video-EEG monitoring.

Results.—Areas of hyperperfusion were localized with SISCOM images more often than with side-by-side SPECT evaluation (71% vs 47.4%). A comparison of SISCOM with traditional SPECT evaluation techniques showed greater concordance for SISCOM than with side-by-side SPECT evaluation (60.53% vs. 36.84%). There were no differences in localization between images derived from single- and dual-headed cameras, and no difference in concordance of seizure localization, compared with traditional techniques, between the 2 groups.

Conclusions.—SISCOM is a useful technique for preoperative evaluation in patients with partial epilepsy and improves the sensitivity and specificity of seizure localization of SPECT images derived from both single- and dual-headed SPECT cameras.

▶ This study gets my little girl comment. You remember: "When she was good, she was very, very good, but when she was bad . . . etc." The very, very good part was the increased diagnostic value of the fusion versus the side-by-side technique. I also liked the point that single-headed cameras work well if you make the count differences large enough (>2 SD). On the horrid side, I am back to one of my favorite complaints. The housekeeping details are poorly stated. The technique these authors used is not even briefly detailed, but only referred to in a 4-year-old article in another journal. I believe that with no more than a short paragraph nicely summarizing the subtraction technique the reader could be on board. I was also disturbed to find that the first time the abbreviation SISCOM was used in the abstract, it was not defined. This type of reader abuse is not necessary, and only detracts from the utility some may place on these data.

A. Gottschalk, MD

Neuroimaging Findings of Cortical Dyslamination With Cytomegaly
Lee SK, Choe G, Hong K-S, et al (Seoul Natl Univ, Korea)
Epilepsia 42:850-856, 2001
9–3

Background.—Focal cortical dysplasia (FCD) is probably the most common type of focal developmental disorder in patients who are referred for intractable epilepsy. The most prominent histologic features of FCD are disruption of cortical lamination and the proliferation of large and abnormal cells. The spectrum of pathologic changes in FCD ranges from mild cortical disruption without giant neurons to the most severe forms, in which cortical dyslamination and large, bizarre cells are present. In this study, the characteristic MRI findings of cortical dyslamination with cytomegaly, including dysplastic and destructive lesions, were identified, and the relationship between MRI findings and pathologic characteristics and the diagnostic role of functional neuroimaging studies in patients with these pathologic disorders was also determined.

Methods.—The study group was composed of 232 adult patients with proven cortical dyslamination with cytomegaly. Abnormalities identified on MRI were subdivided on the basis of patterns of involvement and compared with the patients' pathologic characteristics. Visual qualitative analysis, FDG-PET, and ictal SPECT observations were classified as localizing, lateralizing, nonlateralizing, false-localizing, and false-lateralizing. The standard for correct localization of neuroimages was defined as the resected lobe.

Results.—Focal abnormalities were identified by MRI in 14 of 23 patients. Six patients demonstrated typical MRI findings of FCD, that is, focal areas of cortical thickening with or without poor grey–white matter differentiation. Two patients had focal subcortical high signal intensities on T2-weighted images. Balloon cells were seen in 3 of 8 patients with normal MRI findings and in 4 of 8 patients with the nondestructive cortical dysplasia pattern. However, balloon cells were not found in 6 patients with the destructive MRI pattern. FDG-PET localized the pathologic lobe in 13 of 20 patients (65%), whereas ictal SPECT localized the pathologic lobe in 11 of 18 patients (61.1%). The pathologic lobe was also correctly localized by FDG-PET in 4 patients and by ictal SPECT in 2 patients with normal MRI findings.

Conclusions.—This study of the pathologic characteristics of cortical dyslamination with cytomegaly identified 2 distinct patterns of abnormal MRI findings. These distinct patterns may reflect different pathogeneses, such as the time of insult. FDG-PET and ictal SPECT have confirmatory and independent diagnostic roles in the localization of epileptogenic foci.

▶ My bias—clearly stated in past years—that ictal SPECT beats interictal SPECT or PET for localization of epileptogenic foci was tested in this series. I win but not by a whole lot. This series also clearly supports combining anatomical and functional imaging to achieve the best surgical success rate. Although the numbers are small—91% with both versus 33% with only MRI—they are impressive. As is often the case, however, I was not completely sold on the MRI technique. Fast spin-echo fluid attenuated inversion recovery slices were not obtained in this series, and that could put MRI at a serious disadvantage.

A. Gottschalk, MD

Perfusion SPECT Changes After Acute and Chronic Vagus Nerve Stimulation in Relation to Prestimulus Condition and Long-term Clinical Efficacy

Van Laere K, Vonck K, Boon P, et al (Ghent Univ, Belgium)
J Nucl Med 43:733-744, 2002   9–4

Background.—Chronic intermittent left-sided vagus nerve stimulation (VNS) is a cost-effective and safe treatment for patients with refractory epilepsy, but its mechanism of action is not well understood. The acute and chronic effects of VNS were examined by perfusion SPECT in patients with refractory epilepsy.

Study Design.—The study group consisted of 23 adult patients with refractory complex partial seizures with or without secondary generalization. All patients had SPECT studies before and immediately after their initial stimulation. The baseline, prestimulus SPECT scans of these patients were compared to those of age- and sex-matched healthy volunteers. Ten of the patients were restudied by SPECT imaging in the chronic stimulation condition.

Findings.—In the initial acute stimulation phase, the left thalamus, right parahippocampal gyrus, and right hippocampus were significantly deactivated by VNS. Acute stimulation in the chronic phase caused significant left thalamic increase. When chronic perfusion was compared with pre-VNS baseline, both thalami had perfusion decreases. Initial stimulation changes in the right amygdala and right hippocampus were predictive of response to VNS.

Conclusions.—Chronic intermittent left-sided VNS decreased seizure frequency in patients with refractory epilepsy. At the onset of VNS, left thalamic perfusion and contralateral parahippocampal and posterior neocortical perfusion were decreased. After chronic VNS, there was an increase in left thalamic perfusion. Increased perfusion in the contralateral hippocampus and amygdala were associated with therapeutic effectiveness.

► VNS worked (ie, decreased seizures by 50% or more) in 13 (57%) of this series of 23 patients. Trying to analyze what is going on when the acute SPECT perfusion after vagus stimulation and the chronic SPECT perfusion after vagus stimulation involve different anatomic locations makes for some wide error bars around the data. Nevertheless, these authors have at least formulated a hypothesis that acute amygdala and chronic hippocampal perfusion decrease will predict responders. But the responders are an even smaller subgroup, and the numbers cited above indicate that the series needs to be expanded before this conclusion can be etched in stone.

A. Gottschalk, MD

Superiority of HMPAO Ictal SPECT to ECD Ictal SPECT in Localizing the Epileptogenic Zone

Lee DS, Lee SK, Kim YK, et al (Seoul Natl Univ, Korea)

9–5

Epilepsia 43:263-269, 2002

Objective.—Previous studies have reported both Tc-99m hexamethyl-propylene amine oxime (HMPAO) and Tc-99m electron capture detection (ECD) ictal SPECT to be effective in localizing epileptogenic zones in the brains of patients with epilepsy. However, no studies have compared the performance of the 2 techniques. The 2 SPECT methods were compared for their ability to localize the epileptogenic zone in patients with 2 forms of epilepsy.

Methods.—The study included 24 patients with mesial temporal lobe epilepsy (TLE) and 30 with neocortical epilepsy (NE). Ictal SPECT was performed using stabilized Tc-99m HMPAO in 17 patients with TLE and 23 with NE, and ictal Tc-99m ECD SPECT was performed in 7 patients in each group. In each case, the epileptogenic zone was localized by visual interpretation in single-blind fashion. Asymmetric indexes were calculated, and subtraction ictal SPECT was coregistered with MRI. In all patients, the location of the epileptogenic zone was confirmed by invasive electroencephalographic or surgical results.

Results.—Diagnostic sensitivity in patients with TLE was 82% for Tc-99m HMPAO SPECT and 71% for Tc-99m ECD SPECT. Asymmetric index values were 25 and 13, respectively. In patients with NE, sensitivity was 70% with Tc-99m HMPAO SPECT versus just 29% with Tc-99m ECD SPECT. Again, the asymmetric index was larger with Tc-99m HMPAO: 15 versus 4.8. The results of coregistration to MRI scans were consistent with the SPECT visual assessments.

Conclusions.—For patients with TLE, ictal Tc-99m HMPAO and Tc-99m ECD SPECT offer comparable sensitivity in localizing the epileptogenic zone. However, Tc-99m HMPAO is associated with greater ictal hyperperfusion. In NE, Tc-99m HMPAO SPECT is more sensitive than Tc-99m ECD SPECT and offers greater ictal hyperperfusion. Head-to-head comparisons of the 2 SPECT techniques in the same patients are needed to confirm these results.

▶ These data seem counterintuitive to me, even though the authors stress that HMPAO is a perfusion tracer whereas ECD depends on both perfusion and metabolism. The NE group with ECD is so small (7 patients) that I could not make the differences statistically significant. I accept this as a hypothesis and recognize the trend. But, I hope for a larger (or expanded) series in the future. And you are right to wonder why ECD is called electron capture detection in this paper when the rest of us call it ethylcysteinate dimer. Are these authors confused, or are we confused? You choose.

A. Gottschalk, MD

Low Incidence of Abnormal [18]FDG-PET in Children With New-Onset Partial Epilepsy: A Prospective Study

Gaillard WD, Kopylev L, Weinstein S, et al (George Washington Univ, Washington, DC; NIH, Bethesda, Md)
Neurology 58:717-722, 2002

9–6

Introduction.—Patients with refractory partial epilepsy often demonstrate regional hypometabolism. It is not known whether these metabolic abnormalities are present at the start of seizures or develop over time. A cohort of 40 children with recent-onset complex partial seizures at risk for continued seizures were examined with [18]FDG PET to determine the prevalence of metabolic abnormalities.

Methods.—The mean age at seizure onset was 6.0 years (range, 0.9-11.9) and at evaluation was 7.0 years (range, 2.3-12.9 years). The mean duration of epilepsy was 1.1 years (range, 0.3-2.3 years), and the mean number of seizures per year was 30 (range, 3-200). Children with abnormal structural findings on MRI were excluded, except 4 with mesial temporal sclerosis and 2 with subtle hippocampal dysgenesis. A region-of-interest template was used to assess [18]FDG PET. An absolute asymmetry index greater than .15 was defined as abnormal.

Results.—Thirty-three patients had a presumptive temporal seizure focus based on seizure semiology, interictal electroencephalogram, video-electroencephalogram, and MRI; 5 had a frontotemporal focus, and 2 had a probable frontal lobe focus. The mean asymmetry index for all regions did not vary from that of 10 normal young adults, even when the children who were less likely to have a temporal focus were excluded. Eight children (20%) had focal hypometabolism restricted to the temporal lobe, particularly the inferior mesial and inferior lateral regions. Abnormal findings were ipsilateral to the presumed temporal lobe ictal focus.

Conclusion.—Abnormalities of glucose utilization may be less frequent and profound in children with new-onset partial seizures compared with adults with chronic partial epilepsy. If hypermetabolism develops in these participants in the future, metabolic dysfunction may be associated with persistent epilepsy rather than being present at seizure onset.

▶ I have noted before that interictal FDG-PET scanning or interictal anything scanning is not as good a diagnostic test as ictal SPECT. These authors indicate interictal PET does not work well in the pediatric patient. Their hypothesis that more patients will develop future hypometabolism related to persistent epilepsy is intriguing. They hope follow-up studies will clarify this hypothesis. I hope good therapy will make this a difficult series to obtain.

A. Gottschalk, MD

[¹²³I]β-CIT SPECT Imaging Assessment of the Rate of Parkinson's Disease Progression

Marek K, Innis R, van Dyck C, et al (Yale Univ, New Haven, Conn; Univ of Rochester, NY)
Neurology 57:2089-2094, 2001   9–7

Background.—The clinical progression of Parkinson's disease is highly variable and unpredictable. The relentless clinical decline experienced by patients is a reflection of ongoing nigrostriatal degeneration, but it is unclear whether symptoms of Parkinson's disease arise from age-related neuronal loss in association with a transient neurodegenerative insult or from an ongoing neurodegenerative process. [¹²³I]β-CIT (2β-carboxymethoxy-3β[4-iodophenyl tropane]) and SPECT imaging of the dopamine transporter has been shown to be a sensitive biomarker of the onset and severity of Parkinson's disease. The rate of progression of the dopaminergic terminal loss in patients with Parkinson's disease was assessed by examination of the change in [¹²³I]β-CIT uptake in sequential scans.

Methods.—Thirty-two patients with Parkinson's disease and 24 healthy control subjects were recruited from the Yale Movement Disorders Center to

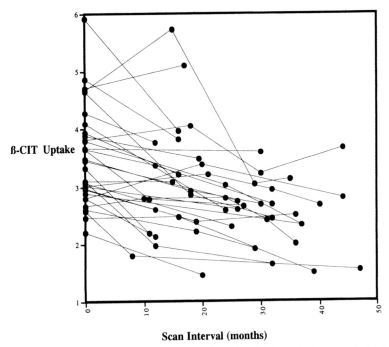

Scan Interval (months)

FIGURE 2.—Striatal β-CIT uptake (specific/nondisplaceable activity) seen in the scans of all patients with Parkinson's disease demonstrates marked intersubject variability in the rate of change of dopamine transporter density. (Courtesy of Marek K, Innis R, van Dyck C, et al: [¹²³I]β-CIT SPECT imaging assessment of the rate of Parkinson's disease progression. *Neurology* 57:2089-2094, 2001. Copyright American Academy of Neurology. Used with permission of Lippincott-Raven Publishers.)

undergo repeated [^{123}I]β-CIT SPECT imaging during a 1- to 4-year period. The primary imaging outcome was the ratio of specific to nondisplaceable striatal activity. The severity of the disease was assessed by Hoehn and Yahr staging and by the Unified Parkinson Disease Rating Scale 12 hours after discontinuing drug use.

Results.—The sequential SPECT scans obtained from patients with Parkinson's disease showed a decline in the striatal uptake of [^{123}I]β-CIT of about 11.2% per year from the baseline scan compared with 0.8% per year in the healthy control subjects. [^{123}I]β-CIT striatal uptake in the patients with Parkinson's disease was correlated with the severity of clinical symptoms of the disease, but the annual percentage loss of [^{123}I]β-CIT striatal uptake was not correlated with the annual loss in measures of clinical functioning (Fig 2).

Conclusions.—The rate of dopaminergic loss in Parkinson's disease is significantly greater than the rate seen in healthy control subjects. [^{123}I]β-CIT SPECT imaging provides a quantitative biomarker for the progressive nigrostriatal dopaminergic degeneration in Parkinson's disease. Dopamine transporter imaging offers the potential for an objective end point in therapeutic trials of novel protective and restorative therapies for patients with Parkinson's disease.

▶ The idea that the decline in [^{123}I]β-CIT in patients with Parkinson's disease can be rigorously quantified is both exciting and laudable. Clearly, if it can be done, any intervention could then be measured precisely. My problem—looking at Fig 2—is that some patients show an initial rise in uptake followed by a precipitous fall, some drop their uptakes slightly and then stabilize, and at least 1 shows no change. It seems there may be mud in these analytical waters.

A. Gottschalk, MD

Beta-CIT-SPECT Combined With UPDRS Appears to Distinguish Different Parkinsonian Conditions
Sjøholm H, Sundsfjord J, Mellgren SI (Univ Hosp, Tromsø, Norway)
Acta Neurol Scand 105:5-7, 2002   9–8

Background.—It would seem relatively simple to make a clinical diagnosis of idiopathic Parkinson's disease using established criteria, but 2 postmortem studies have shown that, even among specialists, about 25% of patients diagnosed with idiopathic Parkinson's disease had other parkinsonian conditions. These findings point out the need for improved diagnostic accuracy both for primary diagnosis and also as a basis for monitoring therapeutic effects. In recent years, neuroimaging methods such as PET measuring either metabolism of f-dopa or the presynaptic dopamine transporter and beta-CIT-SPECT measuring the presynaptic dopamine transporter have shown different degenerative patterns in the basal ganglia when idiopathic Parkinson's disease is compared with other parkinsonian conditions. An earlier study found a linear relationship between nigro-striatal degeneration as measured with beta-CIT-SPECT and motor scores in the Unified Parkinson's

Disease Rating Scale (UPDRS) in patients with idiopathic Parkinson's disease. Whether patients with poor or no response to l-dopa treatment, who were likely not to have idiopathic Parkinson's disease, deviated from that linear relationship was determined.

Methods.—PET imaging was performed 20 hours after injection of beta-CIT in 6 l-dopa poor/non-responding patients. These patients were compared with the l-dopa responding patients with idiopathic Parkinson's disease from the earlier study mentioned above.

Results.—The patients in the present study showed less nigro-striatal degeneration in relation to UPDRS motor scores than the patients with idiopathic Parkinson's disease.

Conclusions.—The findings of this study suggest that the combination of beta-CIT-SPECT and UPDRS motor scores may differentiate idiopathic Parkinson's disease from other parkinsonian conditions.

▶ In the past, I have selected articles indicating that Parkinson's can be separated from parkinsonism by the relative decrease in the putamen compared to the caudate in the former, but not in the latter, when using presynaptic dopamine transporter tracers.[1] These authors present another technique for doing this if you want a double check or if (for some reason) you cannot quantify caudate and putamen uptake.

A. Gottschalk, MD

Reference

1. Snow BJ, Vingerhoets FJG, Langston JW, et al: Pattern of dopaminergic loss in the striatum of humans with MPTP induced parkinsonism. *J Neurol Neurosurg Psychiatry* 68:313-316, 2000. 2001 YEAR BOOK OF NUCLEAR MEDICINE, pp 212-213.

Striatal Dopamine Transporter Function in Dementia With Lewy Bodies and Parkinson's Disease

Ransmayr G, Seppi K, Donnemiller E, et al (Univ Hosp, Innsbruck, Austria)
Eur J Nucl Med 28:1523-1528, 2001   9–9

Background.—Patients with Parkinson's disease are at a significantly increased risk of dementia, and this risk rises exponentially between 65 and 85 years of age. In most of these patients, dementia develops years after the onset of parkinsonian motor symptoms; however, in a small proportion of patients, the onset of both dementia and parkinsonian motor symptoms occurs within 1 year and is accompanied by pronounced fluctuations in cognitive functions, visual hallucinations, depression, postural instability, abnormal rapid eye movement sleep behavior, and urinary incontinence. Postmortem studies in these patients had revealed conspicuous Lewy body pathologic features and neuronal loss in the brainstem, neocortex, archicortex, amygdala, and nucleus basalis of Meynert. This syndrome has been designated "dementia with Lewy bodies." Parkinsonian features and loss of striatal dopamine transporter function in patients with dementia with Lewy bodies (DLB) were compared with those in patients with Parkinson's disease.

Methods.—Twenty patients with DLB and 24 patients with Parkinson's disease were matched for age and disease duration, and 10 control subjects were matched for age. Patients and control subjects were examined with use of SPECT, a dual-head camera, and the dopamine-transporter ligand ^{123}I-β-CIT. In a subgroup of 16 patients with DLB and 20 patients with Parkinson's disease, subscores of the Unified Parkinson's Disease Rating Scale (UPDRS)–motor examination (ME) subscale were obtained 12 hours after withdrawal of antiparkinsonian therapy.

Results.—Compared with the control subjects, striatal/cerebellar ratios of dopamine transporter bindings were significantly reduced in both patients with DLB and in patients with Parkinson's disease. The reductions were more pronounced in the patients with DLB. Side-to-side differences in the striatal/cerebellar ratios were lower in the DLB group and in the control subjects than in the patients with Parkinson's disease, and the total UPDRS-ME scores 12 hours after withdrawal of antiparkinsonian therapy were significantly higher in the DLB group than in the Parkinson's disease group.

Conclusions.—The implication from these findings is that parkinsonism has a largely symmetric evolution and progresses more rapidly with more severe loss of striatal dopamine transporter function in patients with dementia with Lewy bodies than it does in patients with Parkinson's disease. Further studies are needed to determine whether these findings will aid in the differential diagnosis of DLB and Parkinson's disease.

▶ If we get serious therapy for Parkinson's disease, then efforts to sort out subsets of patients with various types of parkinsonism will become very important. It is encouraging to know that use of ^{123}I-β-CIT is likely to be of great value in this regard.

A. Gottschalk, MD

Changes in Regional Cerebral Blood Flow Caused by Deep-Brain Stimulation of the Subthalamic Nucleus in Parkinson's Disease

Sestini S, di Luzio AS, Ammannati F, et al (Univ of Florence, Italy)
J Nucl Med 43:725-732, 2002
9–10

Background.—Idiopathic Parkinson's disease (PD) is usually treated with dopamine replacement therapy, which is only effective temporarily. An alternative treatment is implantation of electrodes for chronic high-frequency deep-brain stimulation. The effect of deep-brain stimulation of the subthalamic nucleus (STN) on regional cerebral blood flow (rCBF) and which areas correlated with improvement was investigated by SPECT perfusion in patients with PD.

Study Design.—The study group consisted of 10 consecutive patients with medically intractable PD. Before scanning and while unmedicated, study participants were evaluated with the motor unified PD rating scale, the Hoehn and Yahr disability scale, and the Schwab and England activities-of-

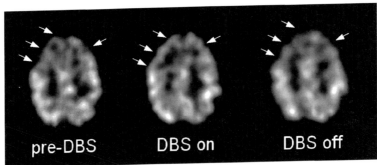

FIGURE 3.—Transaxial brain SPECT section of patient 2 during each scanning condition: preoperatively (*left*), postoperatively with STN stimulatory on (*middle*), and postoperatively with STN stimulators off (*right*). Arrows show rCBF increase in right frontal cortex and, to a lesser extent, left frontal cortex and ACC during STN stimulation in comparison with preoperatively and during no STN stimulation. (Reprinted by permission of the Society of Nuclear Medicine from Sestini S, Di Luzio AS, Ammannati F, et al: Changes in regional cerebral blood flow caused by deep-brain stimulation of the subthalamic nucleus in Parkinson's disease. *J Nucl Med* 43:725-732, 2002.)

daily-living scale. All patients had rCBF SPECT scanning before surgery, after surgery with STN stimulators on, and with STN stimulators switched off.

Findings.—STN stimulation significantly changed rCBF in the right presupplementary motor area (pre-SMA), anterior cingulate cortex, dorsolateral prefrontal cortex, and medial Brodmann's area 8. The rCBF increased with STN stimulation and decreased after stimulation was shut off (Fig 3). There was a significant correlation between motor score improvement and rCBF increase in the right pre-SMA and in the anterior cingulate motor area.

Conclusions.—Stimulation of the STN leads to rCBF increases in the motor, associative, and limbic areas of the frontal cortex of patients with PD. There was a significant correlation between motor improvement and rCBF increase in the pre-SMA and in the anterior cingulated motor area during STN stimulation. Perfusion SPECT is useful for analyzing the neural correlates of disease and the effects of therapy on the living brain.

▶ The apparent unerring results presented here cause me to wonder about 2 things: first, based on the article cited about vagus nerve stimulation, will the long-term chronic results be the same? These patients were studied at about 5 to 6 months. The median time for the chronic examination in the vagus stimulation patient was 15 months. Perhaps these authors will get some longer-term data. Next, all these patients improved medically. If they ever see a nonresponder, what will the blood flow to the pre-SMA cortex be? These data suggest it should be normal or decreased, but we do not know that.

A. Gottschalk, MD

Dopamine Transporter Brain Imaging to Assess the Effects of Pramipexole vs Levodopa on Parkinson Disease Progression

Marek K, for the Parkinson Study Group (Inst for Neurodegenerative Disorders, New Haven, Conn; et al)
JAMA 287:1653-1661, 2002

9–11

Background.—Parkinson disease (PD) is characterized clinically by bradykinesia, tremor, rigidity, and gait dysfunction. The clinical decline in PD reflects ongoing nigrostriatal dopaminergic degeneration. Pramipexole and levodopa are effective medications for the treatment of motor symptoms of early PD. Findings in animal and in vitro studies have suggested that pramipexole may protect dopamine neurons and that levodopa may either protect or damage dopamine neurons. The use of neuroimaging may provide an objective biomarker of dopamine neuron degeneration in patients with PD. The rates of dopamine neuron degeneration after initial treatment with pramipexole or levodopa were studied in patients with early PD by dopamine transporter imaging with SPECT with 2β-carboxymethoxy-3β(4-iodophenyl)tropane (β-CIT) labeled with iodine 123.

Methods.—This parallel group, double-blind, randomized clinical trial involved 82 patients with early PD at 17 sites in the United States and Canada. All the patients required dopaminergic therapy for the treatment of emerging disability from PD. The patients were randomly assigned to pramipexole with levodopa placebo 0.5 mg 3 times per day or carbidopa/levodopa with pramipexole placebo 25/100 mg 3 times per day. The dosage was escalated during the first 10 weeks for patients with residual disability, and open-label levodopa could be added subsequently. The dosage of study drug could be further modified after 24 months of follow-up. The primary outcome variable was the percentage change from baseline in striatal [^{123}I]β-CIT uptake after 46 months. Clinical severity of PD was assessed with the Unified Parkinson Disease Rating Scale (UPRDS) 12 hours off anti-PD medications.

Results.—A decline in mean (SD) [^{123}I]β-CIT striatal uptake was seen on nonsequential SPECT imaging, from a baseline of 10.3% (9.8%) at 22 months, 15.3% (12.8%) at 34 months, and 20.7% (14.4%) at 46 months, for a decline of about 5.2% per year. This decline in [^{123}I]β-CIT striatal uptake from baseline was significantly reduced in the pramipexole group compared with the levodopa group: 7.1% (9%) versus 13.5% (9.6%) at 22 months, 10.9% (11.8%) versus 19.6% (12.4%) at 34 months, and 16% (13.3%) versus 25.5% (14.1%) at 46 months. The percentage loss from baseline in [^{123}I]β-CIT striatal uptake correlated with the change in baseline in UPDRS at the 46-month evaluation.

Conclusions.—Patients with early PD treated initially with pramipexole showed a reduction compared with levodopa treatment in the loss of [^{123}I]β-CIT striatal uptake, which is a marker of dopamine neuron degeneration.

These data underscore the need for further comparison of imaging and clinical end points of PD progression in long-term studies.

▶ Another effective use of [^{123}I]β-CIT. Because all the patients in this study were imaged at Yale, it is fair to assume the imaging technique was consistent. Therefore, the results are believable. I am disappointed that no clear clinical correlation exists between the 2 drugs. In short, good news, but not great news.

A. Gottschalk, MD

Blinded Positron Emission Tomography Study of Dopamine Cell Implantation for Parkinson's Disease
Nakamura T, Dhawan V, Chaly T, et al (New York Univ; Columbia College of Physicians and Surgeons, New York; Univ of Colorado Health Sciences Ctr, Denver)
Ann Neurol 50:181-187, 2001   9–12

Background.—Nigrostriatal dopaminergic functioning was assessed in patients with Parkinson's disease in a double-blind placebo-controlled surgical trial of embryonic dopamine cell implantation. The clinical results of this surgical trial were reported in a previous study. Four twist drill holes penetrating the forehead were placed in 40 patients with Parkinson's disease. The patients had been randomly assigned to either tissue implant or placebo surgery. It was found that patients receiving the transplants improved significantly in standardized motor ratings, whereas no change was noted in the placebo group. In the present study, nigrostriatal dopaminergic functioning at baseline and at 12 months after surgery was assessed with PET and [^{18}F]fluorodopa (FDOPA).

Methods.—Of the 40 patients, 39 survived to 1 year after surgery and were rescanned with FDOPA/PET. These images were then quantified by investigators unaware of the treatment status and clinical outcome. After the treatment status and outcome were revealed, the effects of treatment status and age on the interval changes in the FDOPA/PET signal were evaluated.

Results.—Without knowing the treatment status or outcome, the investigators identified a significant increase (40.3%) in FDOPA uptake in the putamen of the implant group compared with the placebo group. These increases in putamen FDOPA uptake were similar in both the younger (≤ 60 years) and older (>60 years) patients receiving transplants. Significant decrements in putamen uptake were evident in younger patients undergoing placebo surgery (-6.5%) but not in the older patients undergoing placebo surgery.

Conclusions.—The correlations between the PET changes and clinical outcome were only significant in the subgroup of younger patients. The implication from these findings is that the age of the patient does not influence the viability of the graft or its development in the first postoperative year.

However, the age of the host may influence the time course of the downstream functional changes that are required to obtain a clinical benefit.

▶ I have often complained about the lack of "housekeeping details" in the past. The description of the experimental method in this article was superb. This series brings together PET/MRI fusion, statistical parametric mapping, and the use of before and after (rather than single absolute) changes to define the data. Great care to avoid bias was used as well. I congratulate the authors. I really liked this article, and I hope they continue to enlarge the patient database. Because of the number of subgroups, patient numbers in each subgroup are small and could be expanded.

A. Gottschalk, MD

Striatal and Extrastriatal Dysfunction in Parkinson's Disease With Dementia: A 6-[¹⁸F]fluoro-L-dopa PET Study
Ito K, Nagano-Saito A, Kato T, et al (Natl Inst for Longevity Sciences, Obu, Japan; Imperial College School of Medicine, London; Inst of Neurology, London)
Brain 125:1358-1365, 2002   9–13

Background.—In Parkinson disease, 6-[18F]fluoro-L-dopa (¹⁸F-dopa) has been used with PET to obtain a measure of disease severity and to identify persons with early, and even preclinical, disease. Although the main dopaminergic projections are nigrostriatal, extrastriatal dopamine terminals are also involved to varying degrees in the different phenotypes of idiopathic Parkinson disease and other parkinsonian syndromes. Previous studies have reported the association between cognitive impairment and dopaminergic dysfunction in Parkinson disease by using ¹⁸F-dopa PET and conventional region-of-interest analysis, but these methods are unreliable for the detection of dopaminergic changes in cortical and brain stem areas. A newly developed normalization and statistical parametric mapping (SPM) approach was applied to patients with Parkinson disease without dementia and with dementia to localize relative differences in their pathophysiologic processes on a voxel-by-voxel basis.

Methods.—A total of 20 patients with Parkinson disease, 10 with dementia and 10 without dementia, were evaluated with ¹⁸F-dopa PET. A group of 15 normal age-matched persons were also evaluated, and the ¹⁸F-dopa influx constant (Ki) images of the patients and normal controls were transformed into standard stereotactic space. Significant differences between the groups were localized with SPM on a voxel-by-voxel basis.

Results.—In comparison with the normal group, SPM localized declines of the ¹⁸F-dopa Ki bilaterally in the putamen, the right caudate nucleus, and the left ventral midbrain in patients with Parkinson disease without dementia. In comparison with the normal group, patients with Parkinson disease with dementia demonstrated reduced ¹⁸F-dopa Ki bilaterally in the striatum, midbrain, and anterior cingulate area. A relative difference in ¹⁸F-dopa uptake between patients with Parkinson disease without dementia and those with dementia was the bilateral decline in the anterior cingulate area and ventral striatum and in the right caudate nucleus in the patients with dementia.

Conclusions.—Dementia in patients with Parkinson disease is significantly associated with impaired mesolimbic and caudate dopaminergic function.

▶ An interesting study with both physiologic and therapeutic implications.

A. Gottschalk, MD

Longitudinal PET Evaluation of Cerebral Metabolic Decline in Dementia: A Potential Outcome Measure in Alzheimer's Disease Treatment Studies
Alexander GE, Chen K, Pietrini P, et al (Arizona Alzheimer's Research Ctr, Tucson; Arizona State Univ, Tucson; Univ of Arizona, Tucson; et al)
Am J Psychiatry 159:738-745, 2002   9–14

Background.—Regional cerebral metabolic rates for glucose determined by FDG PET, evaluated during a mental resting state with eyes and ears covered, are a sensitive in vivo test of the neurophysiologic effects of Alzheimer's disease. Longitudinal declines due to dementia have not been as well studied with PET. FDG PET and a statistical brain mapping algorithm were used to examine cross-sectional and longitudinal reductions in regional cerebral glucose metabolism on a voxel basis in 14 patients with Alzheimer's disease. These patients were examined at baseline and at 1-year follow-up.

Study Design.—The study group consisted of 14 otherwise healthy patients with mild to moderate dementia. There were 12 men and 2 women, with an average age of 65. Their average score on the Mini-Mental State Examination (MMSE) was 20 at baseline. At baseline, PET scans in the patients were compared with a group of 34 age- and sex-matched volunteers. The patient group was restudied at 1 year. Power analyses for voxels revealing maximal 1-year rates of decline in regional cerebral glucose metabolism and for annual decline rates in cognitive test scores were calculated for the patient group to estimate sample size needed to detect significant treatment response.

Findings.—Patients with Alzheimer's disease had significantly lower glucose metabolism than healthy control subjects in parietal, temporal, occipital, frontal, and posterior cingulate cortices at baseline. At 1-year follow-up, the patients had significant declines in glucose metabolism in all areas except the occipital. Power analysis estimated that a PET study would require as few as 24 patients per group when the voxel value for the left midfrontal cortex was used and from 58 to 89 patients per group when voxel values from the left inferior parietal, left midtemporal, and posterior cingulate cortices were used to detect a significant effect of treatment with 80% power compared with placebo.

Conclusions.—These findings support the use of FDG PET during mental rest for evaluating the longitudinal progression of Alzheimer's disease on a voxel-by-voxel basis. It would also be useful in the assessment of therapies designed to slow or prevent the progression of Alzheimer's disease.

▶ The conclusion that Alzheimer's gets worse and that FDG can show it is not news. But the authors are to be complimented for bringing this up to date within the confines of a potential therapy evaluation trial.

A. Gottschalk, MD

The Neural Substrates of Episodic Memory Impairment in Alzheimer's Disease as Revealed by FDG-PET: Relationship to Degree of Deterioration
Desgranges B, Baron J-C, Lalevée C, et al (EMI INSERM-Unive Laboratoire de Neuropsychologie, Caen Cedex, France; Univ of Cambridge, England)
Brain 125:1116-1124, 2002   9–15

Introduction.—The precise association between lesions and memory impairment in patients with Alzheimer disease (AD) are elusive since available postmortem data have been obtained from patients with extensive impairment in several different cognitive domains. Story Recall test scores and PET measurements of synaptic integrity were obtained in 40 patients with AD to determine whether cerebral structures implicated in episodic memory deficits differ by the severity of cognitive impairment.

Methods.—A classic 12-item Story Recall task was used to evaluate verbal episode memory. Patients underwent PET measurements of resting cerebral glucose utilization, a measure of synaptic integrity. The cerebral metabolic rate for glucose was evaluated at rest with ^{18}FDG. By using statistical parametric mapping 1996 software, positive correlations between the 2 sets of data were calculated on a voxel basis, initially in the whole patient sample, then separately in 2 subgroups of 20 patients who differed in the Mini-Mental State Examination score (less severe vs more severe subgroups).

Results.—Significant correlations in the whole sample ($P < .05$, corrected for multiple tests) involved several limbic structures (hippocampal/rhinal cortex regions, posterior cingulate gyrus, and retrosplenial cortex) bilaterally and, less expectedly, some temporal occipital association areas. Subgroup analysis showed that all significant correlations ($P < .005$, uncorrected) in the less severe subgroup were limited to the parahippocampal gyrus and retrosplenial cortex, in accordance with both the distribution of changes in tau in early AD and the known involvement of this network in normal and impaired memory function. In the more severe subgroup, the left temporal neocortex was primarily involved, which is known to be implicated in semantic memory.

Conclusion.—When episodic memory is mildly impaired, limbic functions are still adequate to subserve the remaining performance. With more severe memory deficit resulting from accumulated pathology, the neocortical areas that are usually involved in semantic memory are recruited, possibly as a form of (inadequate) compensatory mechanism.

▶ These data remind us again that the classic temporoparietal defect we all recognize as AD is a relatively late state of the disease. I first learned this from the late, great Niels Lassen about a decade ago while visiting his laboratory in Copenhagen. When treatment for AD is available, we will all have to know what these early imaging patterns look like.

A. Gottschalk, MD

Longitudinal Evaluation of Both Morphologic and Functional Changes in the Same Individuals With Alzheimer's Disease
Matsuda H, Kitayama N, Ohnishi T, et al (Natl Ctr Hosp for Mental Nervous and Muscular Disorders, Tokyo; Univ of Washington, Seattle; Showa Univ, Tokyo; et al)
J Nucl Med 43:304-311, 2002   9–16

Background.—MRI and PET or SPECT are useful for diagnosis and evaluation of the progression of Alzheimer's disease (AD). However, morphologic and functional imaging studies have not always provided concordant results regarding the brain areas that show atrophic changes and reduced flow or metabolism in patients with AD. For example, patients with mild AD have been reported to show significant atrophy in the medial temporal structures, but recent studies have found significantly decreased glucose metabolism or perfusion not in the medial temporal structures but in the posterior cingulate gyrus and precuneus. The purpose of this study was to determine the initial abnormality and the longitudinal changes in both morphologic and functional measurements for the same patients with AD.

Methods.—A group of 15 patients with mild AD and a control group of 25 age-matched healthy volunteers were studied. The patients with AD underwent 3 evaluations with both MRI and SPECT at approximately 1-year intervals. The gray matter volume, as segmented from MRI, and the regional cerebral blood flow (rCBF) as measured by SPECT, in patients with AD were compared with those of the healthy volunteer group. Statistical parametric mapping, a voxel-based analysis in stereotactic space, was used in the comparisons.

Results.—There was a considerable degree of discordance between areas of regional atrophy and areas of decreased rCBF. The medial temporal areas demonstrated a faster and more extensive reduction of gray matter volume than of rCBF. Compared with baseline values, rCBF in the posterior cingulate gyrus and precuneus and the associative parietal cortex was extensively decreased. In contrast, however, the extent of significant decrease in this area continued to be much narrower for gray matter volume than for rCBF, even in follow-up studies.

Conclusions.—The results of this study indicated a distinct discordance between morphologic and functional changes in a longitudinal study of AD.

The functional changes seen in these patients may be the result, at least in part, of remote effects from the morphologically involved areas, with increased connectivity and also to some degree, the result of a compensatory response by neuronal plasticity.

▶ I have been pushing the need to correlate morphologic brain volume studies with their functional nuclear medicine counterpart for years. These authors have provided a superb sophisticated example of just what I hoped for in patients with early Alzheimer's. Any effort to provide therapy should only be assessed by an effect on data like these. I congratulate the authors. If you have any interest in this subject, I urge you to read this article. Because the illustrations contain color, we cannot reproduce them here.

A. Gottschalk, MD

Positron Emission Tomography in Evaluation of Dementia: Regional Brain Metabolism and Long-term Outcome
Silverman DHS, Small GW, Chang CY, et al (Univ of California, Los Angeles; Kaiser Permanente, Los Angeles; NIH, Bethesda, Md; et al)
JAMA 286:2120-2127, 2001   9–17

Background.—The optimal management of patients with dementia depends on the early recognition and accurate assessment of their cognitive and behavioral symptoms. Patients with cognitive dysfunction attributed to a variety of disease processes have been found to have deficits in cerebral glucose utilization, but the prognostic and diagnostic value of these observations has not been determined. The sensitivity and specificity with which cerebral metabolic patterns at a single point in time forecast subsequent documentation of progressive dementia were assessed.

Methods.—PET studies with [^{18}F]FDG were conducted in 146 patients who were undergoing evaluation for dementia with at least 2 years' follow-up for disease progression at the University of California, Los Angeles, from 1991 to 2000. PET studies were also conducted at several international facilities from 1984 to 2000, and histopathologic diagnoses were made an average of 2.9 years later. The main outcome measures were regional distribution of [^{18}F]FDG in each patient, classified on the basis of criteria established as positive or negative for the presence of a progressive neurodegenerative disease in general and of Alzheimer's disease specifically, compared with results of longitudinal or neuropathologic analyses.

Results.—PET had 93% sensitivity and 76% specificity in the detection of progressive dementia. Among patients with neuropathologically based diagnoses, PET identified patients with Alzheimer's disease and those with any neurodegenerative disease with a sensitivity of 94% and a specificity of 73% and 78%, respectively.

Conclusions.—Regional brain metabolism is a sensitive indicator of Alzheimer's disease and of neurodegenerative disease in general in patients seen with cognitive symptoms of dementia. Negative findings on PET indicated that pathologic progression of cognitive impairment was unlikely during the mean 3-year follow-up.

▶ Vive la negative PET.

A. Gottschalk, MD

Combined Analysis of CSF Tau Levels and [^{123}I]Iodoamphetamine SPECT in Mild Cognitive Impairment: Implications for a Novel Predictor of Alzheimer's Disease
Okamura N, Arai H, Maruyama M, et al (Tohoku Univ, Sendai, Miyagi, Japan)
Am J Psychiatry 159:474-476, 2002   9–18

Background.—Mild cognitive impairment is defined as an intermediate or transitional state from a normal cognitive state to one of dementia. However, it is likely that mild cognitive impairment may represent a complex heterogeneous condition and that some patients with mild cognitive impairment will not have Alzheimer's disease or other dementing disorders develop. As new drugs are introduced that may delay the progression of Alzheimer's disease, the early and accurate detection of elderly patients with mild cognitive impairment who are destined to have Alzheimer's disease develop is particularly important. The goal of this study was to develop an objective and reliable index to predict the development of Alzheimer's disease in a large pool of elderly patients with mild cognitive impairment.

Methods.—The study group consisted of 23 patients with probable Alzheimer's disease, 22 patients with mild cognitive impairment who eventually had Alzheimer's disease develop, 8 patients with mild cognitive impairment who did not have dementia develop, and 19 cognitively normal subjects. The study authors constructed a new diagnostic index, the CSF-CBF index, based on CSF tau level divided by regional cerebral blood flow (CBF) in the posterior cingulate cortex.

Results.—Analysis by receiving operator characteristics demonstrated that applying a cutoff value of 296.0 for the CSF-CBF index achieved a sensitivity of 88.5% and a specificity of 90% in discriminating mild cognitive impairment that progressed to Alzheimer's disease from mild cognitive impairment that did not progress to Alzheimer's disease.

Conclusions.—The CSF-CBF described in this report is a useful tool for the prediction of future development of Alzheimer's disease in patients with mild cognitive impairment.

▶ I worry when 1 of the key groups has only 8 patients (cognitive impairment who did not have Alzheimer's disease develop), so I accept these data as a hypothesis and hope these authors will expand the series. However, the idea of linking tests together thereby making the combo more robust than the separate parts appeals to me.

A. Gottschalk, MD

Tc-99m Ethylcysteinate Dimer Brain SPECT Perfusion Imaging in Ictal Nonepileptic Visual Hallucinations

Lorberboym M, Lampl Y, Gilad R, et al (Tel Aviv Univ, Israel)

Clin Nucl Med 27:87-91, 2002   9–19

Background.—Visual hallucinations may be associated with a variety of conditions, particularly in epilepsy, cerebrovascular disease, the withdrawal state after chronic alcohol intoxication, Alzheimer's and Lewy body disease, and in diseases of the occipitoparietal or occipitotemporal cortex. Acute hallucinations may occur within the CNS without a localizing focus and may be associated with a lesion anywhere along the visual pathway. "Ictal" regional cerebral blood flow was assessed with technetium 99m (^{99m}Tc)–ethylcysteinate dimer SPECT in patients experiencing acute hallucinations. Findings in these patients were compared with findings in the "interictal" state.

Methods.—In this prospective study, patients admitted to the neurology department with nonpsychiatric and nonepileptic visual hallucinations were evaluated with CT scans and thorough neurologic and psychiatric evaluations. Electroencephalographic (EEG) recordings were made during the patients' hallucinations. All patients also underwent a brain SPECT evaluation during acute hallucinations (ictal SPECT) and a follow-up scan 2 to 3 weeks later.

Results.—A total of 9 patients were evaluated, and all had normal ictal EEG findings during their hallucinations. Seven of the 9 patients had increased perfusion in 1 or more regions on the SPECT studies, and the mean lesion-to-contralateral ratio was 2.1 (range, 1.5- 2.7). Of these 7 patients, 3 had findings consistent with a cerebrovascular accident (Fig 1). After treatment, the hallucinations disappeared in 2 patients, and the motor deficit improved dramatically. The follow-up SPECT study also showed significant improvement in all patients 1 week later. Charles Bonnet syndrome, frontal lobe dementia, and Anton's syndrome were each diagnosed in 1 patient. The last patient had no identifiable background disease. All these patients had normal finding on EEG, CT, and MRI examinations. All patients responded well to carbamazepine therapy, and the follow-up study showed resolution of the findings. Posterior cortical hyperperfusion was demonstrated in 2 of 9 patients, and Lewy body disease was eventually diagnosed in these patients. The SPECT examination showed no evidence of hyperperfusion.

Conclusions.—Findings in this preliminary prospective study indicate that brain imaging with SPECT may aid in the identification of the mechanisms involved in visual hallucinations and the evolution of blood flow abnormalities in certain subgroups of patients and may aid in the selection of specific therapeutic approaches for these patients.

▶ This was an interesting series and had good outcomes after treatment in most cases. The authors note that CT in these patients was virtually no help but do not mention MRI. I suspect that diffusion-weighted MRI axial slices

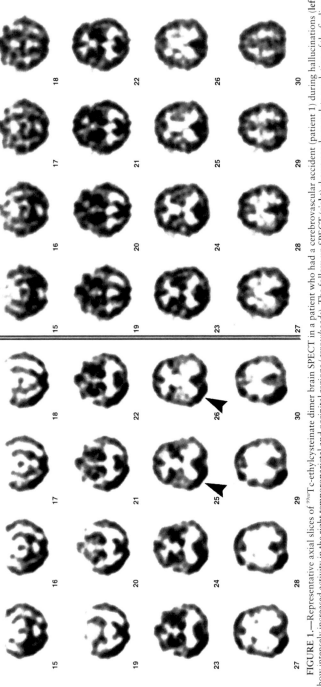

FIGURE 1.—Representative axial slices of ^{99m}Tc-ethylcysteinate dimer brain SPECT in a patient who had a cerebrovascular accident (patient 1) during hallucinations (**left**) show intensely increased activity in the right temporoparietal and occipital regions (*arrowheads*). The follow-up SPECT (**right**) shows nearly complete resolution of the findings. (Courtesy of Lorberboym M, Lampl Y, Gilad R, et al: Tc-99m Ethylcysteinate dimer brain SPECT perfusion imaging in ictal nonepileptic visual hallucinations. *Clin Nucl Med* 27(2):87-91, 2002.)

might show virtually identical initial findings. If so, because it is often part of a routine brain MRI series, MRI might replace SPECT in these patients.

A. Gottschalk, MD

Very Early and Standard Tc-99m Ethyl Cysteinate Dimer SPECT Imaging in a Patient With Reperfusion Hyperemia After Acute Cerebral Embolism
Ogasawara K, Konno H, Yasuda S, et al (Iwate Med Univ, Morioka, Japan)
Clin Nucl Med 27:105-108, 2002   9–20

Background.—Technetium 99m (^{99m}Tc)–ethyl cysteinate dimer (ECD) was developed as a retained-type brain perfusion tracer and has been widely used in clinical practice to visualize regional blood flow in the human brain with SPECT. Studies have demonstrated the correlation of the distribution of ^{99m}Tc-ECD in the brain with regional brain perfusion in healthy volunteers and in patients with chronic strokes. However, other studies have indicated that ^{99m}Tc-ECD SPECT imaging may not demonstrate reperfusion hyperemia in patients with subacute strokes, and the distribution of tracer may reflect not only perfusion but also the metabolic status of brain tissue. A patient had embolic middle cerebral artery occlusion and was examined with xenon-133 and consecutive dynamic and standard ^{99m}Tc-ECD SPECT immediately after early recanalization.

Case Report.—Man, 61, with atrial fibrillation suddenly had left hemiparesis. CT of the brain 3 hours after the onset of symptoms revealed no lesions that might be implicated. An embolic occlusion of the horizontal portion of the right middle cerebral artery was revealed on cerebral angiography. Local intra-arterial thrombolysis was performed, the occluded vessel was recanalized, and blood flow was re-established 4.5 hours after the onset of symptoms. Fifteen minutes after recanalization, xenon-133 and dynamic and standard ^{99m}Tc-ECD SPECT images showed hypoactivity in the area of the ipsilateral middle cerebral artery. However, the dynamic ^{99m}Tc-ECD SPECT images from the first scan 36 seconds after injection showed hyperactivity in the same region and provided imaging contrast comparable to the contrast obtained with xenon-133 tomography. The patient became comatose 12 hours later, and CT showed that hemorrhagic transformation had developed in this region.

Conclusions.—Images obtained from very early dynamic ^{99m}Tc-ECD SPECT of areas with irreversible changes caused by an acute stroke can demonstrate reflow hyperemia that may not be visualized on standard ^{99m}Tc-ECD SPECT images.

▶ This is an elegant use of ECD with an ugly patient outcome. We are now left with a dilemma. If we see early reperfusion with dynamic ECD that indicates recanalization, does that mean subsequent hemorrhagic transformation will occur or only that recanalization was successful? Clearly, we need more data.

A. Gottschalk, MD

Prognostic Value of Subacute Crossed Cerebellar Diaschisis: Single-Photon Emission CT Study in Patients With Middle Cerebral Artery Territory Infarct
Takasawa M, Watanabe M, Yamamoto S, et al (Osaka-Minami Natl Hosp, Japan; Osaka Univ, Japan)
AJNR Am J Neuroradiol 23:189-193, 2002   9–21

Background.—The mechanism that underlies crossed cerebellar diaschisis (CCD) in patients with supratentorial infarction is reported to consist of interruption of the cerebropontocerebellar pathway, which causes deafferentiation and transneural metabolic depression of the contralateral cerebellar hemisphere. Chronic CCD is associated with neurologic improvement after infarct in the middle cerebral artery territory. It has been reported in some studies that CCD seems to be prominent in patients with severe hemiparesis in various stages. However, the prognostic value of early-stage CCD remains controversial. Whether determination of CCD in the acute and subacute stages by SPECT can facilitate the prediction of a stroke outcome was evaluated.

Methods.—Technetium 99m (^{99m}Tc)–hexamethylpropyleneamine oxime (^{99m}Tc-HMPAO) SPECT was used to evaluate the pattern of cerebral blood flow changes after acute middle cerebral artery ischemia with severe cortical symptoms in 15 patients with unilateral ischemia in the early subacute stage (10 ± 5 days). SPECT was performed in 11 patients in both the acute (16 ± 10 hours) and subacute stages. The asymmetry index (AI) was calculated from the total counts obtained from each cerebellar hemisphere. The clinical outcome was assessed at 60 days with the Scandinavian Stroke Scale and the Barthel Index.

Results.—No significant correlation was found between AIs in the acute stage and clinical outcome, but the severity of AI in the early subacute stages showed a significant correlation with both the final Scandinavian Stroke Scale and Barthel Index scores.

Conclusions.—In patients with supratentorial infarct, a worse clinical outcome is indicated by cerebellar hypoperfusion detected with ^{99m}Tc-HMPAO SPECT in the early subacute stage.

▶ CCD has been discussed in the YEAR BOOK OF NUCLEAR MEDICINE in the past, as has cerebral diaschisis after a cerebellar stroke. The interested reader may wish to look up the these articles.[1,2]

A. Gottschalk, MD

References

1. 1998 YEAR BOOK OF NUCLEAR MEDICINE, pp 260-261.

2. 1996 YEAR BOOK OF NUCLEAR MEDICINE, pp 257-259.

Reversible Ischemia Around Intracerebral Hemorrhage: A Single-Photon Emission Computerized Tomography Study

Siddique MS, Fernandes HM, Wooldridge TD, et al (Univ of Newcastle, England; Newcastle Gen Hosp, Newcastle-upon-Tyne, England; Univ of Western Ontario, Toronto)

J Neurosurg 96:736-741, 2002   9–22

Background.—Evidence suggests that a zone of ischemia develops around intracerebral hemorrhage (ICH). Whether cerebral blood flow (CBF) in these areas of perilesional oligemia can improve over time was examined with the use of technetium-99m-labeled hexamethylpropyleneamine oxime SPECT (^{99}Tc-HMPAO SPECT).

Methods.—The subjects were 11 patients (6 men and 5 women; mean age, 62 years) with spontaneous supratentorial ICH. None of the patients was treated surgically. All patients underwent ^{99}Tc-HMPAO SPECT studies within days of the ICH and again 6 to 9 months later. To account for absorption of hematoma over time, the late images were registered to the acute images and aligned to a common 3-dimensional orientation. Count differences were minimized by normalizing images to the maximal counts. Then the late images were compared voxel by voxel with the acute images, and the region-growing algorithm was used to identify perihematoma regions with an improvement in radiotracer uptake of 15% or more on the late images. A signal improvement of 15% corresponds to an improvement in CBF of up to 12 mL/100 gm/min and thus reflects reperfusion.

Results.—All 11 patients had discrete perihematoma regions that had 15% or more improvement in radiotracer uptake on the late images compared with the acute images. The volume of brain with 15% or more improvement in perfusion ranged from 7.2 to 71.3 cm³ (mean, 34.8 cm³). These regions represent a zone of tissues that were underperfused in the acute stage of ICH but that were subsequently reperfused.

Conclusion.—[99]Tc-HMPAO SPECT identified discrete perihematoma regions with 15% or more improvement in CBF over time in all of these patients with ICH. These areas may constitute a zone of reversible perilesional oligemia, or a so-called penumbra, around ICH. It may be possible that medical or surgical interventions could increase the volume of perilesional brain that recovers after ICH and, therefore, improve outcomes and reduce neurologic deficits after ICH.

▶ The idea that penumbra really exists and that if you work to increase it by early interventions after a stroke, you may do the patient some good appeals to me. These authors make their point by normalizing the early and late HMPAO SPECT studies to each other. That bothers me. I would have preferred they compare early and late slices with fusion to an intermediate (like MRI) first. I think the fusion comparison would be more accurate. However, because all 11 patients in this series provided data showing that penumbra was present, it seems my objection above would be unlikely to change the conclusion that penumbra exists.

A. Gottschalk, MD

Combination of Early and Delayed SPET Imaging Using Technetium-99m Ethyl Cysteinate Dimer Immediately After Local Intra-Arterial Thrombolysis

Ogasawara K, Ogawa A, Konno H, et al (Iwate Med Univ, Morioka, Japan; Tohoku Univ, Sendai, Japan)

Eur J Nucl Med 28:498-505, 2001   9–23

Background.—Thrombolytic therapy for acute ischemic stroke is based on the rationale that the resultant recanalization of occluded arteries increases cerebral perfusion and thus reestablishes normal brain metabolism and function by saving viable brain tissue before brain damage becomes irreversible. Intra-arterial thrombolytic therapy has been shown to be beneficial for the treatment of acute ischemic stroke within 6 hours of the onset of symptoms. However, this therapy is also associated with significant morbidity and mortality. The most significant problem is reported to be hemorrhagic transformation, which may result in a rapid deterioration of the patient's neurologic condition. Several radiotracers have been developed over the past decade for imaging cerebral blood flow (CBF) with SPET. The prognostic use of posttreatment technetium (Tc) 99m ethyl cysteinate dimer (^{99m}Tc-ECD) SPET for predicting ischemic outcome in patients with middle cerebral artery occlusion treated with local intra-arterial thrombolysis was investigated.

Methods.—Posttreatment ^{99m}Tc-ECD SPET studies were performed immediately after thrombolysis in 25 patients with a moderately ischemic area determined by using pretreatment ^{99m}Tc-hexamethylpropylene amine oxime (HMPAO). All the patients underwent complete recanalization within 6 hours. The extent of the affected area outlined on pretreatment ^{99m}Tc-HMPAO SPET was used for the posttreatment early and delayed ^{99m}Tc-ECD SPET images, and the ratio of affected regional activity to cerebellar activity (AR/CE ratio) was calculated. Twelve patients without infarction or with small subcortical/basal ganglial infarction, 10 with medium or large cortical infarction, and 3 with hemorrhage were identified by follow-up CT.

Results.—Although the AR/CE ratio in posttreatment early ^{99m}Tc-ECD SPET images was significantly higher in the hemorrhagic group than in the cortical infarction group, this value was not useful in differentiating the reversible ischemia group from either the cortical infarction or the hemorrhagic group. The AR/CE ratio in posttreatment delayed ^{99m}Tc-ECD SPET images differentiated the reversible ischemia group from both the cortical infarction and the hemorrhagic group, but the differences between the cortical infarction and hemorrhagic groups were not statistically significant. The washout index of ^{99m}Tc-ECD statistically differentiated all 3 groups.

Conclusions.—These findings indicate that a combination of early and delayed ^{99m}Tc-ECD SPET imaging obtained immediately after thrombolysis is predictive of ischemic tissue outcome.

▶ When I think about therapy for acute stroke, I worry about questions like, "can the penumbra be preserved; is the 6-hour window for thrombolysis too long; or can the area of the infarct be reduced?" These authors use very large regions of interest in this study, and therefore, I worry that they paint with brush strokes that are too big. But they are painting, and that is a start.

A. Gottschalk, MD

Serial [^{18}F]Fluorodeoxyglucose Positron Emission Tomography After Human Neuronal Implantation for Stroke
Meltzer CC, Kondziolka D, Villemagne VL, et al (Univ of Pittsburgh, Pa; Layton BioScience, Sunnyvale, Calif)
Neurosurgery 49:586-592, 2001   9–24

Background.—The incidence of stroke is incredibly high in the United States: approximately 750,000 occur annually. A stroke is the third leading cause of death, and the most common cause of disability in the United States. Efforts to decrease the incidence of strokes through the control of risk factors have been counterbalanced by the effects of an aging population. Recently, acute strokes have been the focus of efforts to develop effective therapeutic approaches, but these have typically short peri-infarct time windows for the administration of therapy. At this point, there is no known effective treatment for a chronic stroke with fixed neurologic deficit. In this study, PET with [^{18}F]FDG was used to map the metabolic brain response to neuronal cell implantation in the first neuroimplantation trial for strokes in human beings.

Methods.—A total of 12 patients (9 men and 3 women) with chronic basal ganglia infarction and persistent motor deficit underwent FDG PET within 1 week before and 6 to 12 months after stereotactic implantation of human neuronal cells. The patients had a mean age of 60.8 ± 8.3 years. Serial neurologic evaluations during a postoperative period of 1 year included the National Institutes of Health stroke scale and the European stroke scale.

Results.—No difference in the postimplantation change in metabolic activity was observed in patients who received 2 million or 6 million cells. A positive correlation was observed between motor performance measures and alterations in glucose metabolic activity in the stroke area and surrounding tissue at 6 and 12 months after implantation (Fig 2).

Conclusions.—In an open-label trial of implanted human neuronal cells for chronic stroke, FDG PET demonstrated a relationship between relative regional metabolic changes and clinical performance measures. These pre-

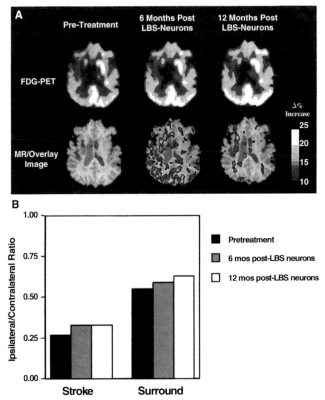

FIGURE 2.—Patient 4, a 61-year-old man with chronic right putamen infarct. **A,** FDG PET; selected serial images obtained before and 6 and 12 months after implantation of human neuronal cells. Overlay of normalized subtraction PET data (posttreatment scans relative to the baseline study) onto co-registered MRI showing localized relative increases in metabolic activity in the peristroke area and ipsilateral temporal cortex. **B,** Bar graph demonstrating a marked and sustained rise in relative glucose metabolic activity in the stroke territory and milder progressive increases in the surrounding regions. (Courtesy of Meltzer CC, Kondziolka D, Villemagne VL, et al: Serial [18F]fluorodeoxyglucose positron emission tomography after human neuronal implantation for stroke. *Neurosurgery* 49(3):586-592, 2001.)

liminary findings indicate the potential for improved local cellular function or engraftment of implanted cells in some patients.

▶ This is an exciting idea. The editorial comments to this article point out that it is an uncontrolled anecdotal series. Only 2 of the 12 patients improved significantly, and many more scores declined. However, as we have nothing else to offer these patients with ischemic strokes, let us hope this group continues this work expeditiously.

A. Gottschalk, MD

Cerebral Perfusion and Haemodynamics Measured by SPET in Symptom-Free Patients With Transient Ischaemic Attack: Clinical Implications
Martí-Fàbregas J, Catafau AM, Marí C, et al (Universitat Autònoma de Barcelona)
Eur J Nucl Med 28:1828-1835, 2001   9–25

Background.—Transient ischemic attacks (TIAs) are episodes of focal brain dysfunction of ischemic origin that last for less than 24 hours. TIAs share risk factors and mechanisms with cerebral infarction, and a focal lesion compatible with an infarct can often be detected on structural neuroimaging examinations in patients with TIA. These findings make it difficult to distinguish between cerebral infarct and TIA beyond the duration of symptoms. Because the symptoms of TIA are of relatively short duration, most patients are asymptomatic when evaluated by the neurologist. Thus, the diagnosis of TIA is subject to considerable interobserver variation. SPET may help in defining the vascular topography and suggesting the probable mechanism in patients with TIA. However, the variables predictive of focal regional cerebral blood flow (rCBF) and cerebrovascular reserve (CVR) abnormalities on SPET and their clinical correlation are poorly understood. The value of rCBF and CVR measured by SPET in patients in the subacute stage after a first-ever TIA was assessed.

Methods.—Two SPET examinations, baseline and after acetazolamide administration, were performed in a prospective series of 42 patients with recent (within the past 30 days) first-ever TIA. Region/reference ratios were obtained with the use of an irregular region of interest method. The relationship of SPET findings with clinical data and results of complementary examinations was assessed.

Results.—Most patients (98%) had abnormal findings on either baseline (43%) or after acetazolamide (19%) studies or on both (36%) SPET studies. Thus, hypoperfusion on baseline SPET was identified in 33 patients. Twenty-three patients (55%) had a poor response to acetazolamide. No predictors for rCBF or CVR impairment were found.

Conclusions.—Most patients who have experienced a first-ever TIA episode present focal hypoperfusion on SPET, either with or without correlation with TIA symptoms. SPET evaluation after acetazolamide administration increased the probability of finding cerebrovascular abnormalities and focuses attention on a hemodynamic compromise. A finding of focal hypoperfusion on SPET in these patients should not be seen as clinically insignificant because it is likely reflective of previous or ongoing clinical and/or subclinical episodes of cerebral ischemia.

▶ Patients with TIA continue to be a challenge for all the modalities I know that seek to diagnose what is going on. MRI, for example, even with the newer diffusion sequences that show ischemia acutely, commonly show only relatively nonspecific "chronic small vessel ischemic change" without much in the way of localizing findings. These authors suggest the SPET findings may show a vascular territory at risk for future cortical infarct. I suspect it will take many patients and much hard work to prove or disprove this hypothesis.

A. Gottschalk, MD

Evaluation of Delayed Appearance of Acetazolamide Effect in Patients With Chronic Cerebrovascular Ischemic Disease: Feasibility and Usefulness of SPECT Method Using Triple Injection of ECD

Murakami M, Yonehara T, Takaki A, et al (Saiseikai Kumamoto Hosp, Japan; Daiichi Radioisotope Labs Ltd, Tokyo; Kumamoto Univ, Japan)

J Nucl Med 43:577-583, 2002   9–26

Background.—Acetazolamide (ACZ) is a potent and fast-acting cerebral vessel dilator. Some patients have a delayed or reduced cerebral vasoreactivity to ACZ and these patients are at increased risk of ischemic attack. A new SPECT method, TIE or triple injection of technetium Tc 99m-ethyl-cysteinate dimer (ECD), was evaluated for the investigation of delayed or poor response to ACZ in patients with cerebral ischemic disease.

Study Design.—The study group consisted of 12 healthy volunteers who were IV injected with saline solution as a negative control, 12 healthy volunteers who were IV injected with ECD as a positive control, 9 patients with complete internal carotid artery (IC) occlusion, and 6 patients with cervical carotid artery stenosis. Three equal volume splits of ECD were IV injected and ACZ was used as a vasodilator. A middle cerebral artery territory in the lateral ventricle was the region of interest. The data at rest and at 7.5 and 20 minutes after ACZ administration were obtained by dynamic SPECT.

Findings.—In the negative control, the value at rest was 100%, at ACZ-7.5 was 100.4%, and at ACZ-20 was 99.6%, indicating the accuracy of TIE. In the positive control, ACZ-7.5 was 124.5%, indicating rapid vasoreactivity. ACZ-20 was 130.1% indicating continuous vasoreactivity. Patients with complete IC occlusion had a poor response at ACZ-7.5, but a normal response at ACZ-20, indicating a delayed response. Patients with severe IC stenosis had restoration of ACZ-7.5 response after carotid endarterectomy.

Conclusions.—The efficacy of TIE, a new SPECT method, for analysis of delayed or poor response to ACZ in patients with chronic cerebral ischemic disease was demonstrated.

▶ OK—we see the potential. Now we need a series to see whether the technique really works.

A. Gottschalk, MD

Imaging Atherosclerotic Plaque Inflammation With [¹⁸F]-Fluorodeoxy-glucose Positron Emission Tomography

Rudd JHF, Warburton EA, Fryer TD, et al (Univ of Cambridge, England)
Circulation 105:2708-2711, 2002   9–27

Background.—Inflammation plays an important role in both the pathogenesis and outcome of atherosclerosis. Plaques containing numerous inflammatory cells, particularly macrophages, have a high risk of rupture, while plaques with few inflammatory cells have a lower risk of rupture. X-ray contrast angiography is the current gold standard imaging technique for atherosclerosis and provides high-resolution definition of the site and severity of luminal stenoses. However, this technique cannot provide information regarding plaque inflammation. The glucose analog ¹⁸FDG can be used to image inflammatory cell activity noninvasively by PET. The potential utility of ¹⁸FDG-PET in identifying inflammation within carotid artery atherosclerotic plaques was explored.

Methods.—The study group comprised 8 patients with symptomatic carotid atherosclerosis and an internal carotid artery stenosis of at least 70%. The patients were examined with ¹⁸FDG-PET and coregistered CT.

Results.—Symptomatic carotid plaques were evident in the ¹⁸FDG-PET images acquired 3 hours after ¹⁸FDG injection. The estimated net ¹⁸FDG accumulation rate (plaque/integral plasma) in symptomatic lesions was 27% higher than in contralateral asymptomatic lesions. No measurable ¹⁸FDG uptake into normal carotid arteries was observed. Autoradiography of excised plaques confirmed the accumulation of deoxyglucose in macrophage-rich areas of the plaque.

Conclusions.—It would appear from these findings that ¹⁸FDG-PET can provide adequate visualization of atherosclerotic plaque inflammation, and that ¹⁸FDG accumulation is greater in symptomatic, unstable plaques than in asymptomatic lesions.

▶ This is an interesting study. I suppose the next step will be to examine patients at risk without a recent transient ischemic attack and randomize to those treated with statins versus those treated some other way or not treated at all to see if a medical management change is possible based on PET findings.

A. Gottschalk, MD

SPECT Imaging in Head Injury Interpreted With Statistical Parametric Mapping

Stamatakis EA, Wilson JTL, Hadley DM, et al (Univ of Stirling, Scotland; Southern Gen Hosp, Glasgow, Scotland)
J Nucl Med 43:476-483, 2002   9–28

Background.—The use of SPECT in the assessment of head injury may reveal abnormalities that are not detected by CT or MRI. The interpretation of SPECT images has frequently involved blind reading by experienced practi-

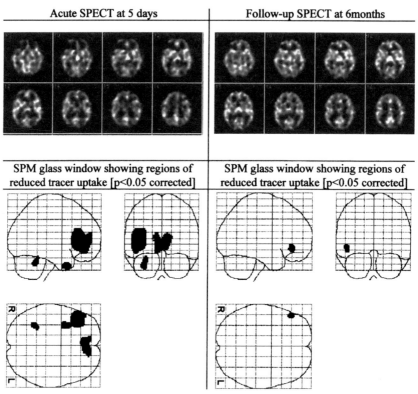

| Acute SPECT at 5 days | Follow-up SPECT at 6months |

| SPM glass window showing regions of reduced tracer uptake [p<0.05 corrected] | SPM glass window showing regions of reduced tracer uptake [p<0.05 corrected] |

FIGURE 1.—SPECT (midsections) and SPECT statistical parametric mapping (*SPM*) images of 33-year-old man after sports injury. He had Glasgow Coma Scale (GCS) rating of 15 on admission. Patient was from focal injury group. (Reprinted by permission of the Society of Nuclear Medicine, from Stamatakis EA, Wilson JTL, Hadley DM, et al: SPECT imaging in head injury interpreted with statistical parametric mapping. *J Nucl Med* 43:476-483, 2002.)

tioners, using a visual grading scheme based on color scales, visual assignment of scores, or classification into categories such as nonfocal, meningeal, or focal lesions and, in other cases, diffuse or focal lesions. However, there are problems associated with this type of SPECT interpretation, such as operator subjectivity, low reproducibility, and extensive time expenditure in analyzing images. Regional cerebral blood flow was investigated in head-injured patients by using statistical parametric mapping (SPM) to detect hypoperfusion on ^{99m}Tc-hexamethylpropyleneamine oxime (HMPAO) SPECT scans.

Methods.—Acute and follow-up SPECT and MRI scans were obtained from 61 patients admitted to a regional neurosurgical unit. All the patients had acute MRI and SPECT performed at 2 to 18 days after injury and follow-up imaging at 130 and 366 days after injury. A separate SPECT control group comprised 32 scans from non–head-injured patients. The SPECT images were aligned to the Talairach-Tournoux atlas and then analyzed statistically with SPM.

Results.—SPECT detected more extensive abnormalities than MRI in both acute and follow-up imaging studies (Fig 1). This effect was more pronounced on follow-up of patients with diffuse injury. Examination of a focal injury group showed the involvement of frontal and temporal lobes and the anterior cingulate. Follow-up scans showed persistence of blood flow abnormalities to a lesser extent. The diffuse group manifested low blood flow in the frontal and temporal lobes, including cingulate involvement, which persisted at follow-up with additional involvement of the thalamus.

Conclusions.—The use of SPM in SPECT image interpretation allows better visualization than other methods of quantitative analysis of the spatial distribution of abnormalities in focal and diffuse head injury. Frontal lobe blood flow abnormality is a common manifestation after head injury, particularly in the anterofrontal regions and mesiofrontal areas.

▶ As an extension of the article below (Abstract 9–34), this article looks specifically at SPM and serves as an example illustrating 3-dimensional localization of perfusion deficits in patients' brain scans. We see that additional image processing techniques can be applied to improve diagnostic image analysis and to sometimes portray the clinical information in a way that is not often obvious to the human eye when viewing reconstructed transverse, sagittal, and/or coronal slices.

I. G. Zubal, PhD

▶ These authors used and love the 1996 version of SPM. They point out previous work they did on "synthetic lesions" and in essence indicate they normalized the SPM technique to their needs in this study. They also stated that SPECT found more lesions than MRI, but most of the MRI was performed on a 0.15T unit. That is barely a low-field MRI—not much stronger than a refrigerator door magnet. Did they use gradient echo cardiography or diffusion or fluid attenuation inversion recovery images? They do not say. However, they also used the old Strichman brain scanner, not a triple-head modern camera. Thus, I take all modality comparisons with a teaspoon (ie, many grains) of salt. Nevertheless, the concept that SPM is more objective than visual inspection is probably correct. Please read on.

A. Gottschalk, MD

Combined Encephaloduroarteriosynangiosis and Bifrontal Encephalogaleo(periosteal)synangiosis in Pediatric Moyamoya Disease

Kim S-K, Wang K-C, Kim I-O, et al (Seoul Natl Univ, Korea)
Neurosurgery 50:88-96, 2002   9–29

Background.—The most common pediatric cerebrovascular disease in eastern Asia is moyamoya disease (MMD). MMD is characterized by progressive occlusion of the internal carotid artery or its terminal branches, along with the formation of extensive collateral vessels at the base of the brain. This disease is usually seen clinically as repeated transient ischemic attacks in children and as intracranial hemorrhaging in adults. There is no known cure, but the benefits of surgery for the ischemic type of MMD have been established. The goal of bypass surgery in patients with MMD is to establish adequate collateral circulation to ischemic brain tissue. The results of simple encephaloduroarteriosynangiosis (EDAS) were compared with the results of EDAS with bifrontal encephalogaleo(periosteal)synangiosis for the treatment of MMD in children.

Methods.—Data were retrospectively analyzed for 159 children (76 boys and 83 girls up to 15 years of age) who underwent indirect revascularization for the treatment of MMD from 1987 to 1998. Patients in group A underwent simple EDAS, and group B patients underwent EDAS with bifrontal encephalogaleo(periosteal)synangiosis. Surgical results for each group were compared in terms of clinical outcomes, neuroimaging changes, extent of revascularization evident on angiograms, and hemodynamic changes evident on SPECT scans. The average follow-up was 45 months for group A and 22 months for group B.

Results.—Overall, group B patients tended to have better clinical outcomes and neuroimaging changes. In terms of SPECT changes of the whole brain after surgery, patients in group B had more favorable outcomes than did group A patients (62% vs 36%). Surgical results for the territory of the anterior cerebral artery were significantly better for group B than for group A with regard to outcomes of anterior cerebral artery symptoms (81% vs 40%), revascularization on angiograms (79% vs 16%), and hemodynamic changes on SPECT scans (70% vs 52%). No significant difference was found between the 2 groups in the incidence of postoperative infarction.

Conclusions.—EDAS with bifrontal encephalogaleo(periosteal)synangiosis is a more effective technique than simple EDAS for the treatment of pediatric moyamoya disease because the former covers both the middle cerebral artery and anterior cerebral artery territories of the brain.

▶ The concept that the more brain you revascularize in MMD the better the clinical outcome makes sense to me. I am glad it worked out this way. The SPECT scan in this article was impressive, but it was also in color, so I could not reproduce it for you.

A. Gottschalk, MD

Metabolic Network Abnormalities in Early Huntington's Disease: An [¹⁸F]FDG PET Study
Feigin A, Leenders KL, Moeller JR, et al (North Shore Univ, Manhasset, New York; Columbia College of Physicians and Surgeons, New York; Groningen Univ, The Netherlands; et al)
J Nucl Med 42:1591-1595, 2001   9–30

Background.—The hereditary neurodegenerative disorder Huntington's disease (HD) is characterized by progressively worsening abnormalities of movement and cognition. PET has been used to identify functional abnormalities in the brains of HD gene carriers preclinically and after symptoms have developed. An important component to increasing our understanding of the pathophysiologic mechanisms of this disorder is the identification of discrete patterns of altered functional brain circuitry in presymptomatic HD gene carriers; these patterns could serve as a biological marker of disease. Abnormal networks of brain regions that are specifically related to the preclinical phase of HD were identified with use of PET imaging of regional cerebral glucose metabolism.

Methods.—A group of 18 presymptomatic HD gene carriers, 13 patients with early-stage HD, and 8 age-matched gene-negative relatives underwent PET scanning with [¹⁸F]FDG to quantify regional glucose use. A network modeling strategy was then applied to the data to identify disease-related regional metabolic covariance patterns in the preclinical group. The main outcome measures were the region weights that defined the metabolic composition of the HD gene carriers and the subject scores quantifying the expression of the pattern in individual research subjects.

Results.—The network analysis showed a significant metabolic covariance pattern that was characterized by caudate and putamental hypometabolism and included mediotemporal metabolic reductions and relative metabolic increases in the occipital cortex. The subject scores for this pattern among the preclinical group were significantly elevated compared with those for the control group. The subject scores for this pattern were also significantly elevated in the early symptomatic group compared with the presymptomatic group.

Conclusions.—FDG PET with network analysis is useful in identifying specific patterns of abnormal brain functioning in individuals with preclinical HD. Findings of discrete patterns of metabolic abnormality in presymptomatic individuals with the HD gene may have applications for the quantification of disease progression during the earliest phases of HD.

▶ If I were asymptomatic but possibly had HD, I am not sure I would want to know whether my condition was in the preclinical stage. Finding out that your life is going to be ruined is not something everyone would gladly volunteer to know. However, once you know it, the possibility of using that knowledge to help monitor any treatment likely to come along or to see how "badly" you were doing could be useful. The PET data seem to fill this niche.

A. Gottschalk, MD

Seizures in Paediatric Chiari Type I Malformation: The Role of Single-Photon Emission Computed Tomography
Iannetti P, Spalice A, Ciccoli CDF, et al ("La Sapienza" Univ, Roma, Italy; Regina Elena Hosp, Roma, Italy)
Acta Paediatr 91:313-317, 2002   9–31

Background.—Chiari malformations are thought to be a pathological continuum of hindbrain maldevelopment characterized by downward herniation of cerebellar tonsils. These malformations have increasingly been identified with the aid of MRI, but little is known of the clinical manifestations of Chiari malformations during childhood. There are 4 types of Chiari malformations, which are referred to as the Chiari complex because they share many common features. The pathogenesis of Chiari malformations is unclear, but different mechanisms, such as traction, hydrocephalus, and maldevelopment, have been suggested. The Chiari I type of malformation is a congenital abnormality in which there is a displacement of deformed cerebral tonsils below the foramen magnum with normal intracranial pressure and no other posterior fossa or supratentorial abnormalities. Different clinical manifestations have been observed in patients with Chiari type I malformation. Seizures have been sporadically signaled in several studies, but since cerebral MRI demonstrated a normal structure, this technique would not appear to aid the clarification of seizure manifestation. SPECT was used in the evaluation of seizures in children with Chiari type I malformation.

Methods.—SPECT studies were performed on 4 patients with epilepsy and Chiari type I malformation to determine the pathogenesis of seizures. There was no cortical structural involvement observed in these children.

Results.—In all 4 patients the area of hypoperfusion on SPECT correlated with EEG focal abnormalities. These hypoperfusions may represent the functional aspect of a cerebral microdysgenesis; thus seizures and EEG epileptic anomalies may be associated to the complex network connection between cortices and cerebellar hemispheres. In 2 patients, a cerebellar hypoperfusion was also detected, indicating a functional or structural involvement.

Conclusions.—This study demonstrated the usefulness of interictal SPECT scans for the clarification of seizures in patients with Chiari type I malformation.

▶ As the authors note, MRI finds many Chiari I malformations that otherwise go undiagnosed. Seizures rarely go undiagnosed. Put the 2 concepts together, and is it fair to ask if the association described above is pure coincidence?

A. Gottschalk, MD

Brain PET and Technetium-99m-ECD SPECT Imaging in Lhermitte-Duclos Disease
Ogasawara K, Yasuda S, Beppu T, et al (Iwate Med Univ, Morioka, Japan)
Neuroradiology 43:993-996, 2001   9–32

Introduction.—Lhermitte-Duclos disease is a rare condition that may be caused by a hamartomatous overgrowth of cerebellar ganglion cells, which replace granular cells and Purkinje cells. Two cases involving patients with Lhermitte-Duclos disease were reported, in which hyperperfusion was identified on cerebral blood flow images obtained by PET, and hyperactivity was identified by technetium-99m-ethyl cysteinate dimer (^{99m}Tc-ECD) SPECT.

Case 1.—Woman, 25, was seen for a 2-month history of occasional headaches. Medical history was otherwise unremarkable, and she was free of neurologic deficits on physical examination. MRI demonstrated the presence of a well-defined lesion with an abnormal laminated pattern of cortical architecture in the right cerebellar hemisphere. There was no apparent enhancement with IV contrast agents. Histologic analysis of surgically excised tissue revealed the classic characteristics of Lhermitte-Duclos disease.

Case 2.—Boy, 17, had a 1-month history of gait impairment. He had exhibited a global developmental delay since childhood. An ataxic gait was observed on neurologic examination. An MRI showed the presence of a well-defined lesion with an abnormal laminated pattern of cortical architecture in the left cerebellar hemisphere that extended to the vermis with no apparent enhancement with IV contrast agents. The mass was resected, and a diagnosis of Lhermitte-Duclos disease was verified.

Imaging Studies.—Brain PET and SPECT were performed preoperatively by using the same procedures in both patients. Regional cerebral blood flow was determined with a 4-ring PET scanner. An autoradiographic approach with 90-second scanning after IV administration of 1110 MBq of ^{15}O-water was used. Patients underwent dynamic and standard ^{99m}Tc-ECD SPECT studies 3 days after PET. The dynamic ^{99m}Tc-ECD SPECT images revealed a plateau of activity in each lesion.

Conclusion.—Lesions in Lhermitte-Duclos disease have a retention mechanism for ^{99m}Tc-ECD similar to that of normal neural tissue.

▶ Finding comparisons of PET and SPECT in the same patients is more difficult than I would like it to be. It should be no surprise that increased blood flow and metabolism go together.

A. Gottschalk, MD

Sturge-Weber Syndrome: Correlation Between Clinical Course and FDG PET Findings

Lee JS, Asano E, Muzik O, et al (Wayne State Univ, Detroit)
Neurology 57:189-195, 2001   9–33

Introduction.—The pathophysiology of Sturge-Weber syndrome (SWS) is not well understood. The clinical severity of seizures and the degree of cognitive, visual, and motor deficits varies greatly with SWS. It is challenging to predict the neurologic outcome for individual patients. The association between the degree and extent of focal asymmetric cortical metabolism on glucose PET and seizure characteristics, cognitive function, and interictal electroencephalogram (EEG) abnormalities was examined in children with unilateral cerebral involvement of SWS and epilepsy.

Methods.—Thirteen children with unilateral SWS, aged 0.7 to 15.1 years, underwent FDG PET. All children were taking antiepileptic medications at the time of PET scanning. Based on asymmetries between homologous cortical areas in FDG-PET images, cortical areas of mildly (10%-20% reduction) and severely (>20% reduction) asymmetric cortical metabolism were determined. These areas were normalized to the size of the ipsilateral hemisphere and correlated with clinical seizure characteristics, full-scale IQ, and abnormal interictal EEG findings.

Results.—Both seizure frequency ($P = .027$) and lifetime number of seizures ($P = .017$) demonstrated a positive relationship with the area (expressed as the percentage of cortical area of ipsilateral hemisphere) of mildly asymmetric cortical metabolism. Patients with higher IQ experienced a shorter duration of epilepsy ($P = .044$) and a greater area of severely asymmetric cortical metabolism ($P = .044$). Patients with bilateral interictal EEG abnormalities had a greater number of lifetime seizures ($P = .042$), lower IQ ($P = .024$), and a smaller region of severely asymmetric cortical metabolism ($P = .019$) compared with those with only ipsilateral EEG abnormalities.

Conclusion.—The correlation between severely asymmetric cortical metabolism and relatively preserved cognitive function in SWS indicates that functional reorganization occurs more readily when the cortex is severely rather than mildly damaged. The area of mildly asymmetric cortical metabolism may have a nociferous influence on the rest of the brain. The extent and degree of glucose asymmetry identified by PET are sensitive markers of seizure severity and cognitive decline in SWS.

▶ In short, the worse the cortical metabolism, the higher the IQ. If that is not contraintuitive, what is?

A. Gottschalk, MD

Analysis of Clinical Brain SPECT Data Based on Anatomic Standardization and Reference to Normal Data: An ROC-Based Comparison of Visual, Semiquantitative, and Voxel-Based Methods
Van Laere KJ, Warwick J, Versijpt J, et al (Ghent Univ, Belgium; Univ of Stellenbosch, Matieland, South Africa)
J Nucl Med 43:458-469, 2002 9–34

Background.—Anatomic standardization and comparison of individual patient studies with normal templates is increasingly used in clinical practice for SPECT of the brain. This technique allows automated, operator-independent volume-of-interest (VOI) or voxel-based analysis of whole-brain data. Such automated assessment of brain perfusion deficits lowers variability across institutions and enhances the consistency of image interpretation independent of reader experience. Among the software packages available to allow automated whole-brain analysis of tomographic functional radionuclide brain scans on the basis of anatomic standardization are statistical parametric mapping (SPM) using SPM99, and brain registration and analysis of SPECT studies (BRASS). SPM99, BRASS, and a predefined VOI approach were compared in the evaluation of SPECT brain perfusion deficits in 2 distinct clinical populations with severe traumatic brain injury and cognitive impairment.

Methods.—A total of 74 persons were studied, including 14 patients with severe, traumatic brain injury (group 1) and 15 patients with cognitive impairment (group 2). Data from these patients were compared with data

FIGURE 3

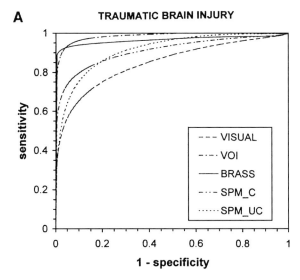

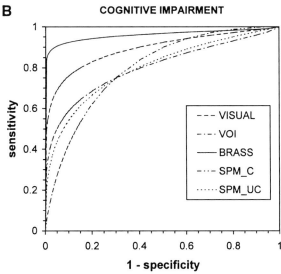

(*Continued*)

FIGURE 3 (cont.)

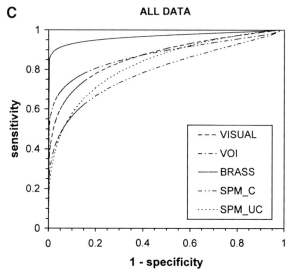

FIGURE 3.—Receiver operating characteristic (ROC) curves for traumatic brain injury (TBI) group (A), cognitive impairment group (B), and total population (C). Curves represent visual scoring, predefined volume-of-interest (*VOI*) analysis, voxel-based region growing (*BRASS*), and statistical parametric mapping (SPM99), both uncorrected (*SPM_UC*) and corrected for multiple comparisons (*SPM_C*). (Reprinted by permission of the Society of Nuclear Medicine, from Van Laere KJ, Warwick J, Versijpt J, et al: Analysis of clinical brain SPECT data based on anatomic standardization and reference to normal data: An ROC-based comparison of visual, semiquantitative, and voxel-based methods. *J Nucl Med* 43:458-469, 2002.)

from, respectively, 25 and 20 age- and sex-adjusted healthy volunteers. All the data were analyzed in 4 ways: with SPM99, BRASS, a predefined VOI approach, and visual analysis based on consensus reading by 3 experienced nuclear medicine physicians. Receiver operating characteristic (ROC) analysis was performed at various statistical cutoffs.

Results.—In both study groups, BRASS voxel-based analysis was most accurate, as defined by the area under the ROC curve (Fig 3). VOI assessment was slightly more accurate than visual consensus analysis, whereas SPM demonstrated a lower area under the ROC curve. SPM analysis was also significantly less sensitive at thresholds corresponding to low false-positive fractions. Regional analysis showed 83% to 92% agreement between all methods.

Conclusions.—The classification of brain SPECT studies can be significantly improved by anatomic standardization techniques and reference to normal data. SPM had a lower sensitivity than VOI or voxelwise region-growing techniques, particularly at low false-positive fractions.

▶ This excellent article emphasizes that brain imaging continues to develop new and interesting techniques. Several methods of analyzing perfusion scans are evaluated in this application of finding perfusion deficits in clinical studies. From an image processing point of view, one would emphasize that software tools (like SPM, VOI analysis, and registration techniques) deliver improved receiver operator charcteristics when compared with visual reading.

I. G. Zubal, PhD

▶ The good news is that these data show diagnosis can be helped by using automated computerized techniques compared with a normal database. The bad news is that the widely used SPM method (these authors used the 1999 version) did not do too well. I could worry about the lack of a gold standard, or the degrees of smoothing used here by SPM, but I think the bottom line is that before you use SPM (or any quantitative aid), try it with phantoms, patients with diagnosis, or whatever, and be sure SPM functions as you need it to.

A. Gottschalk, MD

Transfer of Normal ^{99m}Tc-ECD Brain SPET Databases Between Different Gamma Cameras
Van Laere K, Koole M, Versijpt J, et al (Ghent Univ, Belgium)
Eur J Nucl Med 28:435-449, 2001   9–35

Background.—Advances in methodology and instrumentation are expected to result in more accurate and widespread diagnostic use of brain perfusion SPET. The use of fan-beam collimation has led to improved resolution and sensitivity, allowing the acquisition of technetium (Tc) 99m-labeled radioligands with a resolution of 7 to 8 mm full width at half-maximum, whereas correction algorithms for physical factors that degrade image quality have become commercially available. There has also been much progress toward the automated analysis of functional imaging data involving operator-independent retrospective intramodality as well as intermodality coregistration. A stereotactic, normal perfusion database is imperative for optimal clinical brain SPET. However, accurate transferability of these datasets is necessary for interdepartmental use of normal data. The transfer of 3 normal perfusion databases obtained in the same large population of healthy volunteers who underwent sequential scanning using multihead gamma cameras with different resolution was investigated.

Methods.—The study group comprised 89 healthy adults (46 women and 43 men) age 20 to 81. The participants were screened by history, biochemistry, physical and neurologic examinations, neurophysiologic testing, and MRI. A total of 101 scans were acquired from all participants after injection of 925 MBq Tc 99m-labeled ethyl cysteinate dimer under standard conditions with a triple-head Toshiba GCA-9300A camera. Ninety-one sequential scans were obtained with a dual-head Elscint Helix camera, and 22 participants also underwent imaging with a triple-head Prism 3000. All the images were transferred to the same processing platform and reconstructed by filtered back-projection with the same Butterworth filter and uniform Sorensen attenuation correction. After registration, all participants were automatically reoriented to a stereotactic template by a 9-parameter affine transformation.

Results.—Between-camera reproducibility was 2.5% and 2.7% for the Toshiba camera versus the Helix and the Prism database, respectively. The greatest reduction in between-camera variability was obtained by resolution adjustment in combination with linear washout correction and a Hoffmann phantom-based correction.

Conclusions.—It is possible to accurately achieve the transfer of normal perfusion data between multihead gamma cameras. Widespread interdepartment use of the data is therefore possible, which is likely to have a positive effect on the diagnostic capabilities of clinical brain perfusion SPET.

▶ Good news. But the authors also show that you need to know about and correct for many variables before just accepting a normal brain SPECT database "off the shelf."

A. Gottschalk, MD

Brain Perfusion SPECT: Age- and Sex-Related Effects Correlated With Voxel-Based Morphometric Findings in Healthy Adults
Van Laere KJ, Dierckx RA (Ghent Univ, Belgium)
Radiology 221:810-817, 2001   9–36

Background.—Technological advancements in the instrumentation and analysis software associated with functional brain SPECT have increased the clinical utility of this technique. However, optimal clinical and research analysis sensitivity relies on the detailed characterization of covariate factors such as age and sex, which may affect interindividual physiologic uptakes of technetium 99m (^{99m}Tc)–labeled ethylene cysteine dimer (ECD). Many studies have indicated that aging changes both regional blood flow and glucose metabolism with a specific frontotemporal pattern, but none of these functional topographic studies have included regional structural data in the analysis. This is an important point because both CT and MRI studies have demonstrated an age-related decrease in brain size, an enlargement of cortical sulci, and an increase in the CSF space after age 30 years. Age is, therefore, considered a confounding variable in functional studies. Brain perfusion was investigated with SPECT as a function of age and sex in healthy adult volunteers, and perfusion was correlated with other gray matter concentration determined by the use of voxel-based morphometry (VBM).

Methods.—A group of 81 healthy volunteers underwent both ^{99m}Tc ECD SPECT and 3-dimensional magnetization preparation rapid acquisition gradient-echo MRI. Statistical parametric mapping was used for VBM analysis of the morphological data. These morphological data were compared voxel by voxel with the results of a similar analysis of the perfusion data and were compared more specifically in brain areas that demonstrated significant changes in perfusion.

Results.—VBM data, when compared with perfusion changes, demonstrated a more symmetric age-related decrease in gray matter volume along the Sylvian fissure and in subcortical regions. The combination of functional and structural changes indicated a relatively lower functional decrease with aging compared with the structural atrophy demonstrated in visual, parietal, sensorimotor, and right prefrontal cortices. Significant morphological sex-based differences were observed in the cerebellar and temporal cortices, but no significant differences were found between the functional and morphometric data.

Conclusions.—Age-related changes in perfusion are accompanied by similar, more symmetric changes in gray matter concentration. These changes are more prominent than the perfusion changes observed in some regions. No sex-based differences between perfusion and gray matter concentration were found.

▶ Without this detailed map of the normal aging brain, subtle changes in future functional SPECT studies would be obscured by the subtle changes from the aging and sex differences described above. As I understand it, changes in brain volume (shown on the MRI) were not calculated. This would make these data more precise, but they would be more difficult to use.

A. Gottschalk, MD

10 Cardiovascular Nuclear Medicine

Introduction

This year has seen further refinement of cardiovascular imaging. Though there has been little progress in the development of new radiopharmaceuticals, improvements in techniques and enhanced understanding of the importance of specific scan findings continue to add to the clinical utility of nuclear cardiology. In 2002, more than 700 articles were published about the myocardial perfusion agents, more than 100 on specific applications of gated SPECT, and more than 500 on the detection and quantitation of myocardial ischemia. From this literature, a small sample of 53 important articles was selected for inclusion in this section of the YEAR BOOK. The selected articles include technical points on study performance and patient preparation, such as optimizing patient preparation for viability studies with FDG, as well as new insights into the importance of specific scan findings.

As in previous editions, the combined determination of myocardial perfusion and ventricular function, the mainstay of nuclear cardiology practice, has the largest number of selections. Several articles describe the importance of key observations when perfusion imaging is used in specific circumstances, such as in patients immediately post coronary stent placement. There is further validation of tetrofosmin as a perfusion agent and its value in dual tracer imaging. In addition, there are studies describing the duration of ischemic left ventricular dysfunction, confirmation of the low event rate in patients studied with "stress only" imaging, and the relationship of severe coronary stenosis to the location of myocardial perfusion defects.

Overall, this has been a good year. The coming year promises even more applications of positron imaging. The growth of PET imaging in the community will lead to use of this technology in cardiac patients. Applications of FDG for identifying coronary disease, PET perfusion agents, and the use of PET-CT to define coronary lesions, assure the future growth of nuclear cardiology.

H. William Strauss, MD

Early Prediction of Regional Functional Recovery in Reperfused Myocardium Using Single-Injection Resting Quantitative Electrocardiographic Gated SPET

Kurihara H, Nakamura S, Hatada K, et al (Kansai Med Univ, Osaka, Japan; Kochi Med School, Japan)

Eur J Nucl Med 29:458-464, 2002

10–1

Background.—After an acute myocardial infarction, regional wall motion in reperfused myocardial tissues may not recover for several weeks. Myocardial perfusion and regional function can both be estimated by using quantitative ECG gated single-injection photon emission tomography (SPET) with technetium-99m compounds. The use of resting ECG gated SPET to estimate perfusion and systolic wall thickening patterns allows the classification of pathologic conditions of the myocardium that show differing functional recovery rates after revascularization. This method has not previously been used to predict regional functional recovery after primary percutaneous transluminal coronary angioplasty (PTCA). Its ability to predict improved regional wall motion after successful PTCA was evaluated.

Methods.—Twenty-six patients successfully underwent PTCA, then were evaluated at 3 days and 3 weeks with ECG gated SPET and ^{99m}Tc-tetrofosmin. Regional functional parameters were calculated automatically with a 20-segment model on the third day image. Myocardial segments where there was a perfusion/thickening mismatch were characterized as showing preserved perfusion in the absence of systolic wall thickening.

Results.—For all 20 segments, the average score of regional ^{99m}Tc-tetrofosmin uptake was 70%. Variations were considerable for regional systolic wall thickening, ranging from 17.1% in the basal slice to 51.3% in the midventricular slice, to 66.0% in the apical slice. However, regional wall motion showed relative uniformity from the apex to the base, with mean scores of 7.6 (basal slice), 7.9 (midventricular slice), and 8.4 (apical slice). A moderate but significant correlation was noted between regional systolic wall thickening and wall motion scores throughout the 20 slices. On the third day, the combination of myocardial perfusion and systolic wall thickening characteristics led to 37 segments being classified as mismatched, 41 as matched normal, and 108 as matched abnormal. Systolic wall thickening increased significantly between 3 days and 3 weeks in all areas. After 3 weeks, the regional wall motion score in mismatched segments was significantly higher than that in matched abnormal segments. At the same time, regional wall motion scores were significantly greater for mismatched segments than for matched normal and matched abnormal segments. Wall motion scores improved at 3 weeks for 30% of the segments, with 73% of those with perfusion/thickening mismatching having significant wall motion improvement; only 20% of the matched abnormal segments and 15% of the matched normal segments improved in wall motion scores.

Conclusions.—The recovery of regional wall motion after successful PTCA could be predicted from the early use of the resting ECG gated SPET imaging method with ^{99m}Tc-tetrofosmin.

▶ Three days after PTCA, segments with relative perfusion of greater than 55% of peak normal value and reduced thickening had a higher likelihood of improved function at 3 weeks. Although this report is interesting, it would have been helpful to know the change in perfusion resulting from the PTCA.

H. W. Strauss, MD

Tetrofosmin Imaging in the Detection of Myocardial Viability in Patients With Previous Myocardial Infarction: Comparison With Sestamibi and Tl-201 Scintigraphy

Acampa W, Cuocolo A, Petretta M, et al (Univ Federico II, Napoli, Italy; IRCCS Neuromed, Pozzilli, Italy; IRCCS Ospedale Maggiore, Milano, Italy)
J Nucl Cardiol 9:33-40, 2002   10–2

Background.—The myocardial perfusion agent technetium 99m tetrofosmin has shown the ability to identify patients with coronary artery disease at levels similar to those of thallium 201 and sestamibi. A same-patient comparison of the abilities of tetrofosmin and sestamibi imaging to detect reversible left ventricular (LV) dysfunction has not been accomplished. Patients with previous myocardial infarction were used to compare the efficacy of tetrofosmin, thallium, and sestamibi SPECT at rest.

Methods.—For each of the 17 patients (15 men and 2 women) who had come for coronary revascularization, echocardiography, and SPECT at rest were done at baseline and after 3 months to assess the degree of recovery attained in LV function. Coronary revascularization was performed within 3 weeks of the baseline studies.

Results.—None of the patients had indications of recurrent ischemia. Normal LV function was found in 47% of segments before revascularization, and abnormal wall motion was found in 53%. Functional improvement was found in 39% of the 77 akinetic or dyskinetic segments, and 61% remained nonviable. Tetrofosmin and both thallium and sestamibi uptake were significantly correlated, with even better correlation between the 2 agents labeled with technetium 99m. Mean tracer activity values differed significantly both in segments that improved in function and in those that did not improve. For the improved segments, the uptake of tetrofosmin was 53%, that of sestamibi was 52%, and that of thallium was 61%. In those remaining nonviable, the tetrofosmin uptake was 40%, sestamibi was 39%, and thallium was 46%. For akinetic or dyskinetic segments the best cutoff point to identify reversible LV dysfunction was 60% for thallium activity and 55% for both tetrofosmin and sestamibi. The extent of dysfunctional viable myocardium did not differ significantly between tetrofosmin, sestamibi, and thallium. A significant relationship was noted between probability that akinetic or dyskinetic segments represented viable myocardium and quantitative level of regional tracer activity for the 3 agents (Fig 2). The areas under the receiver operating characteristic curves were 0.74 for tetrofosmin, 0.75 for thallium, and 0.74 for sestamibi activity. Ten regions of the 77 akinetic or dyskinetic segments were discordant, and thallium

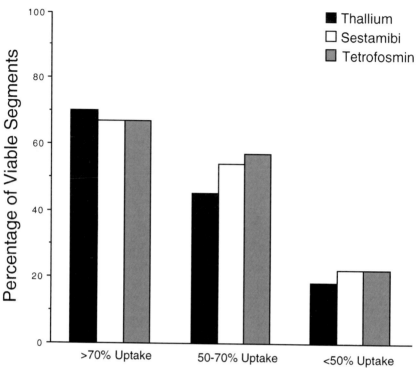

FIGURE 2.—Bar graph showing percentage of akinetic or dyskinetic segments that represent viable myocardium (defined as improved wall motion after revascularization) in normal segments (>70% uptake at quantitative analysis) and in segments with moderate (50%-70% uptake) and severe (<50% uptake) reduction of tracer uptake. The probability of dysfunctional segments at baseline to represent viable myocardium is related to the magnitude of regional activity at quantitative analysis for all tracers. (Courtesy of Acampa W, Cuocolo A, Petretta M, et al: Tetrofosmin imaging in the detection of myocardial viability in patients with previous myocardial infarction: Comparison with sestamibi and Tl-201 scintigraphy. *J Nucl Cardiol* 9:33-40, 2002.)

showed viable myocardium in 4 not detected on tetrofosmin SPECT, 1 of which ultimately showed functional improvement after revascularization. Six regions appeared viable on tetrofosmin but not thallium imaging, and 4 improved functionally after revascularization. Tetrofosmin results were concordant with those of sestamibi in 90% of the regions.

Conclusions.—There was a significant correlation between the tetrofosmin myocardial activity at rest and thallium and sestamibi uptake values in patients who had previous myocardial infarction and impaired LV function. Among these patients, the use of tetrofosmin imaging led to accurate diagnoses at rates comparable with those of redistribution thallium and resting sestamibi SPECT.

▶ In spite of the lower extraction fraction, tetrofosmin imaging compares favorably with sestamibi and thallium for the identification of viable ischemic tissue.

H. W. Strauss, MD

Incremental Prognostic Value of Myocardial SPET With Dual-Isotope Rest ^{201}Tl/Stress ^{99m}Tc-Tetrofosmin

Groutars RGEJ, Verzijlbergen JF, Zwinderman AH, et al (St Antonius Hosp, Nieuwegein, The Netherlands; Univ Hosp, Leiden, The Netherlands)
Eur J Nucl Med 29:46-52, 2002
10–3

Background.—Determining which patients have a high risk and which have a low risk of having a future cardiac event is important to the management of individuals who have or are suspected to have coronary artery disease. Myocardial perfusion scintigraphy has been performed over a 2-day period with excellent prognostic value. Because the 2-day protocol can be difficult for some patients, a 1-day, dual-isotope, rest thallium 201/stress technetium 99m tetrofosmin sestamibi SPET protocol was developed that combines the desirable physiologic attributes of the 2 radionuclides. The prognostic value of the dual-isotope, rest ^{201}Tl/stress ^{99m}Tc-tetrofosmin protocol was evaluated in light of the prognostic value of clinical and exercise variables.

Methods.—The 348 men ranged in age from 27 to 85 years (mean, 60 years), and the 249 women ranged in age from 23 to 84 years (mean, 63 years); all had known or suspected coronary artery disease. Tests included a rest ^{201}Tl study, exercise electrocardiography, and SPET imaging. Postexercise test likelihood of coronary artery disease was calculated based on age, sex, symptoms, and response of the electrocardiographic ST segment. Follow-up lasted a mean of 23 months. A semiquantitative visual analysis was used to express the summed stress score, summed rest score, and summed difference score with a 5-point scoring system.

Results.—During follow-up, 46 hard cardiac events were documented, with 16 deaths from cardiac causes and 30 nonfatal myocardial infarctions. The value with the most predictive power was the postexercise test likelihood of coronary artery disease. Of those undergoing the bicycle exercise test the significant predictors were peak heart rate and percentage of maximal heart rate achieved. On multivariate analysis, the significant independent predictors of hard cardiac events were abnormal SPET results and summed stress score. Patients who had normal scintigraphic results had a low rate of cardiac death and of nonfatal myocardial infarction, whereas those with mild to moderately or severely abnormal results had a significant increase in both cardiac death and nonfatal myocardial infarction. The combined hard cardiac event rate in patients with a low postexercise test likelihood of coronary artery disease of 1.1% per year was significantly lower than that for patients who had intermediate or high postexercise test likelihood of coronary artery disease. A favorable prognosis was found in patients who had normal images; the prognoses for those with mildly to moderately or severely abnormal scintigraphic images were essentially the same.

Conclusions.—The performance of nuclear imaging added incremental prognostic information that is of value in determining the correct management of patients with known or suspected coronary artery disease.

▶ This study demonstrates that tetrofosmin can provide prognostic data similar to sestamibi. The investigators observed 46 events in 597 patients over a 2-year follow-up interval. The event rate correlated with the severity of the perfusion abnormality. The stress imaging data provided more information than the conventional stress test variables. These data confirm the value of perfusion imaging using tetrofosmin for the stress portion of the dual-tracer protocol.

H. W. Strauss, MD

Assessment of Transient Left Ventricular Dilatation on Rest and Exercise on Tc-99m Tetrofosmin Myocardial SPECT
Kinoshita N, Sugihara H, Adachi Y, et al (Kyoto Prefectural Univ, Japan; Matsushita Mem Hosp, Osaka, Japan)
Clin Nucl Med 27:34-39, 2002   10–4

Background.—When multiple vessels are involved in coronary artery disease (CAD), the diagnosis may be difficult on myocardial perfusion imaging. Patients with multiple-vessel disease can be identified if transient left ventricular (LV) dilatation is found on Tl-201 myocardial SPECT. Transient LV dilatation may be detected on exercise myocardial perfusion imaging. The usefulness of Tc-99m tetrofosmin myocardial SPECT in measuring transient LV dilatation as a means of detecting multiple-vessel CAD was investigated.

Methods.—Fifty-five patients with CAD and 20 controls had Tc-99m tetrofosmin myocardial SPECT imaging under conditions of exercise and rest. The exercise images were obtained 30 minutes after the patient received an injection of 370 MBq (10 mCi) of Tc-99m tetrofosmin. An intravenous injection of 740 MBq (20 mCi) of Tc-99m tetrofosmin was administered 210 minutes after the previous injection, and resting images were taken 30 minutes later. The LV transient dilatation index (TDI) was calculated for the apical, middle, and basal myocardial short-axis images.

Results.—At peak exercise the rate-pressure product of the control subjects was significantly higher than that of the patients with CAD. None of the patients with CAD and 40% of the controls reached target heart rate. Angiography showed that 17 patients had single-vessel disease, 25 had 2-vessel disease, and 13 had 3-vessel disease. The degree of stenosis detected in the 165 coronary vessels of the CAD patients was at least 99% in 19 patients, 90% in 37 patients, and 75% in 51 patients. Control subjects had a TDI of 0.970, patients with 1-vessel disease had a TDI of 1.034, patients with 2-vessel disease had a TDI of 1.093, and patients with 3-vessel disease had a TDI of 1.131 (Fig 3). Coronary flow reserve was assessed by using a Doppler guidewire in 18 patients; their TDI correlated with the coronary flow reserve

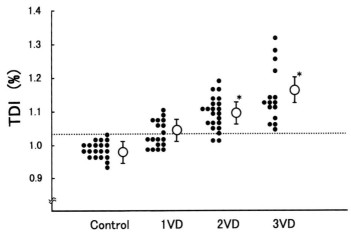

FIGURE 3.—The relation between the transient dilatation index (*TDI*) and the number of narrowed coronary vessels. Mean ± SD values are shown at the right of the individual values for each group. The *dotted line* is the normal upper limit for the TDI. *Asterisk, P* < .01 vs. normal control. *Abbreviations: 1VD,* One-vessel disease; *2VD,* two-vessel disease; *3VD,* three-vessel disease. (Courtesy of Kinoshita N, Sugihara H, Adachi Y, et al: Assessment of transient left ventricular dilatation on rest and exercise on Tc-99m tetrofosmin myocardial SPECT. *Clin Nucl Med* 27:34-39, 2002.

measurement. Assuming that the normal upper limit is equal to the mean plus 2 standard deviations of the TDI in normal persons, the sensitivity of this method for detecting 2- or 3-vessel disease was 91.4%, its specificity was 76.9%, and its accuracy was 84%.

Conclusions.—Determination of the TDI with Tc-99m tetrofosmin SPECT during exercise and rest proved useful in evaluating patients for the presence of multiple-vessel disease. TDI values were significantly higher in patients who had more occluded coronary artery vessels, and obtaining them is easy enough to allow the method to be used routinely for patients who have subendocardial ischemia.

▶ This article demonstrates that early imaging does make a difference. With a 30-minute interval between exercise and SPECT imaging, the authors observed a striking impact of residual ischemia–induced LV dysfunction. Imagine what their results would be if the images were recorded immediately after stress!

H. W. Strauss, MD

Effects of Adjustment for Referral Bias on the Sensitivity and Specificity of Single Photon Emission Computed Tomography for the Diagnosis of Coronary Artery Disease

Miller TD, Hodge DO, Christian TF, et al (Mayo Clinic, Rochester, Minn)
Am J Med 112:290-297, 2002　　　　　　　　　　　　　　　　　10–5

Background.—Referrals for testing are influenced by the results of diagnostic tests, which generally identify 2 populations: those with a normal test result, who are generally not referred, and those with an abnormal result, who are referred. Thus, any evaluation of test performance will underestimate the prevalence of true-negative and false-negative results. Sensitivity is increased and specificity is decreased. Although mathematical formulas have been developed to adjust for referral bias, few studies have used them. The apparent accuracy of stress SPECT imaging in diagnosing coronary artery disease was compared with the test accuracy after correction was made for referral bias.

Methods.—Stress SPECT was used for 14,273 patients with no known coronary artery disease during the course of 10 years. For 1853 patients, coronary angiography was done within 3 months of the stress test. The sensitivity, specificity, and likelihood ratios of SPECT were evaluated; then 2 formulas to eliminate referral bias were used.

Results.—Patients who had angiography tended to be older and male, to carry more risk factors for coronary artery disease, and to have typical angina at greater rates than did patients who did not have angiography. Abnormal SPECT images were found in 6745 patients, but greater evidence of ischemia was present in patients who were referred to undergo angiography. Ninety-seven patients who had normal images also were referred for angiography. Coronary artery disease was found in 76% of the men and 62% of the women referred for angiography. Men also had severe disease (left main involvement, 3 vessels affected, or both) more commonly than women, and severe disease was more common in patients who had pharmacologic stress tests than in those having exercise stress testing. Adjustment for referral bias produced lower sensitivity and higher specificity in all subgroups of patients except men who had pharmacologic Tc-99m sestamibi SPECT with the Diamond method. The effects of adjustment were greater for women than for men. Apparent sensitivity was 98% and specificity was 13%. Adjustment resulted in a sensitivity of 67% and a specificity of 75%.

Conclusions.—The effects of posttest referral bias in test performance are significant. When adjustment is made, the estimate of test performance is more accurate and realistic.

▶ Evaluating diagnostic procedures presents a very complex problem once the procedure has been enrolled in the pantheon of procedures. Once the test is accepted, referral bias will inevitably occur, making it difficult to determine whether improvements in technique really enhance the results. These authors provide 2 approaches to "correct" for referral bias, which may be applied in ongoing evaluations to determine the ongoing utility of the procedure.

H. W. Strauss, MD

Low Event Rate for Stress-Only Perfusion Imaging in Patients Evaluated for Chest Pain
Gibson PB, Demus D, Noto R, et al (Brown Univ, Providence, RI)
J Am Coll Cardiol 39:999-1004, 2002   10–6

Background.—Typically myocardial perfusion SPECT is performed under resting and stress conditions, because attenuation artifacts on the stress images obscure interpretation. Whether testing under the stress condition only with attenuation correction (AC) would be an effective and safe method for evaluating coronary artery disease (CAD) was examined.

Methods.—The subjects were 652 patients (224 men and 428 women; mean age, 52) being evaluated for chest pain. All patients were at low to medium risk of CAD. On the first day of a planned 2-day test, patients underwent stress technetium (Tc) 99m sestamibi SPECT to evaluate cardiac perfusion. A gadolinium (Gd) 153 scanning line source was used for AC. In each case, the stress scan was normal without AC or was normal with AC, and according to protocol the patient did not need to return for testing at rest. Patients were monitored for a mean of 22.3 months to identify occurrences of cardiac death, nonfatal myocardial infarction, and disease progression.

Results.—Of these 652 patients, 409 (63%) had normal stress scans without AC, and 243 (37%) had non-AC images that had significant artifacts; however, all of these latter images corrected completely with AC. During follow-up, there were 2 noncardiac deaths, no cardiac deaths, and 1 nonfatal acute myocardial infarction. Three patients developed unstable chest pain and underwent coronary angiography; all 3 were found to have significant CAD. Thus, the overall cardiac event rate was 0.6% (4 of 652 patients).

Conclusion.—In patients with a low to moderate prescan probability of CAD, stress-only SPECT ^{99m}Tc sestamibi myocardial imaging with AC is effective and safe, and avoids the inconvenience and costs of rest imaging in select patients.

▶ These data suggest that the rest study may be unnecessary in the majority of patients. However, the certainty of diagnosis is increased when rest and stress studies are evaluated on the same patient. An ideal solution would be to develop the techniques to correct for scatter so that a dual-tracer rest/stress study could be recorded with a single data acquisition.

H. W. Strauss, MD

Value of Stress Myocardial Perfusion Single Photon Emission Computed Tomography in Patients With Normal Resting Electrocardiograms: An Evaluation of Incremental Prognostic Value and Cost-effectiveness
Hachamovitch R, Berman DS, Kiat H, et al (Univ of California, Los Angeles; Atlanta Cardiovascular Research Inst, Ga)
Circulation 105:823-829, 2002   10–7

Background.—The use of a modality to assess coronary artery disease (CAD) in specific patient groups must be justified by offering evidence that added value is achieved in the areas of prognostic information, risk stratification, and cost. Stress SPECT has not been evaluated in this respect in comparison with clinical and exercise treadmill testing (ETT) information for patients who have normal resting ECGs, who are usually at lower risk for CAD. Exercise stress myocardial perfusion SPECT was evaluated in patients with normal resting ECG results to determine its incremental prognostic value over pre-SPECT information, its ability to accurately stratify patients according to risk in a clinically relevant way, and its cost-effectiveness as part of a testing strategy.

Methods.—A total of 3058 patients had exercise dual-isotope SPECT. Seventy hard events occurred, specifically 16 cardiac deaths and 58 myocardial infarctions (the 4 patients who had both were only counted as cardiac deaths). Survival analysis and cost-effectiveness determinations were performed.

Results.—Patients who had hard events tended to be significantly older; had previous catheterizations, myocardial infarctions, or percutaneous interventions more frequently; experienced more anginal symptoms; carried more cardiac risk factors; and had a higher pre-ETT likelihood of CAD than those who did not have hard events. Patients who had normal studies had an extremely low hard-event rate of 0.4% annually. Risk increased significantly as a function of the SPECT result, which also significantly stratified patients according to sex and history if previous CAD was present. Women and those without previous CAD had a lower risk than men and patients with previous CAD when a normal stress SPECT result was obtained (Fig 3). Adjusting for pre-SPECT information, an incremental value for the prediction of hard events was found for exercise stress SPECT. For patients who had an intermediate to high risk of CAD after ETT, the cost-effectiveness ratio was $25,134 per hard event detected. With SPECT, 300 patients were correctly reclassified and 138 were incorrectly reclassified. Eliminating the patients who were at low risk after ETT, for each reclassification of patient risk the cost was $5417.

Conclusions.—For predicting adverse events in patients with normal resting ECGs, exercise stress myocardial perfusion SPECT was found to offer incremental prognostic value to the clinical and ETT data obtained. All the clinical risk subgroups showed clinically relevant risk stratification with stress SPECT. For patients with intermediate to high risk of CAD after ETT, SPECT proved to be cost-effective.

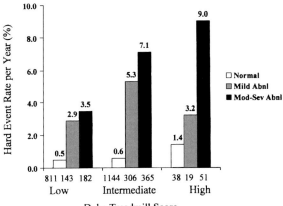

FIGURE 3.—Rates of hard events per year as a function of the result of stress SPECT in patients with low, intermediate, and high Duke treadmill scores groups. *Asterisk, P < .05* across SPECT categories in all Duke treadmill score subgroups. *Abbreviations: Abnl,* Abnormal; *Mod-Sev,* moderately to severely. (Courtesy of Hachamovitch R, Berman DS, Kiat H, et al: Value of stress myocardial perfusion single photon emission computed tomography in patients with normal resting electrocardiograms: An evaluation of incremental prognostic value and cost-effectiveness. *Circulation* 105:823-829, 2002.)

▶ Myocardial perfusion imaging adds important information to that available from exercise testing alone, even in patients with normal ECGs. One feature of this investigation is that even with the predictive power of the perfusion scan, the overall hard event rate in this study was 2% over 1.6 years.

H. W. Strauss, MD

Frequency and Clinical Significance of Myocardial Ischemia Detected Early After Coronary Stent Implantation

Rodés-Cabau J, Candell-Riera J, Domingo E, et al (Hosp Gen Universitari Vall d'Hebron, Barcelona)
J Nucl Med 42:1768-1772, 2001   10–8

Background.—The 30% to 50% incidence of early ischemic defects occurring after successful coronary balloon angioplasty suggests the presence of either a temporary defect in the autoregulation of distal vessels or a local arterial wall spasm at the point of dilatation. Some evaluations suggest that better coronary flow reserve is present after coronary stent implantation than after balloon dilatation because of the larger residual luminal area. The incidence of early ischemic defects after optimal percutaneous transluminal coronary angioplasty (PTCA) with stent placement was evaluated by using simultaneous maximal subjective exercise and ^{99m}Tc-tetrofosmin SPECT. In addition, early detection of ischemic defects after coronary stent implantation was investigated for its ability to predict the occurrence of late restenosis and clinical events.

Methods.—Single-vessel coronary angioplasty with stent implantation was carried out in 30 patients (mean age, 60 years) who had no history of previous myocardial infarction. Coronary angiography and PTCA were done in 19 (63%) of the patients for their unstable angina. After approximately 6 days, maximal-exercise ^{99m}Tc-tetrofosmin SPECT was performed along with dipyridamole if exercise was below optimal levels. Follow-up evaluations were carried out about 8 months later, at which time 77% of the patients had angiography.

Results.—The mean minimal luminal diameter was 0.89 mm and mean stenosis grade was 68.5% before the intervention. These values were 2.82 mm and 9.3% after the intervention. On myocardial SPECT exercise testing, mild or moderate defects in the area of the dilated artery were present in 5 patients; 5 additional patients had mild myocardial perfusion defects distant from the point of dilatation. No differences relating to the angiogram or the procedure were found between these patients and those without defects. Target lesion revascularization was required by 4 patients because of clinical restenosis, but none of the patients died before follow-up. The restenosis rate for those who had ischemic defects and follow-up angiography was 75%; that for patients with no ischemic defects who had follow-up angiography was 16%. Forty percent of patients who had early myocardial defects needed target lesion revascularization, whereas only 8% of those without early ischemic defects required revascularization. No clinical events occurred in the patients who had significant ECG changes during exercise testing. In predicting restenosis, the specificity of maximal-exercise (plus dipyridamole) ^{99m}Tc-tetrofosmin myocardial SPECT performed early after stent implantation was 94%; the sensitivity was 50%; and the positive and negative predictive values were 75% and 84%, respectively. These values were 88%, 50%, 40%, and 92%, respectively, for target lesion revascularization.

Conclusions.—Myocardial perfusion returns to normal in most patients who undergo coronary stent implantation, but although their stent implantation was successful and their angiographic results were good, 17% of those studied had persistent myocardial defects. Detecting these defects early is linked to a high rate of restenosis. Patients who have normal myocardial perfusion results are at low risk for restenosis.

▶ These data suggest that even stent placement does not totally eliminate postprocedure lesions on perfusion scans. However, the follow-up data suggest that those patients with ischemia have a high incidence of restenosis.

H. W. Strauss, MD

Early Detection of Myocardial Ischaemia in the Emergency Department by Rest or Exercise ^{99m}Tc Tracer Myocardial SPET in Patients With Chest Pain and Non-diagnostic ECG
Conti A, Gallini C, Costanzo E, et al (Careggi Gen Hosp, Florence, Italy)
Eur J Nucl Med 28:1806-1810, 2001   10–9

Background.—Patients come to emergency departments (EDs) frequently for the evaluation of chest pain, which generally yields a nondiagnostic

ECG. High costs are incurred in this evaluation, and there remains the risk of missing coronary artery disease (CAD) or acute myocardial infarction. Acute rest myocardial scintigraphy (rest SPET) has been performed because of its high sensitivity, but rest SPET can also underestimate the extent of perfusion deficits or not detect myocardial ischemia when the patient is seen more than 3 hours after the onset of symptoms. Exercise myocardial scintigraphy (exercise SPET) may offer the ability to screen patients within 24 hours of the onset of symptoms. Rest SPET in patients with early presentation at the ED was compared with exercise SPET in patients with delayed presentation. The patients were screened to distinguish those at risk for coronary events, requiring aggressive management, from those at very low risk for coronary events, who can be discharged early.

Methods.—The 231 patients came to the ED within 24 hours of having their first episode of chest pain. They all had a negative first-line evaluation, including ECG, troponins, creatine kinase-MB, and echocardiography, and were considered to be at low risk for short-term coronary events. Patients initially seen within 3 hours of the onset of chest pain were studied with rest SPET; those seen more than 3 hours after the onset of chest pain underwent exercise SPET. Study end points were the angiographic detection of significant CAD, and major coronary events or death from cardiac causes within 6 months.

Results.—Thirty-one percent of patients had myocardial perfusion defects and 15% had CAD. Eighty patients underwent rest SPET and 151 patients had exercise SPET. For 159 patients, the SPET study was negative (48 rest SPET and 111 exercise SPET); 2 of these patients (one in the rest SPET group and one in the exercise SPET group) had a coronary event during follow-up. Of the 72 patients who had positive SPET results (32 rest SPET and 40 exercise SPET), 34 had CAD confirmed, with 18 from the exercise group and 16 from the rest SPET group. No angiographic evidence of coronary stenosis was found in the remaining 38 patients. Thirteen of the 18 patients who had positive exercise SPET and CAD on angiography had normal exercise tolerance tests. However, excercise tolerance testing demonstrated features of myocardial ischemia in 7 patients with a negative scan and negative angiographic results, and exercise SPET scans were positive in 22 patients with no confirming angiographic findings. The number of false-negative results on exercise SPET was less than that with the standard ECG tolerance test, but the proportion of false-positive results was higher.

Conclusions.—Performing an exercise SPET on patients who came for evaluation within 24 hours of the onset of chest pain and had a nondiagnostic ECG yielded the same accuracy as performing a rest SPET in patients who came within 3 hours of the pain's onset. Exercise SPET had a negative predictive value of 99%, so it is particularly useful in screening to exclude coronary heart disease in patients who do not come to the ED immediately. Exercise SPET showed an incremental diagnostic value over the exercise tolerance test that was both significant and clinically important.

▶ The results are impressive. Within 24 hours of an ED visit for chest pain, in a patient considered to have a low likelihood of coronary disease, stress perfusion imaging with bicycle exercise is safe and has a surprisingly high diagnostic yield.

H. W. Strauss, MD

Selective Dual Nuclear Scanning in Low-Risk Patients With Chest Pain to Reliably Identify and Exclude Acute Coronary Syndromes

Fesmire FM, Hughes AD, Stout PK, et al (Univ of Tennessee, Chattanooga)
Ann Emerg Med 38:207-215, 2001
10–10

Background.—Identifying acute coronary syndromes (Acss) in patients seeking emergent care for chest pain is essential. Acute coronary syndromes include acute myocardial infarction, recent myocardial infarction, and unstable angina. The routine use of selective nuclear cardiac scanning in low-risk patients with chest pain during the emergency department evaluation was reported.

Methods.—The prospective observational study included 1775 low-risk patients with chest pain seen over 13 months. All had intermediate- and high-risk Acss excluded by a 2-hour protocol consisting of automated serial 12-lead ECG monitoring along with baseline and 2-hour creatine kinase MB and troponin I measurements. Patients classified as low risk were further categorized as level III, indicating possible ACS, or level IV, probable non-ACS chest pain. Category III patients had immediate dual nuclear scanning, including rest thallium and stress sestamibi scanning. Category IV patients were discharged directly from the emergency department, unless another serious non-ACS condition was suspected. A board-certified radiologist interpreted the rest and stress scans as patient evaluations were completed. Thirty-day follow-up data were obtained.

Findings.—Eight hundred five patients (45.4%) had immediate dual nuclear scanning. The sensitivity and specificity of a positive stress nuclear scan result for 30-day ACS were 97.3% and 87.7%, respectively, compared

TABLE 2.—Thirty-Day Outcome According to 2-Hour Chest Pain Category in the 1775 Study Patients

30-Day Outcome	Category III Patients (n=828) (%)	Category IV Patients (n=947) (%)	*P* Value
AMI on presentation	2 (0.2)	0	.42 (NS)
30-day PTCA	30 (3.6)	1 (0.1)	<.0001
30-day CABG	18 (2.2)	1 (0.1)	.0001
30-day stenosis*	24 (2.9)	0	<.0001
30-day life-threatening complication	4 (0.5)	0	.1 (NS)
30-day death	1 (0.1)	0	.94 (NS)
30-day ACS	74 (9.1)	2 (0.2)	<.0001

*Stenosis 70% or greater not amenable to percutaneous transluminal coronary angioplasty/coronary artery bypass grafting (*PTCA/CABG*).

Abbreviation: NS, Not significant.

(Courtesy of Fesmire FM, Hughes AD, Stout PK, et al: Selective dual nuclear scanning in low-risk patients with chest pain to reliably identify and exclude acute coronary syndromes. *Ann Emerg Med* 38(3):207-215, 2001.)

with 71.2% and 72.6% for a positive resting nuclear scan result. The protocol of selective dual nuclear scanning had sensitivities and specificities of 93.4% and 94.7%, respectively, for 30-day ACS (Table 2).

Conclusion.—Stress nuclear scanning is more sensitive and specific than resting nuclear scanning for detecting ACS in low-risk patients seeking emergency department care for chest pain. After high- and intermediate-risk ACS have been excluded by the 2-hour evaluation, selective dual nuclear scanning reliably identifies and excludes 30-day ACS.

▶ In a population that has ruled out acute myocardial infarction, 74 of 828 (approximately 9%) patients have a positive stress myocardial perfusion scan. The scan has important prognostic information, which confirms that these patients are at high risk for acute events in the next 30 days. Performing the stress myocardial perfusion scan in parallel with the clinical evaluation allows the imaging procedure to play an important role in patient management.

H. W. Strauss, MD

Consideration of Perfusion Reserve in Viability Assessment by Myocardial Tl-201 Rest-Redistribution SPECT: A Quantitative Study With Dual-Isotope SPECT

Paeng JC, Lee DS, Cheon GJ, et al (Seoul Natl Univ, Korea)
J Nucl Cardiol 9:68-74, 2002   10–11

Background.—Hibernating myocardium and chronic stunned myocardium are believed to represent a continuum of disease, in which chronic stunned myocardium has preserved resting perfusion and impaired perfusion initially, but then resting perfusion gradually declines as disease progresses to hibernating myocardium. Myocardial SPECT has shown that delayed redistribution of thallium (Tl) 201 is a significant predictor of myocardial viability. SPECT was used to examine differences in perfusion reserve (ie, difference between perfusion at rest and perfusion during stress) before and after coronary artery bypass grafting (CABG), and to investigate whether delayed Tl-201 redistribution can predict functional improvement according to differences in perfusion.

Methods.—The subjects were 20 patients (17 men and 3 women; mean age, 59) with unstable angina, left ventricular dysfunction, and coronary artery disease. All patients underwent Tl-201 rest-dipyridamole stress technetium (Tc) 99m sestamibi-gated SPECT/Tl-201 24-hour redistribution SPECT before and 3 months after CABG. A 20-segment computer model was used to quantify segmental stress perfusion, rest perfusion, and segmental wall thickening. Perfusion was defined as the average percentage of maximal radiotracer uptake. Perfusion reserve was evaluated by a perfusion difference score (PDS; calculated as rest perfusion minus stress perfusion); thus, a high PDS indicated inducible ischemia, whereas a low PDS reflected little or no inducible ischemia. Viability was defined as a 10% or greater improvement in thickening of dysfunctional segments after CABG. The ability of delayed Tl-201 redistribution to predict viability was examined by receiver operating characteristic (ROC) analysis.

Results.—There were 270 segments subtended by vascular territories undergoing CABG; of these, 109 were dysfunctional. Every parameter examined differed significantly between the dysfunctional and nondysfunctional segments, and before and after CABG. The area under the curve (AUC) in ROC analysis of the overall sensitivity of Tl-201 redistribution in predicting viability was 0.709 (Fig 1). With the use of a cutoff value of 7, 57 of the 109 dysfunctional segments had high PDS, whereas 52 of the segments had low PDS. The ability of delayed Tl-201 redistribution to predict viable myocardium was significantly better in segments with a low PDS (AUC = 0.785) than in those with a high PDS (AUC = 0.582).

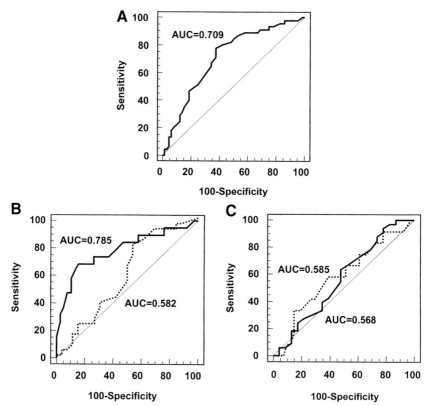

FIGURE 1.—ROC analyses on prediction of viability by Tl-201 redistribution. **A**, Analysis in all dysfunctional segments. **B**, Analysis in the high (*dotted line*) and low (*solid line*) PDS group after classification of dysfunctional segments by PDS of 7, which showed a significant difference in area under the curve (*AUC*). **C**, Analysis in the high (*solid line*) and low (*dotted line*) resting perfusion group after classification of dysfunctional segments by resting perfusion of 50%, which showed no significant difference in AUC. (Courtesy of Paeng JC, Lee DS, Cheon GJ, et al: Consideration of perfusion reserve in viability assessment by myocardial Tl-201 rest-redistribution SPECT: A quantitative study with dual-isotope SPECT. *J Nucl Cardiol* 9:68-74, 2002.)

Conclusion.—The ability of Tl-201 rest-redistribution SPECT to predict viable myocardium after CABG differed according to perfusion reserve. Predictability was significantly better when examining dysfunctional myocardial segments that had a persistent perfusion decrease between rest and stress measures (ie, the low PDS group). Thus, Tl-201 rest-redistribution SPECT would be useful for predicting myocardial viability in patients after CABG who do not have marked stress-induced changes in perfusion.

► Perfusion reserve can be added to the parameters of redistribution and rest perfusion 50% as indicators of viability.

H. W. Strauss, MD

Effect of Primary Coronary Angioplasty on Left Ventricular Function and Myocardial Perfusion as Determined by Tc-99m Sestamibi Scintigraphy
Castro PF, Corbalan R, Baeza R, et al (Hosp Clínico de la Pontificia Universidad Católica de Chile, Santiago)
Am J Cardiol 87:1181-1184, 2001   10–12

Background.—Few data are available about changes in lesion size after acute myocardial infarction (AMI) and the evolution of left ventricular (LV) function over time after primary angioplasty. Evaluation of these parameters may provide additional insight into the mechanisms of myocardial recovery and the possible additional benefits of adjunctive therapy after primary angioplasty. SPECT scintigraphy with technetium 99m–sestamibi can be used to quantify AMI lesion size. Changes in LV function and AMI lesion size were evaluated with SPECT scintigraphy in patients who underwent primary angioplasty to treat AMI. SPECT scintigraphy was performed in these patients at admission and again at 72 hours and 3 months after primary angioplasty.

Methods.—Twenty-four consecutive patients with a first AMI were included in the study. The diagnosis of AMI was made on the basis of the classic criteria of chest pain and ST-segment elevation (≥ 1 mm in 2 or more contiguous ECG leads). All patients were seen within 6 hours of the onset of chest pain. The patients received 740 to 1110 MBq IV bolus doses of ^{99m}Tc-sestamibi before primary angioplasty and during the chest pain episode. SPECT was performed within 6 hours after primary angioplasty. Resting ^{99m}Tc-sestamibi injection and imaging were repeated at 72 hours and 3 months after primary angioplasty. LV volume, LV ejection fraction (LVEF), and size of the uptake defect were determined in the short axis, long horizontal axis, and bull's-eye images in all studies.

Results.—The mean time to satisfactory coronary patency was 4.1 ± 2.4 hours from onset of symptoms. Primary angioplasty was successful in all but 2 patients (92%), and 14 patients (58%) underwent stent implantation. β-blockers were used in 75% of patients, and angiotensin converting enzyme (ACE) inhibitors in 37%. There was a significant increase in LVEF at 3 months (50% $\pm$ 10%), but no differences in LVEF between baseline and 72

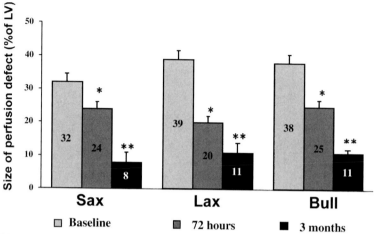

FIGURE 4.—Change in time in the size of the perfusion defect of the left ventricle after primary angioplasty. This is expressed as a percentage of the total left ventricular mass in the short axis (*Sax*), long horizontal axis (*Lax*), and bull's-eye (*Bull*). The size of the defect decreased significantly at 72 hours. *$P < .05$ compared with baseline and at 3 months. **$P < .05$ compared with baseline. (Reprinted from *American Journal of Cardiology*, from Castro PF, Corbalan R, Baeza R, et al: Effect of primary coronary angioplasty on left ventricular function and myocardial perfusion as determined by Tc-99m sestamibi scintigraphy. *Am J Cardiol* 87:1181-1184, 2001. Copyright 2001 with permission from Excerpta Medica, Inc.).

hours. A significant reduction in size of the myocardial perfusion defect was found at 72 hours after primary angioplasty, and an even greater reduction after 3 months (Fig 4). Average myocardial salvage at 72 hours was 30% of the area of risk, and increased to 65% at 3 months. The correlation between LVEF and myocardial defect size was similar at baseline, 72 hours, and 3 months. The increase in LVEF from baseline to 3 months was similar in patients who did and did not receive ACE inhibitors.

Conclusions.—Primary angioplasty is associated with reduction in myocardial perfusion defect size within the first few days, and even greater reduction at 3 months. LV function improves significantly over time, in association with a progressive decrease in LV volume and favorable LV remodeling.

▶ Recovery of perfusion and function following prolonged myocardial ischemia can take months. The reduction in lesion size can be attributed to both a gradual return of perfusion and scar formation, with shrinkage of the lesion. The result is a modest improvement in global function and a striking reduction in lesion size.

H. W. Strauss, MD

Absolute Quantification of Regional Myocardial Uptake of 99mTc-Sestamibi With SPECT: Experimental Validation in a Porcine Model

Da Silva AJ, Tang HR, Wong KH, et al (Univ of California, San Francisco; Univ of California, Berkeley)

J Nucl Med 42:772-779, 2001   10–13

Background.—SPECT imaging has been used for 2 decades in the noninvasive study of myocardial perfusion. Current techniques for the assessment of myocardial perfusion studies rely mainly on visual interpretation and an analysis of relative tracer activity within the myocardial regions defined by an individual SPECT study. There are limitations, however, to making only a relative measurement of the radionuclide distribution. The ultimate goal is to obtain absolute quantification, an absolute measurement of becquerels of tracer per gram of tissue in a specified region of the left ventricular myocardium. A method for making absolute in vivo quantification of 99mTc-sestamibi uptake in myocardium in a porcine model is described.

Methods.—Correlated CT and radionuclide images were obtained from 8 adult pigs with a combined CT-SPECT imaging system (Fig 6). In each case, the CT image was used to generate an object-specific attenuation map.

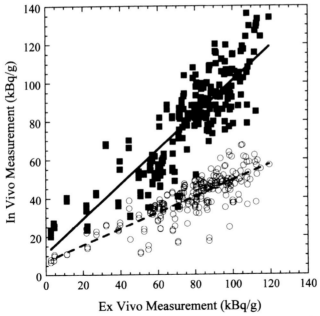

Ex Vivo Measurement (kBq/g)

FIGURE 6.—In vivo versus ex vivo activity concentration measurement for 8 pigs included in study. *White circles* indicate activity concentration measured in every myocardial segment with only attenuation correction applied. *Dashed line* is least-squares linear fit to data with slope of 0.421 and offset of 7.09 kBq/g (*r* = 0.821). *Black squares* indicate activity concentration measured in every myocardial segment with both attenuation and partial-volume corrections applied. *Solid line* is least-squares linear fit to data with slope of 0.901 and offset of 11.17 kBq/g (*r* = 0.863). (Reprinted by permission of the Society of Nuclear Medicine, from Da Silva AJ, Tang HR, Wong KH, et al: Absolute quantification of regional myocardial uptake of 99mTc-sestamibi with SPECT: experimental validation in a porcine model. *J Nucl Med* 42:772-779, 2001.)

This attenuation map was then incorporated into an iterative algorithm, which was used for the reconstruction and attenuation correction of the radionuclide image. Anatomical data obtained from the correlated CT image was used to correct for partial-volume errors in the radionuclide image by mathematical modeling of the radionuclide imaging process. A template that approximated the geometric extent of the myocardium was defined from the CT image. The template was projected with a realistic physical model of the radionuclide imaging process, including nonideal collimation and object-specific attenuation, and was then reconstructed. The reconstruction of the template yielded a pixel-by-pixel partial-volume correction for the myocardium in the radionuclide image. The anatomical boundaries of the myocardium were determined with the CT image for quantification of the radionuclide images. Finally, the pixel intensities in the corrected radionuclide images were calibrated in activity concentration (MBq/g) and compared with the ex-vivo activity concentration measured in the excised myocardium.

Results.—Before correction, the in vivo activity concentration in the pig myocardium was measured at only 10% of the true value. After correction for object-specific attenuation, accuracy of this measurement improved but was only 42% of the true value. When correction was made for both attenuation and partial-volume errors, however, absolute quantification with an accuracy error of approximately 10% was obtained.

Conclusions.—In a porcine model, the application of object-specific attenuation corrections and appropriate partial volume corrections enables the accurate determination of absolute regional activity concentration in the myocardium.

▶ The investigators clearly demonstrate the importance of measuring attenuation and correcting for partial volume as key components to the calculation of absolute myocardial uptake. When this problem is solved, we will minimize false-negative perfusion scans and eliminate attenuation artifacts.

H. W. Strauss, MD

Relationship Between the Location of the Most Severe Myocardial Perfusion Defects, the Most Severe Coronary Artery Stenosis, and the Site of Subsequent Myocardial Infarction
Candell-Riera J, Pereztol-Valdés O, Santana-Boado C, et al (Hosp Universitari Vall d'Hebron, Barcelona)
J Nucl Med 42:558-563, 2001   10–14

Background.—The findings of some angiographic studies have suggested that the correlation between the site of acute myocardial infarction (AMI) and the severity of preexisting anatomical coronary artery disease is not high. The conclusion of these studies has been that non–flow-limiting stenoses are a common site of subsequent plaque rupture and thrombotic occlusion. Other studies using myocardial perfusion SPECT have demon-

SPECT-AMI (n=31)

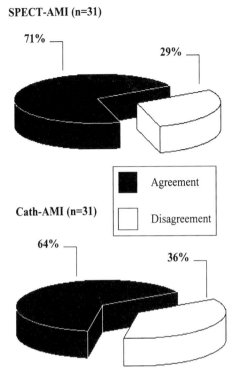

FIGURE 1.—Agreement between site of most severe reversible defects detected by SPECT, most severe stenosis detected by coronary angiography, and subsequent AMI location. *Abbreviation: Cath,* Catheterization. (Reprinted by the Society of Nuclear Medicine, from Candell-Riera J, Pereztol-Valdés O, Santana-Boado C, et al: Relationship between the location of the most severe myocardial perfusion defects, the most severe coronary artery stenosis, and the site of subsequent myocardial infarction. *J Nucl Med* 42:558-563, 2001.)

strated a similar correlation between the location of the perfusion defects and the site of the subsequent AMI. These differences may possibly be attributable to a poor relationship between the anatomical descriptors of coronary lesions and the hemodynamic effects on coronary blood flow. The results, however, can be influenced by other factors, such as the time between imaging and infarction, the severity of coronary artery disease, or the presence of previous acute coronary syndromes. The relationship between the location of the most severe myocardial perfusion defects, the most severe coronary artery stenosis, and the site of subsequent AMI was assessed.

Methods.—From a population of 3180 patients who were admitted with a diagnosis of AMI, a group of 44 patients were identified who had undergone previous myocardial perfusion SPECT. The findings in these patients were evaluated to determine the relationship between the location of the perfusion defect, the coronary artery stenosis, and the site of subsequent AMI.

Results.—A concordance of 71% was obtained between the location of the most severe reversible defects detected by SPECT and the site of subsequent AMI, and a concordance of 64% was realized between the most severe stenosis detected by coronary angiography and the site of subsequent AMI. However, good κ values were obtained for SPECT and coronary angiography when the interval between these investigations and subsequent AMI was more than 3 months for moderate-to-severe perfusion defects, and for 90% to 99% coronary stenosis (Fig 1).

Conclusions.—These findings demonstrated that the culprit lesion is not always the lesion that is identified by the most severe reversible perfusion defect or the most critical coronary artery stenosis. Myocardial SPECT can predict the location of a future AMI in 71% of patients, and coronary angiography can predict the location of a future AMI in 64% of patients. Performance is improved, however, when the period between investigations and subsequent AMI is more than 3 months for patients with moderate-to-severe perfusion defects and for patients with 90% to 99% coronary stenosis.

▶ The investigators' 3-way comparison demonstrated a good correlation between the most severe angiographic lesion and the site of infarction, but a better correlation between the perfusion scan and the site of infarction. One possible reason for the higher correlation with SPECT is the potential that vulnerable plaque, which may not cause significant stenosis (and may be considered insignificant angiographically), causes abnormal vasoreactivity (which causes a perfusion abnormality).

H. W. Strauss, MD

Time Course Evaluation of Myocardial Perfusion After Reperfusion Therapy by ^{99m}Tc-Tetrofosmin SPECT in Patients With Acute Myocardial Infarction
Tanaka R, Nakamura T (Kushiroshi Ishikai Hosp, Hokkaido, Japan)
J Nucl Med 42:1351-1358, 2001   10–15

Background.—The extent of myocardial salvage can be underestimated when myocardial perfusion imaging with ^{99m}Tc-labeled agents is used immediately after reperfusion therapy. It is also possible that delayed imaging is useful for assessment of the area at risk. Few previous studies have sequentially evaluated these image changes. ^{99m}Tc-tetrofosmin (TF) and ^{123}I-β-methyl-p-iodophenylpentadecanoic acid (BMIPP) SPECT were used before and after reperfusion for the treatment of acute myocardial infarction. The changes in TF myocardial accumulation and reverse redistribution were then quantified and assessed.

Methods.—Reperfusion was successfully performed in 17 patients with a first myocardial infarction. Investigators evaluated the SPECT images that were obtained at the onset (preimage), at 30 minutes (early image), and 6 hours (delayed image) after TF injection as well as the images that were acquired at 1, 4, 7, and 20 days after reperfusion (post–1-day, post–4-days, post–7-days, and post–20-days image, respectively). BMIPP SPECT images obtained after a mean of 7 days were also examined. Polar maps were divided into 48 segments so that percentage uptake could be calculated. Time course changes in segment numbers below 60% were observed as abnormal area. In addition, cardiac function was analyzed by gated TF SPECT on day 1 and day 20 after reperfusion.

Results.—With respect to the abnormal area seen in the early images, significant improvement was noted in the post–1-day image compared with the preimage. This was also the case with the post–7-days image compared with the post–1-day and post–4-days images. No significant differences were noted, however, between the post–20-days and post–7-days images, which indicates that the improvement of myocardial accumulation reaches a plateau at 7 days after perfusion. In contrast, the abnormal area on the delayed images was much greater in comparison with the abnormal area seen on early images from 4 to 20 days after reperfusion. A very close correlation was observed between the BMIPP image and both the preimage and the post–7-days image.

Conclusions.—The findings in this study suggest that the optimal interval between reperfusion therapy and TF SPECT is 7 days for the evaluation of the salvage effect. Both TF delayed and BMIPP images are useful for estimating the risk area.

▶ MI patients with early successful reperfusion have a significant reduction in lesion extent over the first 20 days. Two potential explanations for this observation are (1) a reduction of edema, resulting in improved peri-infarct perfusion; or (2) scar formation with reduction of lesion extent. The improvement in wall motion suggests that the first explanation is more likely to be correct.

H. W. Strauss, MD

Comparison of 2-Dimensional and 3-Dimensional Cardiac [82]Rb PET Studies
Votaw JR, White M (Emory Univ, Atlanta, Ga)
J Nucl Med 42:701-706, 2001   10–16

Background.—Myocardial perfusion imaging with [82]Rb has been well established for 2-dimensional (2D) PET. The continued development of newer scanners, however, has prompted interest in the effectiveness of [82]Rb when imaged with 3-dimensional (3D) PET. The need for investigation of this potential use of 3D [82]Rb studies has become more urgent as many state-of-the-art scanners are now being sold only with 3D capability. The 3D mode offers the advantage of collecting many more lines of response, which means that less radioactivity is injected into the patient, reducing both the radiation exposure and the amount of [82]Rb needed. A comparison of the results of 2D and 3D data collection for [82]Rb cardiac studies using the ECAT EXACT scanner was made.

Methods.—The study included 33 consecutive patients who underwent resting [82]Rb cardiac studies. The images were then evaluated by 4 experienced physicians, who rated the images to determine if the different acquisition methods would lead to different patient care. A separate quantitative

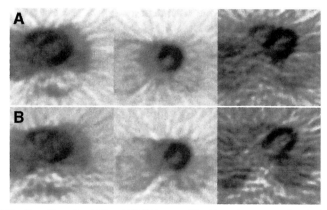

FIGURE 1.—Two-dimensional (**A**) and 3D (**B**) images of 3 subjects show range of results. Left pair represents better-than-average agreement between 2D and 3D scans of 73-kg male with major defect. Note, however, that septal wall is decreased and apex is noisier in 3D study. Middle pair is from 60-kg female and represents best agreement between 2D and 3D scans. Right pair is from 125-kg male. Both images are noisy, but apex is decreased in 3D study. (Reprinted by permission of the Society of Nuclear Medicine, from Votaw JR, White M: Comparison of 2-dimensional and 3-dimensional cardiac ^{82}Rb PET studies. *J Nucl Med* 42:701-706, 2001.)

analysis was performed on data from multiple scans of a thoracic phantom, which was filled to simulate cardiac and background radioactivity corresponding to ^{82}Rb injections ranging from 37 to 1740 MBq.

Results.—Differences between the 2D and 3D studies were significant, with the image quality of the 3D studies being much poorer than the quality of the 2D studies (Fig 1). The scanner collected data at a near-maximal counting rate for 1480-MBq or 37-MBq acquisitions. The 2D acquisitions yielded more detected true events and had a better signal-to-noise ratio, because the data collection is limited by the counting rate in either mode, and more random and scatter events occur in the 3D mode.

Conclusions.—The 2D mode should be used to perform cardiac ^{82}Rb studies with the ECAT EXACT scanner.

▶ PET scanners operating in 2D mode have a lower incidence of random coincident events, which results in higher contrast in the image. However, the 2D mode is associated with lower sensitivity than the 3D mode, requiring either a higher administered dose or longer imaging times to record images of similar count density. Imaging tracers have a short half-life in 3D mode and this presents a substantial challenge. This study confirms that clinically useful data can be recorded in 3D mode with a reduced administered dose of ^{82}Rb. This observation is particularly important, since the new combined PET/CT machines are designed to operate primarily in the 3D mode.

H. W. Strauss, MD

Reduced Myocardial Flow Reserve in Anatomically Normal Coronary Arteries Due to Elevated Baseline Myocardial Blood Flow in Men with Old Myocardial Infarction
Yonekura K, Yokoyama I, Ohtake T, et al (Univ of Toyko)
J Nucl Cardiol 9:62-67, 2002   10–17

Background.—Declines in myocardial flow reserve (MFR) occur in relation to the severity of coronary stenosis but cannot be accurately depicted with conventional angiography. Patients with coronary artery disease may have reduced myocardial blood flow (MBF) in areas supplied by either stenosed or angiographically normal arteries. Patients who have old myocardial infarction (OMI) may also show reduced MFR in normal arteries through undetermined mechanisms. The factors that produce reductions in MFR among patients with OMI were sought, and a comparison was made between them and those present in patients with angina pectoris (AP).

Methods.—The study group consisted of 13 men with AP, 18 men with OMI, and 15 age-matched control subjects, also men. Baseline MBF and MBF during dipyridamole administration were determined by using nitrogen 13 ammonia PET, and the MFR was calculated and compared in areas perfused by nonstenotic arteries.

Results.—Control subjects and patients with AP had significantly lower baseline MBF values than patients with OMI. MBF values during dipyridamole administration were comparable between the two patient groups but significantly lower in the controls. Compared with patients with AP, patients with OMI had significantly decreased ejection fraction and significantly higher left ventricular end-systolic volume index and left ventricular end-diastolic volume index. The additive effects of underlying coronary risk factors were revealed by rating the various factors; results were comparable between the two patient groups. Considering baseline MBF, MBF during dipyridamole administration, ejection fraction, left ventricular end-systolic volume index, left ventricular end-diastolic volume index, blood pressure, cardiac index, wall stress, plasma lipid concentration, hemoglobin A1c level, single- versus multiple-vessel disease, and age, the baseline MBF and ejection fraction were significant factors for the compromised MFR. Analysis revealed ejection fraction to be the most important factor for increased baseline MBF and reduced MFR.

Conclusions.—Patients with OMI had decreased MFR in anatomically normal coronary arteries, and a significant relationship was found between reduced MFR and elevated baseline MBF in these patients when compared with patients with AP. The combination of elevated baseline MBF and decreased ejection fraction played a significant role in the reduction of MFR in patients with OMI and AP.

▶ This study demonstrates a remarkable reduction in flow reserve in nonstenotic vessels of patients with old infarction compared with subjects with angina and compared with normal subjects. The slight elevation of resting perfusion in patients with OMI could be attributable to the compensatory increase in function of the noninfarcted myocardium. A potential confounding problem with this study is the elevation of blood sugar in the OMI group, which suggests the presence of diabetes with its known impairment of vasoreactivity.

H. W. Strauss, MD

Reverse Redistribution on Exercise-Redistribution ^{201}Tl SPECT in Chronic Ischemic Dysfunction: Predictive of Functional Outcome After Revascularization?
Roelants VA, Vanoverschelde J-LJ, Vander Borght TM, et al (Université Catholique de Louvain, Brussels, Belgium; Université Catholique de Louvain, Yvoir, Belgium)
J Nucl Med 43:621-627, 2002   10–18

Background.—Various clinical conditions and imaging protocols produce reverse redistribution (RR), which consists of a worsening perfusion defect or a new perfusion defect on redistribution images obtained with ^{201}Tl scintigraphy. Its clinical significance on stress-redistribution ^{201}Tl SPECT for patients with coronary artery disease is not clear. Whether RR occurring on stress-redistribution ^{201}Tl SPECT images predicts functional outcome after revascularization and whether ^{201}Tl reinjection differentiates viable and nonviable myocardium in RR segments were evaluated.

Methods.—The 62 men and 11 women studied (mean age, 59 years; range, 35-74 years) had chronic coronary artery disease and were scheduled to undergo coronary revascularization. Within 10 minutes of completing a symptom-limited multistep dynamic bicycle exercise test, SPECT images were obtained. Two-dimensional echocardiograms taken before and a mean of 5.5 months after revascularization determined recovery of left ventricular systolic function. Radionuclide ventriculography was also performed. The appearance of a new defect (RR-A pattern) or worsening of a defect apparent on the poststress image (RR-B pattern) was confirmed by a fall of at least 10% on the corresponding circumferential profile (Fig 1). For ^{201}Tl uptake and wall motion analyses, the left ventricle was subdivided into 16 segments.

Results.—Eighteen patients (25%) exhibited RR in 39 segments (3.3% of total). All patients had a reduction in luminal diameter of at least 50% in at least one major vessel, classified as significant coronary stenosis. The proportion of patients who had experienced a myocardial infarction was higher for the RR group than for those not having RR. The ^{201}Tl stress-redistribution study showed RR patients had significantly fewer ischemic segments than non-RR patients. For the non-RR segments of the RR group, poststress uptake was significantly higher than in those of the non-RR group. For RR segments, ^{201}Tl uptake was significantly higher than in non-RR segments and in the normal and dysfunctional regions of non-RR patients. Most of the RR segments followed the RR-B pattern. In RR patients, functional recovery occurred in 8 of 13 dysfunctional RR segments and in 52 of 154 dysfunctional segments without RR, indicating that the RR segments contribute negligibly to functional recovery after revascularization. Defining viability as a mean

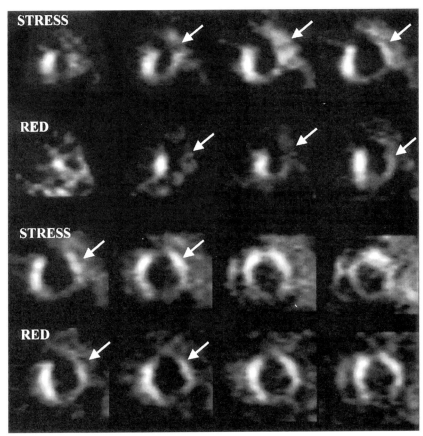

FIGURE 1.—Stress-redistribution ^{201}Tl SPECT: short-axis slices from apex (**upper left corner**) to base (**lower right corner**). *Arrows* indicate regions where RR can be observed (ie, lateral wall). *Abbreviation: RED*, Redistribution. (Reprinted by permission of the Society of Nuclear Medicine, from Roelants VA, Vanoverschelde J-LJ, Vander Borght TM, et al: Reverse redistribution on exercise-redistribution ^{201}Tl SPECT in chronic ischemic dysfunction: Predictive of functional outcome after revascularization? *J Nucl Med* 43:621-627, 2002.)

[201]Tl uptake of more than 54% at reinjection, viable myocardium was detected with a sensitivity of 87%, a specificity of 60%, and an accuracy of 77% in RR segments. For non-RR segments, these values were 75%, 52%, and 60%, respectively, whereas for non-RR patients the values were 72%, 55%, and 62%, respectively. Thirty-four of the 154 dysfunctional segments in the RR group had redistribution, which carried a predictive for outcome sensitivity of 56%, a specificity of 55%, and an accuracy of 55%. Only viable segments showed reinjection uptakes differing significantly from redistribution uptakes. Any artifactual cause of RR was excluded in all but one segment.

Conclusions.—RR on exercise-redistribution ^{201}Tl SPECT studies is found in areas with normal and abnormal wall motion. Dysfunctional segments with RR also often have viable myocardium, but the contribution of this viable tissue to improved function is minimal. RR occurring on ^{201}Tl SPECT is not an artifact, occurring only rarely in myocardium that is functioning normally and in dysfunctional myocardium.

▶ RR is a rare phenomenon, which can be caused by technical problems. It likely does have a physiologic meaning, but it is often difficult to know if the changes seen are real.

H. W. Strauss, MD

Arbutamine Stress Perfusion Imaging in Dogs With Critical Coronary Artery Stenoses: ^{99m}Tc-Sestamibi versus ^{201}Tl
Ruiz M, Takehana K, Petruzella FD, et al (Univ of Virginia, Charlottesville)
J Nucl Med 43:664-670, 2002   10–19

Background.—When patients who require cardiac stress testing cannot exercise adequately, pharmacologic stress imaging nay be substituted. Either a vasodilator or an inotropic agent can be used. When dobutamine is given simultaneously with ^{99m}Tc-methoxyisobutylisonitrile (sestamibi [MIBI]), MIBI uptake in normal myocardium may be reduced. Arbutamine has less inotropic effect than dobutamine and may reduce the MIBI uptake less and improve contrast results, thus reflecting stenosis severity and abnormal flow reserve more accurately.

Methods.—Eight open-chest dogs with critical coronary stenoses that eliminated flow reserve underwent infusions of 0.5 to 250 ng/kg per minute of arbutamine. When peak arbutamine effect was achieved, MIBI, ^{201}Tl, and sodium microspheres were coinjected. After 5 minutes, the dogs were killed and determinations were made of MIBI activity and myocardial blood flow. Heart slices were imaged ex vivo.

Results.—Significant increases were produced by the arbutamine in mean heart rate, peak positive left ventricular pressure and its first time-derivative, and thickening of the myocardium in the normal zone. Flow in the stenotic zone and thickening there did not increase. A lower mean stenotic-to-normal ratio for myocardial flow was associated with greater heterogeneity in flow or MIBI and ^{201}Tl activity between the 2 zones. MIBI activity ratios underestimated the flow disparity at injection significantly. At peak arbutamine stress, the defect count ratios for ^{201}Tl exceeded those for MIBI. The defects appearing on ^{201}Tl images were markedly greater in magnitude (Fig 4). The flow-^{201}Tl uptake link during arbutamine stress is more favorable than the flow-MIBI association.

Conclusions.—Arbutamine-induced flow heterogeneity between normal and stenotic regions was notably underestimated with both ^{201}Tl and MIBI, but the MIBI showed a greater degree of underestimation. The effect of arbutamine-induced hyperemia in normal myocardium was underestimated with MIBI uptake to the same degree as that shown with dobutamine. The physiologic severity of coronary stenoses is thus underestimated by MIBI uptake with arbutamine-induced stress, with the possibility that mild

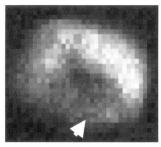 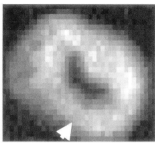

²⁰¹Thallium   Sestamibi
(0.49)   (0.79)

FIGURE 4.—Ex vivo images from representative dog. *Arrows* indicate location of ²⁰¹ Tl and ⁹⁹ᵐTc-MIBI perfusion defects. *Numbers in parentheses* below each image are stenotic-to-normal defect count ratios. (Reprinted by permission of the Society of Nuclear Medicine, from Ruiz M, Takehana K, Petruzella FD, et al: Arbutamine stress perfusion imaging in dogs with critical coronary artery stenoses: ⁹⁹ᵐTc-sestamibi versus ²⁰¹Tl. *J Nucl Med* 43:664-670, 2002.)

stenoses may be missed with either arbutamine or dobutamine. ²⁰¹Tl produced less underestimation and thus offers better accuracy.

▶ Technetium-labeled perfusion agents do not provide the same contrast as thallium. This is an important point to keep in mind when interpreting subtle lesions.

H. W. Strauss, MD

Assessment of Residual Coronary Stenoses Using ⁹⁹ᵐTc-N-NOET Vasodilator Stress Imaging to Evaluate Coronary Flow Reserve Early After Coronary Reperfusion in a Canine Model of Subendocardial Infarction
Takehana K, Beller GA, Ruiz M, et al (Univ of Virginia, Charlottesville)
J Nucl Med 42:1388-1394, 2001   10–20

Background.—Reperfusion after recanalization therapy for acute MI is often incomplete because of the presence of residual stenoses in the infarct-related artery. The detection of mild-to-moderate stenoses necessitates the assessment of coronary flow reserve with vasodilator stress. A new neutral lipophilic myocardial imaging agent, ⁹⁹ᵐTc-(N-ethoxy-N-ethyl-dithiocarbamato)nitrido (N-NOET), is a viability-independent flow tracer that may be useful in the assessment of coronary flow reserve in the acute phase of reperfusion. This potential application of ⁹⁹ᵐTc-N-NOET vasodilator stress imaging was evaluated in a canine model.

Methods.—In 12 open-chest dogs, 60 minutes of total left anterior descending artery (LAD) occlusion was followed by either full reperfusion (group 1, 4 dogs) or reperfusion through a residual critical stenosis (group 2, 8 dogs). ⁹⁹ᵐTc-N-NOET was administered during peak vasodilator stress at 165 minutes after reperfusion, and initial and 60-minute delayed images

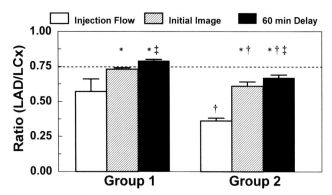

FIGURE 2.—Comparison of mean LAD/LCx defect count ratio obtained from background-subtracted in vivo images. Transmural myocardial blood flow ratio at time when ^{99m}Tc-N-NOET was administered during vasodilator stress is superimposed for comparison. Note that initial and 60-minute delayed defect count ratios were significantly less in group 2 dogs with residual stenoses than those in group 1 dogs with no stenoses, reflecting greater diminution in coronary flow reserve preserved in group 2 dogs. *$P < .05$ vs injection flow ratio; †$P < .01$ vs group 1; ‡$P < .05$ vs initial image. *Abbreviations: LAD,* Left anterior descending coronary artery; *LCx,* left circumflex coronary artery. (Reprinted by the Society of Nuclear Medicine, from Takehana K, Beller GA, Ruiz M, et al: Assessment of residual coronary stenoses using ^{99m}Tc-N-NOET vasodilator stress imaging to evaluate coronary flow reserve early after coronary reperfusion in a canine model of subendocardial infarction. *J Nucl Med* 42:1388-1394, 2001.)

were obtained. Radiolabeled microspheres were used to assess regional blood flow.

Results.—Infarct size was similar in both groups of dogs (9% and 8%, respectively), but the 2 groups were differentiated by both initial and 60-minute defect count ratios, which reflected the greater diminution in coronary flow reserve in the dogs that underwent reperfusion through residual critical stenosis (Fig 2). Of particular interest was the finding that coronary flow reserve in the reperfused zone of dogs that underwent full reperfusion was diminished despite the absence of a stenosis. As a result, a less-than-expected difference in ^{99m}Tc-N-NOET uptake was noted between the 2 groups.

Conclusions.—^{99m}Tc-N-NOET imaging can detect residual coronary stenoses in a canine model of myocardial infarction with some coronary flow reserve preservation. However, in settings of more prolonged occlusion that results in more severe endothelial or microvascular dysfunction, it may be difficult to differentiate varying degrees of vessel patency with any coronary flow reserve technique.

▶ ^{99m}Tc-N-NOET is a perfusion agent with high myocardial extraction, making it a better imaging agent for use with vasodilators. The data demonstrate the ability of the tracer to identify the decrease in perfusion caused by residual stenosis, but it also identifies the minimal amount of redistribution that takes place with the agent.

H. W. Strauss, MD

Risk Stratification in Patients With Remote Prior Myocardial Infarction Using Rest-Stress Myocardial Perfusion SPECT: Prognostic Value and Impact on Referral to Early Catheterization

Zellweger MJ, Dubois EA, Lai S, et al (Univ of California, Los Angeles; Johns Hopkins Univ, Baltimore, Md; Emory Univ, Atlanta, Ga; et al)

J Nucl Cardiol 9:23-32, 2002   10–21

Background.—Myocardial perfusion SPECT is an effective tool for risk stratification and for deciding about the need for catheterization in patients with acute myocardial infarction (MI). Its prognostic value in patients with remote prior MI has received little attention and is the subject of this report.

Methods.—The subjects were 1413 patients (76% men) with a prior MI who underwent their first rest thallium Tl 201/stress technetium Tc 99m sestamibi SPECT imaging 6 or more months after their MI. The extent of perfusion of the left ventricle was evaluated according to a 20-segment, 5-point model (0 = normal, 4 = no uptake). The scores of these 20 segments were combined to determine a summed rest score (SRS) and a summed stress score (SSS). The extent of ischemia was estimated as the difference between stress and rest scores, and expressed as a summed difference score (SDS). Infarct size was estimated by determining the number of nonreversible segments. Patients were monitored for 1 year or more (mean 667 days) to identify the incidence of cardiac death (CD), recurrent nonfatal MI, and early catheterization.

Results.—During follow-up, there were 64 CDs, 54 nonfatal MIs, and 345 early catheterizations. The annual CD and hard event (HE) rates (CD + nonfatal MI) increased significantly as the number of abnormalities on SPECT increased (Fig 4). Annual CD rates were 0.4% of patients with an SSS less than 4, 0.9% for an SSS 4 to 8, 1.7% for an SSS 9 to 13, and 3.5% for an SSS more than 13 ($P = .002$). The HE rate also increased as a function of infarct size. The annual CD rate was 0.6% in patients with a small MI (<4 nonreversible segments) and no or mild ischemia, then increased to 1.6% in patients with a small MI and moderate or severe ischemia. The annual CD rates for patients with a large MI and mild or moderate ischemia was 3.7%, and that for patients with a large MI and extensive ischemia was 6.6%. The need for early catheterization also increased as the number of abnormalities on SPECT increased, both for symptomatic and asymptomatic patients. Ultimately, almost one third of patients with symptoms and an SSS greater than 13 were referred for early catheterization. In multivariate analyses, independent predictors of CD were the presence of symptoms (relative risk [RR] 2.58), infarct size (RR 1.63), age (RR 1.03), and prior coronary artery bypass grafting (RR 0.47). Independent predictors of HEs were the presence of symptoms (RR 3.84), the prescan likelihood of coronary artery disease (RR 2.57), infarct size (RR 1.13), SDS score (RR 1.05), and prior coronary artery bypass grafting (RR 0.56). The SSS was still a significant independent predictor of CD and HE after data adjustment for prescan information. In a cost analysis, a strategy in which only patients with a risk for CD of greater than 1% as determined by myocardial perfusion SPECT were referred for cath-

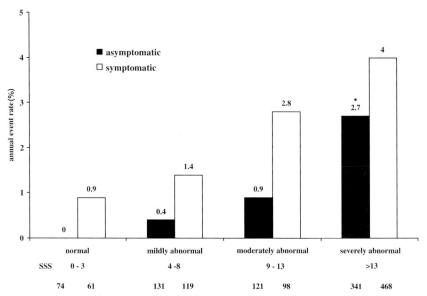

FIGURE 4.—Annual CD rate as a function of SSS and symptoms (n = 1413). A significant increase as a function of scan result was found (*P = .03). (Courtesy of Zellweger MJ, Dubois EA, Lai S, et al: Risk stratification in patients with remote prior myocardial infarction using rest-stress perfusion SPECT: Prognostic value and impact on referral to early catheterization. *J Nucl Cardiol* 9:23-32, 2002.)

eterization would be 41.6% less costly than a strategy in which all patients were referred for catheterization.

Conclusion.—Myocardial perfusion SPECT adds incremental prognostic value in the risk stratification of patients with remote prior MI. It is cost-effective compared with universal catheterization, and can identify patients with a low risk of CD and who thus can probably forego catheterization.

▶ Stress perfusion imaging adds important information about the risk for recurrent events. Even in the high-risk group, however, the annual incidence was only 3.5%, suggesting that a more specific noninvasive test for vulnerable atheromatous plaque could be very cost-effective.

H. W. Strauss, MD

Prognostic Value of Dobutamine Stress Technetium-99m-Sestamibi Single-Photon Emission Computed Tomography Myocardial Perfusion Imaging: Stratification of a High-Risk Population
Calnon DA, McGrath PD, Doss AL, et al (Univ of Virginia, Charlottesville)
J Am Coll Cardiol 38:1511-1517, 2001   10–22

Background.—Dobutamine attenuates myocardial uptake of technetium 99m–sestamibi in animal models, which results in underestimation of coronary stenosis. It was hypothesized that the prognostic value of dobutamine stress ^{99m}Tc-sestamibi SPECT myocardial perfusion imaging might be impaired by the lower rate of detection of coronary stenoses. Intrinsic cardiac risk in patients referred for dobutamine stress perfusion imaging was defined, and whether risk stratification in these patients can be accomplished with use of dobutamine ^{99m}Tc-sestamibi SPECT was determined.

Methods.—Clinical findings were reviewed in 308 patients (166 women, 142 men) who underwent dobutamine stress ^{99m}Tc-sestamibi SPECT at 1 institution from September 1992 through December 1996.

Results.—Average follow-up was 1.9 ± 1.1 years, during which time there were 33 cardiac events (18 nonfatal myocardial infarctions, 15 cardiac deaths), corresponding to an annual cardiac event rate of 5.8% (Fig 3). This rate is significantly higher than that for patients who were referred for exercise SPECT (2.2% per year) at the same institution (Fig 4). The event rate was also higher in patients with abnormal findings (10% per year), even after adjustment for clinical variables. Prognosis for a subgroup of 29 patients with dobutamine-induced ST-segment depression and abnormal SPECT results was poor. In this subgroup the annual cardiac death rate was 7.9%, and the annual rate of nonfatal myocardial infarction was 13.2%.

Conclusions.—Patients referred for dobutamine perfusion imaging represent a population at high risk. In these patients, risk stratification can be attained with ^{99m}Tc-sestamibi SPECT.

▶ Dobutamine stress is not so sensitive as exercise, but appears to be more specific (based on the difference in events in subjects with normal and abnor-

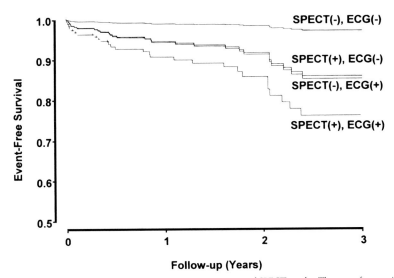

Follow-up (Years)

FIGURE 3.—Event-free survival according to ECG response and SPECT results. The event-free survival was significantly and independently associated with both ECG (P = .035) and SPECT (P = .012) results. Patients with normal ECG responses and normal SPECT results had a very favorable event-free survival (P = .0062 vs other groups). Patients with abnormal ECG responses and abnormal SPECT results had a very high event rate. (Reprinted with permission from the American College of Cardiology, from Calnon DA, McGrath PD, Doss AL, et al: Prognostic value of dobutamine stress technetium-99m-sestamibi single-photon emission computed tomography myocardial perfusion imaging: Stratification of a high-risk population. *J Am Coll Cardiol* 38:1511-1517, 2001.)

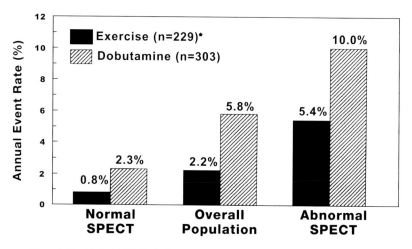

*Am J Cardiol. 1997;79:270-274.

FIGURE 4.—The impact of population risk on the annual cardiac event rates after SPECT perfusion imaging. Excellent risk stratification is achieved with both exercise and dobutamine SPECT imaging as reflected by a roughly 5-fold differential in event rates between patients with normal and abnormal SPECT results. However, regardless of SPECT results, event rates are higher in patients referred for dobutamine stress than they are in those referred for exercise stress, reflecting the higher intrinsic cardiac risk in patients referred for dobutamine perfusion imaging. (Reprinted with permission from the American College of Cardiology, from Calnon DA, McGrath PD, Doss AL, et al: Prognostic value of dobutamine stress technetium-99m-sestamibi single-photon emission computed tomography myocardial perfusion imaging: Stratification of a high-risk population. *J Am Coll Cardiol* 38:1511-1517, 2001.)

mal SPECT studies). These data, however, support the idea that patients with an abnormal dobutamine stress SPECT study, especially when accompanied by an abnormal ECG, have a much higher probability of cardiac events.

H. W. Strauss, MD

Diagnostic Performance of an Expert System for the Interpretation of Myocardial Perfusion SPECT Studies
Garcia EV, Cooke CD, Folks RD, et al (Emory Univ, Atlanta, Ga; Georgia Inst of Technology, Atlanta, Ga)
J Nucl Med 42:1185-1191, 2001   10–23

Background.—Techniques that use artificial intelligence have been investigated as a method, for the development of a tool that can help physicians to interpret more rapidly myocardial perfusion SPECT imaging studies for the assessment of coronary artery disease (CAD). One expert system, PERFEX, is now becoming widely available. A systematic validation of the diagnostic performance of this system for the interpretation of myocardial perfusion SPECT studies is described.

Methods.—A group of 655 stress/rest myocardial perfusion prospective SPECT studies in patients who also underwent coronary angiography were evaluated. Included in this population were 480 CAD patients and 175 healthy volunteers. The group included 449 men and 206 women. Data from a total of 461 other patient studies were used for implementation and refinement of 253 heuristic rules that best correlated the presence and location of left ventricular myocardial perfusion defects on SPECT studies with both angiographically detected CAD and expert visual interpretations. Myocardial perfusion defects were automatically identified as segments with counts less than sex-matched normal limits. The PERFEX system infers the presence and location of CAD from the certainty of the location, size, shape, and reversibility of the perfusion defects. Comparisons between diagnostic approaches were automatically generated on the basis of the visual interpretations of tomograms and polar maps, vessel stenosis from coronary angiography, and PERFEX interpretations.

Results.—The physician's reading was used as a gold standard. The sensitivity and specificity levels of PERFEX were 83% and 73%, respectively, for the detection of CAD; 76% and 66%, respectively, for the anterior descending artery; 90% and 70%, respectively, for the left circumflex artery; and 74% and 79%, respectively, for the right coronary artery.

Conclusions.—This study demonstrated that that diagnostic performance of PERFEX for the interpretation of myocardial perfusion SPECT studies compares well with that of nuclear medicine experts in the detection and localization of coronary artery disease.

▶ These data suggest that we are all replaceable. Though the expert system performed well, it is not quite as good as an expert reader, yet.

H. W. Strauss, MD

The Optimal Reference Population for Cardiac Normality in Myocardial SPET in the Detection of Coronary Artery Stenoses: Patients With Normal Coronary Angiography or Subjects With Low Likelihood of Coronary Artery Disease?

Toft J, Lindahl D, Ohlsson M, et al (Ctr of Imaging, Informatics and Engineering in Medicine, Copenhagen; Lund Univ, Sweden)
Eur J Nucl Med 28:831-835, 2001   10–24

Background.—The optimal reference standard in noninvasive stress testing for ischemic heart disease has long been disputed. Two reference populations, with different criteria of cardiac normality, have been used. One population includes patients with normal coronary angiography, and the other population is composed of subjects whose likelihood of coronary artery disease (CAD) is less than 5%. Both of these criteria have been criticized. These 2 different reference populations were compared by testing the performance of artificial neural networks designed to interpret myocardial scintigrams.

Methods.—The artificial neural networks were trained using either myocardial perfusion scintigrams from 87 patients with angiographically documented CAD or studies from 1 of 2 reference groups. The first reference group comprised 48 patients with no angiographic indications of CAD, and the second reference group consisted of 128 healthy volunteers with a likelihood of CAD of less than 5%. The performance of the 2 different networks was tested, using scintigrams from a separate group of 68 patients in whom coronary angiography was used as the gold standard.

Results.—For the network trained on patients with no angiographic evidence of CAD, the receiver operating characteristic (ROC) area was 93%; for the network trained on healthy volunteers, the ROC area was 72%, a difference that was statistically significant.

Conclusions.—Findings from the use of artificial neural networks in this investigation of the optimal reference population for myocardial scintigraphy suggests that normal angiography should be preferred as the reference standard for a patient who is being evaluated for CAD before possible angiography. This study did not provide any determination as to whether the same is true for other indications, such as prognostic evaluation.

▶ These results are interesting, and counterintuitive. It would seem that patients who have come to coronary angiography generally have some symptoms, perhaps due to coronary spasm, while the normal subjects should be asymptomatic, and less likely to have occult disease in their coronaries. Unfortunately, the investigators do not tell us about potential differences in body habitus, which could partially explain the lack of specificity in the data on low-likelihood subjects.

H. W. Strauss, MD

Comparison of ^{99m}Tc-Sestamibi Lung/Heart Ratio, Transient Ischaemic Dilation and Perfusion Defect Size for the Identification of Severe and Extensive Coronary Artery Disease

Romanens M, Grädel C, Saner H, et al (Rodiag Group, Olten, Switzerland; Univ Hosp Kantonspital, Basel, Switzerland; Cantonal Hosp of Olten, Switzerland)
Eur J Nucl Med 28:907-910, 2001   10–25

Background.—Currently, the ability to identify patients with severe coronary artery disease (CAD) through analysis of perfusion defects is limited. The use of technetium-99m (^{99m}Tc) sestamibi myocardial perfusion scintigraphy, although clinically important, has not been well documented. Transient ischemic left ventricular dilatation (TID) has been proposed as a marker for exercise-induced left ventricular dysfunction, and lung/heart ratio (LHR) as a measure of increased lung uptake has been established as a prognostic marker in thallium-201 perfusion imaging. The role of these parameters, however, in ^{99m}Tc-sestamibi single PET (SPET) imaging has not been clarified. In a single-day rest/stress ^{99m}Tc-sestamibi SPET perfusion protocol, TID and LHR were determined, and the findings were then compared with perfusion defect size (PDS) and angiographic severity of CAD.

Methods.—From a group of 849 patients referred for ^{99m}Tc-sestamibi myocardial perfusion scintigraphy, 120 patients were identified in whom coronary angiography was performed within 3 months of the perfusion study. For these patients, significant coronary stenoses were documented without any coronary events or interventions between the procedures and without left bundle branch block, severe nonischemic heart disease, or a left ventricular ejection fraction of less than 0.45. Diagnostic accuracy and predictive values were compared between 22 patients with severe CAD and 98 patients without severe CAD.

Results.—LHRs demonstrated a higher sensitivity (73%) for the assessment of severe CAD compared with PDS (41%) and TID (23%); however, TID ratio had the highest specificity (95%) compared with PDS (84%) and LHR (82%).

Conclusions.—It appears from these findings that increased lung uptake in ⁹⁹ᵐTc-sestamibi myocardial perfusion imaging can be obtained from a single-day rest/stress study and provides good diagnostic accuracy in the detection of patients with severe CAD.

▶ These investigators recorded an anterior planar image within 4 to 6 minutes of completion of exercise, followed by SPECT. The short interval between completion of the stress test and imaging is the reason these investigators succeeded in detecting the elevated lung/heart ratio.

H. W. Strauss, MD

Myocardial Glucose Utilization and Optimization of ¹⁸F-FDG PET Imaging in Patients With Non–Insulin-Dependent Diabetes Mellitus, Coronary Artery Disease, and Left Ventricular Dysfunction

Vitale GD, deKemp RA, Ruddy TD, et al (Univ of Ottawa, Ont, Canada)
J Nucl Med 42:1730-1736, 2001   10–26

Background.—While cardiac ¹⁸F-FDG PET imaging is useful for patients with reduced left ventricular (LV) function for the evaluation of myocardial viability, with its input having an impact on management choices, patients with non–insulin-dependent diabetes mellitus (NIDDM) do not benefit because FDG is poorly taken up. Thus, patients with NIDDM have been excluded from FDG PET studies. However, defining viability is extremely important in patients with NIDDM, coronary artery disease (CAD), and severe LV dysfunction. Thus, it becomes necessary to define the optimal means of FDG PET imaging.

Methods.—Three imaging protocols were developed: the standard protocol of oral glucose loading, the niacin protocol wherein free fatty acid levels are lowered with nicotinic acid, and the insulin clamp protocol in which a hyperinsulinemic euglycemic clamp is used. The 8 men and 2 women evaluated had NIDDM, CAD with more than 50% stenosis (determined angiographically), and severe LV dysfunction (LV ejection fraction < 40%); their mean age was 59 years. Satisfactory images were obtained with at least one approach in 8 patients. Glucose, insulin, and free fatty acid levels were evaluated also.

Results.—Because 2 patients had poor FDG uptake regardless of technique, the 8 patients with at least one satisfactory image became the primary

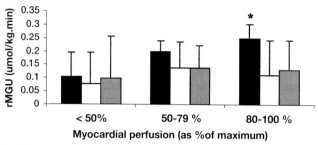

FIGURE 3.—Comparison of rate of myocardial glucose utilization (*rMGU*) among three protocols (insulin clamp [*black bars*], standard [*white bars*], and niacin [*hatched bars*]) for segments of different myocardial perfusion. *P < .05 for insulin clamp vs. niacin and standard protocols. (Reprinted by permission of the Society of Nuclear Medicine, from Vitale GD, deKemp RA, Ruddy TD, et al: Myocardial glucose utilization and optimization of ¹⁸F-FDG PET imaging in patients with non–insulin-dependent diabetes mellitus, coronary artery disease, and left ventricular dysfunction. *J Nucl Med* 42:1730-1736, 2001.)

study group. Both fasting plasma glucose levels and free fatty acid levels were similar between the groups. Insulin levels were minimally altered with the standard and niacin protocols but increased with the insulin clamp protocol. The insulin clamp protocol was also linked to better image quality as expressed in the myocardium–to–blood-pool activity ratio. The rate of myocardial glucose uutilization (rMGU) of the whole myocardium was significantly higher with the insulin clamp when compared with the standard protocol, and trended toward statistical significance in comparison with the niacin protocol. Higher regional rMGU values were also obtained with the insulin clamp protocol than with the others, but no significant differences were found for the 3 protocols between patients with moderate and severe perfusion defects (Fig 3).

Conclusions.—Better image quality, higher FDG uptake rates, and higher rMGU values were found with the insulin clamp protocol than with the standard or the niacin protocols in these patients with NIDDM, CAD, and severe LV dysfunction. Thus, the use of the insulin clamp protocol may offer the best chance to assess myocardial viability for these patients, although predictive accuracy remains to be evaluated.

▶ Optimizing the contrast between ischemic lesions and normal myocardium is difficult. The heterogeneity observed in normal myocardium when patients are fasting resulted in the standard protocol of preparing patients with an oral glucose load. The hyperinsulinemic euglycemic clamp approach extended the glucose loading concept, resulting in higher normal myocardial uptake. These investigators also tested niacin (albeit at a low dose) to reduce fatty acid levels, to (hopefully) enhance glucose uptake.

The results indicate that the hyperinsulinemic clamp approach maximizes uptake in normal myocardium. Now we need to understand whether this approach also enhances identification of viable myocardium.

H. W. Strauss, MD

Feasibility, Safety and Image Quality of Cardiac FDG Studies During Hyperinsulinaemic-Euglycaemic Clamping

Bax JJ, Visser FC, Poldermans D, et al (Leiden Univ, The Netherlands; Free Univ, Amsterdam; ThoraxCenter, Rotterdam, The Netherlands)

Eur J Nucl Med 29:452-457, 2002   10–27

Background.—Metabolic and hormonal circumstances are the most important determinants of image quality during FDG imaging of the heart. Hyperinsulinemic-euglycemic clamping was used in an effort to improve image quality during the assessment of myocardial viability through FDG SPECT.

Methods.—The subjects were 131 patients undergoing FDG SPECT to assess myocardial viability. At time 0, 2 cannula were inserted in the left and right antecubital veins, 1 for infusing glucose and insulin and the other for monitoring plasma glucose, insulin, and free fatty acid (FFA) levels. Insulin in 0.65% sodium chloride was infused at a rate of 100 mU/kg/h to achieve hyperinsulinemia. Glucose was infused as 500 mL 20% glucose with 20 mL 14.9% potassium chloride at a rate of 6 mg/kg/min, with adjustments to maintain normoglycemia. Sixty minutes later, FDG was injected and plasma levels of glucose, insulin, and FFA were again recorded. Forty-five minutes after FDG administration, thallium (Tl) 201 SPECT was performed. Image quality during hyperinsulinemia-euglycemic clamping was evaluated visually and by determining heart-to-lung, head-to-liver, and myocardium-to-background ratios both for the group as a whole and for 19 patients with diabetes mellitus (DM). Viability was defined as 3 or more dysfunctional but viable segments.

Results.—The clamping technique resulted in high levels of insulin, low levels of FFAs, and normal levels of glucose—in other words, the metabolic circumstances were optimal for FDG. Levels of these substrates during FDG imaging were comparable between patients with and without DM. All images were of good quality as assessed visually. The target-to-background ratios were good: the mean heart-to-lung ratio was 2.4, the mean heart-to-liver ratio was 2.3, and the mean myocardium-to-background ratio was 2.2. Overall, 53 patients (40%) were classified as having viable myocardium, including 11 of 19 patients (58%) with DM. The only adverse events were 4 cases of pain at the infusion site.

Conclusion.—FDG imaging of the heart during hyperinsulinemic-euglycemic clamping is safe and effective for assessing myocardial viability. Imaging quality was good, even in patients with DM.

▶ The clamp technique, though more complicated, should standardize the quality and appearance of studies performed for myocardial viability.

H. W. Strauss, MD

Positron Emission Tomography Using [18]**F-Fluoro-Deoxyglucose and Euglycaemic Hyperinsulinaemic Glucose Clamp: Optimal Criteria for the Prediction of Recovery of Post-Ischaemic Left Ventricular Dysfunction: Results From the European Community Concerted Action Multicenter Study on Use of** [18]**F-Fluoro-Deoxyglucose Positron Emission Tomography for the Detection of Myocardial Viability**
Gerber BL, Ordoubadi FF, Wijns W, et al (Hammersmith Hosp, London; Univ of Louvain, Brussels, Belgium; Turku Univ, Finland; et al)
Eur Heart J 22:1691-1701, 2001   10–28

Background.—PET is often viewed as the most accurate technique for the assessment of myocardial viability before surgery, and its accuracy for the prediction of recovery of cardiac function has been evaluated in many studies. In most of these studies, however, recovery of cardiac function was assessed only with respect to improvement of regional wall motion abnormalities. A more quantitative parameter is global left ventricular function, because it correlates better with symptoms of heart failure, physical capacity, and survival. The ability of PET to predict recovery of global cardiac function for patients with coronary artery disease after revascularization was assessed.

Methods.—The study included 178 patients (male, 88%) with coronary artery disease and left ventricular dysfunction who were enrolled in 6 centers in Europe. The mean age of the patients was 58 years. The patients underwent a common protocol using ^{18}F-fluoro-2-deoxyglucose (FDG) PET during a standardized euglycemic hyperinsulinemic glucose clamp before revascularization either surgically (140 patients) or with angioplasty (38 patients). The patients were then classified on the basis of their recovery of global ejection fraction 2 to 6 months after revascularization.

Results.—Of 171 patients who completed the study, 82 (47.9%) experienced an improvement greater than 5% in ejection fraction postoperatively, and 89 (52.0%) patients had no postoperative improvement in ejection fraction. Computation of the optimal cutoff points for postoperative improvement of global cardiac function showed that the highest sensitivity and specificity (79% and 55%, respectively) for predicting postoperative ejection fraction improvement with PET occurred when 3 or more dysfunctional segments had a relative FDG uptake of more than 45% of normal remote myocardium.

Conclusions.—In a large-cohort study, FDG-PET demonstrated high sensitivity and moderate specificity in predicting improvement of cardiac function after coronary revascularization in coronary patients with impaired ejection fraction.

▶ The criteria for viable ischemic tissue is a focal zone of relative increased FDG uptake, in excess of perfusion. Some normal patients injected in the fasting state were found to have irregular myocardial uptake of FDG, leading to the concept that FDG should be injected after glucose loading. The hyperinsulinemic euglycemic clamp technique provides an innovative means of standardizing this important procedure. Although the results are not perfect (sensitivity varied from 74%-87%, and specificity from 45%-58%) the clamp approach offers a significant step forward in evaluating patients with left ventricular dysfunction.

H. W. Strauss, MD

Assessment of Infarct Size by Positron Emission Tomography and [18F]2-fluoro-2-deoxy-D-glucose: A New Absolute Threshold Technique

Chareonthaitawee P, Schaefers K, Baker CSR, et al (Imperial College School of Science Technology and Medicine, London; Queen Elizabeth Med Centre, Birmingham, England; Hammersmith Hosp, London; et al)

Eur J Nucl Med 29:203-215, 2002   10–29

Background.—The total amount of scarred nonviable myocardium determines outcome after an acute myocardial infarction. Both the process of remodeling of the left ventricle (LV) and the progression of congestive heart failure depend on infarct size and hibernating myocardium, as do changes in remote nonischemic tissues. A new technique for quantifying infarct size uses PET with FDG. With a receiver-operating curve, hibernating myocardium has been identified based on the absolute myocardial uptake of FDG as determined by PET under a hyperinsulinemic-euglycemic clamp. This same technique was used to validate a new method for the quantification of infarct size based on an absolute threshold of tracer uptake obtained from a parametric image of the metabolic rate of FDG.

Methods.—Seven pigs with surgically produced acute myocardial infarction and 2 sham-operated pigs, 6 human beings who had ischemic cardiomyopathy and were waiting for cardiac transplantation, and 5 normal volunteers were assessed for myocardial FDG uptake with PET during hyperinsulinemic-euglycemic clamp. Infarct size was quantified, and the estimates were compared with independent ex vivo planimetric measurements from the swine and the patients' hearts at transplantation.

Results.—For the pigs, the LV myocardial volume showed a strong linear relationship between gravimetric and PET-derived estimates. The PET infarct size estimates determined with planimetry and PET showed good agreement, with a mean difference of 0.004% of the LV. For the human patients, PET-derived and planimetric infarct sizes also showed good agreement, with a systematic slight overestimation produced by using PET. The difference between the 2 methods was 0.99% of the LV.

Conclusions.—The PET FDG method proved feasible and accurate in its estimates of infarct size. The measurements were in good agreement with planimetric results both in the animal model of acute infarction and in human beings who had chronic ischemic cardiomyopathy.

▶ Driving FDG into the myocardium with the hyperinsulinemic clamp approach loads viable tissue with glucose, clearly delineating areas of reduced/absent glucose uptake. The model tested produced transmural infarcts under circumstances where collateral flow was minimal. This provides a high-contrast distinction between viable and nonviable tissue. The FDG technique looks excellent under these circumstances. The true test of this approach will occur when nontransmural lesions are evaluated.

H. W. Strauss, MD

Quantification of Myocardial Glucose Utilization by PET and 1–Carbon-11–Glucose

Herrero P, Weinheimer CJ, Dence C, et al (Washington Univ, St Louis)
J Nucl Cardiol 9:5-14, 2002   10–30

Background.—In measuring the rate of myocardial glucose utilization (rMGU) with PET and FDG, the net uptake and phosphorylation of glucose and FDG differ significantly, requiring that a correction factor (the lumped constant) be included in the rMGU determination. Yet even this is not accurate in all cases. Using radiolabeled (carbon 11) glucose as a radiopharmaceutical, with the ^{11}C specifically at the 1-carbon position, may avoid this problem. The quantification of rMGU in dog hearts was attempted with compartmental modeling of myocardial kinetics of 1–C-11–glucose measured by PET.

Methods.—Various interventions were performed on the dogs, including fasting (5 dogs), hyperinsulinemic-euglycemic clamp at rest (6 dogs), clamp and phenylephrine (5 dogs), and clamp and dobutaine (4 dogs). The 20 dogs underwent PET with oxygen-15–water to measure myocardial blood flow and 1–C-11–glucose to measure rMGU. The rMGU measurement was performed on arterial-coronary sinus samples with the Fick method.

Results.—The highest and next highest plasma fatty acid levels occurred in the fasted and clamp/dobutamine groups, with no significant differences in plasma glucose and lactate levels found among the various groups. Differential myocardial uptake of the tracer increased as the rMGU increased. Under the fasting conditions, the myocardium and blood were indistinguishable; during clamp and rest and even more significantly during phenylephrine, they were easily distinguished. While the blood cleared rapidly of tracer, myocardial time-activity curves were higher than the blood curves and showed a distinctive shape. PET-derived values for myocardial extraction of glucose correlated closely with those obtained directly over a wide range of substrate and insulin availability and levels of cardiac work. The PET-derived values for rMGU and directly measured rMGU values also coincided, although PET consistently showed a 15% underestimation of glucose extraction and rMGU. Significant correlations were noted between rMGU that was directly measured and PET-derived and the total C-11–carbon dioxide production. Intraregional variation in rMGU estimates was less than 20% in all cases; interregional variation was less than 17%. The coefficient of variation for regional rMGU estimates was 11.3% for the clamp at rest group (lowest value) and 16.3% for the clamp with phenylephrine group (highest value).

Conclusions.—The quantification of myocardial glucose use is possible with PET and 1–C-11–glucose, with accuracy sustained over a broad range of substrate and insulin availability and levels of cardiac work.

▶ ^{18}F-2-deoxyglucose is used for metabolic imaging because the agent is metabolically trapped and has the disadvantage of a relatively long myocardial residence time and a relatively slow blood clearance. Universally labeled glucose (^{11}C) has the disadvantage of complex catabolism, making quantitation almost impossible. Labeling either the 1 or 6 position of glucose with ^{11}C results in myocardial retention of ^{11}C activity for about 10 minutes before measurable [11]CO_2 is released. Table 2 and Fig 3 in the original article highlight the difficulties of using C-11-1-glucose to determine myocardial metabolism: low extraction of glucose, even under clamp and adrenergic stimulus, and slow blood clearance in the fasting state. It looks as if FDG will continue to be the major agent used to determine myocardial glucose utilization.

H. W. Strauss, MD

Mechanisms of Coronary Microcirculatory Dysfunction in Patients With Aortic Stenosis and Angiographically Normal Coronary Arteries
Rajappan K, Rimoldi OE, Dutka DP, et al (Hammersmith Hosp, London; St Mary's Hosp, London; Royal Brompton Hosp, London; et al)
Circulation 105:470-476, 2002   10–31

Background.—The development of left ventricular hypertrophy (LVH) in patients with aortic valve stenosis is an adaptive response that attempts to reduce wall stress in the left ventricle. The development of LVH also affects the coronary circulation, and patients with aortic valve stenosis have a reduced coronary vasodilator reserve (CVR) despite having angiographically normal coronary arteries. The impairment of CVR is primarily attributable to a reduction in maximal myocardial blood flow which, in the absence of epicardial stenosis, reflects dysfunction of the coronary microcirculation.

Characteristic pathologic changes that contribute to the impairment of microvascular function have been described in the hypertrophied ventricles of patients with aortic valve stenosis. However, the interactions among microvascular dysfunction, severe aortic valve stenosis, hemodynamic overload, and coronary perfusion are poorly understood. PET allows the noninvasive quantification of myocardial blood flow (MBF), but limitations in the spatial resolution of PET have thus far allowed the demonstration of subendocardial hypoperfusion only in massively hypertrophied septa (greater than 25 mm) of hypertrophic cardiomyopathy patients.

However, recent advances in the technology of PET imaging have made possible the study of transmural distribution of MBF in patients with lesser degrees of LVH as in aortic valve stenosis. The purposes of this study were to quantitatively demonstrate differences in subendocardial and subepicardial microcirculation and evaluate the relative contributions of myocyte hyper-

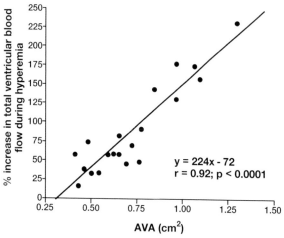

FIGURE 3.—Relationship between percentage increase in total ventricular blood flow during hyperemia and aortic valve area (*AVA*). (Courtesy of Rajappan K, Rimoldi OE, Dutka DP, et al: Mechanisms of coronary microcirculatory dysfunction in patients with aortic stenosis and angiographically normal coronary arteries. *Circulation* 105:470-476, 2002.)

trophy, hemodynamic load, severity of aortic valve stenosis, and coronary perfusion to impairment of microcirculatory function.

Methods.—The study involved 20 patients with isolated moderate-to-severe aortic valve stenosis. The patients underwent echocardiography to determine the severity of the stenosis, cardiovascular MRI to measure left ventricular mass (LVM), and PET to quantify resting and hyperemic MBF and CVR in both the subendocardium and subepicardium.

Results.—In 15 patients with the most severe aortic valve stenosis, the subendocardial to subepicardial MBF ratio decreased from 1.14 ± 0.17 at rest to 0.92 ± 0.17 during hyperemia. Subendocardial CVR (1.43 ± 0.33) was lower than subepicardial CVR (1.78 ± 0.35). Resting total left ventricular flow was linearly related to LVM, while CVR was not linearly related to LVM (Fig 3). The increase of total left ventricular blood flow during hyperemia was linearly related to aortic valve area. The decrease in CVR was related to the severity of aortic valve stenosis, increased hemodynamic load, and reduction in diastolic perfusion time, particularly in the subendocardium.

Conclusion.—Coronary vasodilator reserve was more significantly impaired in the subendocardium of patients with LVH attributable to severe aortic valve stenosis. The severity of impairment was related to aortic valve area, hemodynamic load imposed, and diastolic perfusion but was not related to left ventricular mass.

▶ The investigators performed a multi- measurement determination of myocardial perfusion and mass, which demonstrates a striking relationship between percent increase in ventricular blood flow with hyperemia and aortic valve area: The smaller the area, the lower the increase in blood flow. In other words, the microcirculation fails to respond in those hearts with the greatest hypertrophy. This fact is important because stress perfusion scans in patients with aortic stenosis may be abnormal, particularly in patients' with tight stenosis in the absence of epicardial coronary artery disease.

H. W. Strauss, MD

Passage of Inhaled Particles Into the Blood Circulation in Humans
Nemmar A, Hoet PHM, Vanquickenborne B, et al (Katholieke Universiteit Leuven, Belgium; MRC Toxicology Unit, Leicester, England)
Circulation 105:411-414, 2002   10–32

Background.—When particulate matter air pollution is worst, both morbidity and mortality from respiratory and cardiovascular diseases increase. These particulates, whose diameter is less than 10 μm, may produce inflammation in the lungs, which releases cytokines systemically, and these may affect cardiovascular end points. Alternatively, the pollutants may alter cardiac autonomic function, changing heart rate variability and increasing the risk of sudden cardiac death. Yet another theory proposes that the smallest particles move from the lungs to the circulation and directly influence cardiovascular end points. The extent and rapidity with which inhaled pollutant particles pass into the systemic circulation were determined in healthy volunteers.

Methods.—Five volunteers inhaled "Technegas," an aerosol that contains mainly ultrafine [99m]technetium-labeled carbon particles measuring less than 100 nm. The distribution of radioactivity was then determined.

Results.—Radioactivity was detected in blood after 1 minute, was maximal in 10 to 20 minutes, and remained at maximal levels for as long as 60 minutes. Thin-layer chromatography of blood revealed peak radioactivity at the application point and moving with the solvent front. Thin-layer chromatography of urine principally revealed the latter peak. Bound radioactivity remained at the origin; free pertechnetate moved with the solvent front. Liver radioactivity remained stable at about 8%; bladder radioactivity increased over time.

Conclusions.—Inhaled ultrafine particles diffuse rapidly into the systemic circulation. Thus, ambient particle pollution may directly influence cardiac function.

▶ Inhaled particulates can cross from the airspace to the vasculature in the lungs. These findings suggest that a trip to the country, and the fresh air, may be a healthy idea.

H. W. Strauss, MD

Cost-effectiveness of Preoperative Positron Emission Tomography in Ischemic Heart Disease

Jacklin PB, Barrington SF, Roxburgh JC, et al (Guy's and St Thomas' Hosps, London)

Ann Thorac Surg 73:1403-1410, 2002   10–33

Background.—The poor prognosis for patients with ischemic heart disease and severe left ventricular dysfunction can be improved if the areas of myocardium where significant amounts of viable tissue remain can be identified and targeted for blood flow improvement via revascularization. PET can establish the metabolic integrity of dysfunctional myocardium and can detect hibernating myocardium more accurately than other methods. A model was developed to test the hypothesis that PET would be cost-effective in selecting patients with poor left ventricular function for revascularization. The model was designed to allow changes of input data to reflect differences in key variables such as cost, prevalence of disease, and survival of patients over time and locality, and to take account of new research results, various health care systems, and varying characteristics in referral populations.

Methods.—Three management strategies were compared for cost-effectiveness. One used coronary artery bypass grafting (CABG) for all patients; one used PET to select candidates for CABG, leaving those without hibernating myocardium on medication; and one used medical therapy for all patients. The economic model used data from 1 hospital and from a literature review. The sensitivity of the various approaches was also analyzed.

Results.—Medical therapy alone was the least costly option; the most effective option used PET to select patients for assignment to receive CABG or medical therapy, generating the greatest number of life-years (916 of a possible 1000). Performing revascularization for all patients was more costly and less effective than selecting patients with PET. The sensitivity analysis indicated that the medical therapy option was the least costly regardless of the variables used, and the CABG option without PET was the most costly. The factors most predictive of cost-effectiveness were the prevalence of hibernation and the survival rate of patients who were refused revascularization based on the PET analysis. Sensitivity testing documented the PET option as less costly and gaining more life-years than either of the other options.

Conclusions.—PET showed cost-effectiveness in selecting patients with poor left ventricular function who were referred for CABG. Factors affecting the cost-effectiveness of PET were the prevalence of hibernating myocardium and the survival rate of patients who did not undergo CABG because of the PET recommendations.

▶ The mortality rate of patients with impaired left ventricular ejection fraction subjected to bypass surgery can approach 30%, even in skilled hands. On the other hand, the mortality rate of patients treated medically who could have benefited from surgery is even higher. It is the mortality rate, and the overall quality of life, that should be driving forces determining whether PET is helpful.

H. W. Strauss, MD

Planar Imaging Versus Gated Blood-Pool SPECT for the Assessment of Ventricular Performance: A Multicenter Study

Groch MW, DePuey EG, Belzberg AC, et al (Northwestern Univ, Chicago; Rush-Presbyterian-St Luke's Med Ctr, Chicago; Rush Univ, Chicago; et al)
J Nucl Med 42:1773-1779, 2001   10–34

Background.—Even though planar equilibrium radionuclide angiography (ERNA) provides a fairly simple, noninvasive way to assess ventricular function, especially left ventricular ejection fraction (LVEF), it has limitations because of anatomic considerations. LVEF has recently been calculated from gated myocardial perfusion SPECT, but this also has limitations. Ventricular function can be evaluated well by using gated blood-pool SPECT (GBPS), which is able to isolate the left and right ventricles without overlapping of other cardiac chambers and shows improved evaluation of regional wall motion (RWM). It offers the potential to replace ERNA in evaluating LVEF, RWM, and right heart function. The assessment of ventricular function by these 2 methods was compared in a large, multicenter group of patients.

Methods.—Both ERNA and GBPS were performed in 178 patients referred for nuclear medicine studies. A GBPS acquisition protocol dictated the clinical sites assessed; it included 180° of rotation, a 64 by 64 matrix, and 64 or 32 views with a single-head or double-head camera. A new GBPS program was used to process the GBPS studies and calculate LVEF. For 33 patients, right ventricular ejection fraction (RVEF) was also calculated. Thirty patients also had RWM and image quality from 3-dimensional surface-shaded and volume-rendered cine displays.

Results.—GBPS findings for global LVEF closely matched those obtained with conventional planar methods. Bland-Altman plotting showed higher LVEF values were obtained systematically by using the GBPS system and revealed that as LVEF values increased in magnitude, the GBPS values were increasingly higher than the planar LVEF values. Interoperator agreement was good. Mean global RVEF was 59.8% in patients who had no right ventricular dysfunction, with the average RVEF values in these patients consistently lower than the average LVEF obtained by GBPS but a bit higher than the RVEF values obtained by planar technique. The GBPS RWM value was deemed superior to the planar value in 8 patients, equivalent in 20 patients, and inferior in 2 patients.

Conclusions.—Good correlation was found between GBPS- and planar-derived LVEF values over a large range of LVEF values. The GBPS values for LVEF tended to be higher than planar values, especially at higher values of LVEF. RWM analysis with GBPS was better than or equivalent to planar results in those patients so analyzed. The computation of RVEF requires more experience with the GBPS methods.

▶ Intuitively, 3-dimensional imaging of the heart, which allows the observer to select specific views for evaluation, should provide better information than selected planar images. This new software program appears to provide excellent 3-dimensional renderings of the heart. The site and extent of wall motion abnormalities should be particularly striking. Unfortunately, that was not observed in this study, because the investigators studied patients with near-normal wall motion.

H. W. Strauss, MD

Measurement of Myocardial β-Adrenoceptor Density in Clinical Studies: A Role for Positron Emission Tomography?
de Jong RM, Blanksma PK, van Waarde A, et al (Univ Hosp Groningen, The Netherlands)
Eur J Nucl Med 29:88-97, 2002   10–35

Background.—Among the factors influencing the regulation of heart function is the β-adrenoceptor (β-AR). The downregulation of β-AR density has been assessed during in vitro studies in heart failure and other cardiac conditions that may precede heart failure. Neither longitudinal nor regional assessment of myocardial β-ARs in human beings is possible using in vitro cardiac tissue samples, but PET has been used in vivo.

In Vitro Findings.—The density of β-AR varies from 70 to 100 fmol/mg protein, which may be explained by differences in the circumstances under which tissues are obtained, the methods of transportation, the radioligands used, or the measuring method used. Study of the downregulation of β-ARs reveal that β_1-AR downregulation is more pronounced in patients who have end-stage ischemic cardiomyopathy or hypertension; these patients also have downregulation of β_2-ARs. Both myocardial β_1-ARs and lymphocyte β_2-ARs are downregulated in left ventricular overload disease. Patients with aortic valve regurgitation have more distinct downregulation than those with mitral regurgitation. Lymphocyte β_2-ARs have not proved widely useful for predicting the status of cardiac β-ARs, with cardiac tissue needed to assess cardiac β-AR function.

In Vivo Findings.—PET measurements of β-AR density in vivo show that patients with heart failure clearly differ from those without heart failure and healthy individuals. PET studies require a ligand of high selectivity and affinity for the receptor of interest, and because the changes in density mainly affect the β_1-ARs, it would be best to have a subtype-selective radioligand as well as one that has antagonist action and seroselectivity. [11C]CGP 12177 holds promise as a hydrophilic β-AR antagonist that binds only to functional β-ARs on the cell surface, although the radiochemical synthesis is very demanding for clinical experiments. β-AR density was decreased in vivo in patients with heart failure caused by idiopathic dilated cardiomyopathy.

The measurements on PET correlated with the findings on endomyocardial biopsy and with functional measurements of β-contractile responsiveness to intracoronary dobutamine infusion. Finding myocardial β-AR downregulation in patients with arrhythmogenic right ventricular cardiomyopathy may result from increased local synaptic catecholamine levels, which also occur in patients with heart failure.

Conclusions.—Although in vitro determinations of the role of β-AR in cardiac function are limited, the new in vivo PET methods offer the promise of clarifying the role of β-AR function in heart failure and of aiding in making clinical decisions.

▶ β-Receptor imaging has been used in research studies but has not gained wide clinical acceptance. The procedure is complex, and there are few disorders for which specific information about receptor distribution affects clinical care. However, this review is worth reading because it details the experience of 2 groups of investigators in patients with heart disease and asthma.

H. W. Strauss, MD

Quantification of β-Adrenoceptor Density in the Human Heart With (*S*)-[¹¹C]CGP 12388 and a Tracer Kinetic Model

Doze P, Elsinga PH, van Waarde A, et al (Groningen Univ Hosp, The Netherlands)

Eur J Nucl Med 29:295-304, 2002

10–36

Background.—The distribution of various receptors and the quantitative analysis of the pharmacokinetics and pharmacodynamics of radioligands can be evaluated with PET. Various pathophysiologic conditions alter the β-adrenergic receptor density in the heart. Use of PET to quantify myocardial and pulmonary β-adrenergic receptors allows the investigation of β-adrenergic receptor changes both in disease and through the course of treatment. (*S*)-CGP 12388 can be used in a simplified model because it is equally potent and its procedure is more suited to the clinical setting. The myocardium of healthy volunteers was evaluated by using (*S*)-CGP 12388 PET tracer kinetic modeling to determine all model parameters, especially the density of β-adrenergic receptors and ligand affinity. The goal was to evaluate this method for its application as a gold standard by which to validate other simplified methods.

Methods.—During a period of 60 minutes, dynamic PET data were acquired in 6 healthy volunteers. Varying degrees of specific activity (SA) were applied, producing 3 different injection protocols (high SA, low SA, and unlabeled ligand only). Radial artery blood samples were collected via cannula, and time-activity data for the myocardial tissue were obtained according to regions of interest on short-axis planes. The 2-tissue compartment, 6-parameter model used to analyze data allowed description of the kinetics of both labeled and unlabeled radioligand.

Results.—With the high SA injection, apparent tissue radioactivity levels rose to a maximum, then declined relatively slowly to a plateau at 3 minutes. With the low SA injection at 20 minutes, volunteers showed a very rapid rise in activity, then a rapid fall, with a slight continuing decline that indicated dissociation of the labeled ligand from the receptor. A further decline occurred with the injection at 40 minutes of unlabeled ligand only. Estimates of blood, free and bound concentrations of the labeled ligand, corrected for blood volume, showed that ligand concentrations in blood and free in tissue (labeled or unlabeled) were similar to those noted in plasma. It was clear that unlabeled ligand displaced labeled ligand from receptor sites, with a slight increase in the fraction of unlabeled ligand bound to receptors occurring after coinjection or injection of unlabeled ligand. Then plasma levels of labeled ligand rose. The B_{max} values calculated were 9.74 nM, and the K_D values were 0.58 nM, with no systematic differences between the various injection protocols. The receptor densities were higher in the inferior part of the left ventricle than in the anterior part for all volunteers. A 10% change in B_{max} was detected, especially once the second and third injections were made. The injection protocol of high SA, low SA, and unlabeled ligand was most sensitive to 10% changes in the B_{max} values, whereas the high SA, unlabeled ligand, and low SA protocol was totally insensitive to these alterations.

Conclusions.—The β-adrenergic receptor density of the human heart was obtained accurately by using tracer kinetic modeling with (S)-[^{11}C]CGP 12388. Thus, this method may serve as a gold standard to validate other simplified methods.

▶ This kind of study can be very helpful to define the pharmacokinetics of drugs designed to block the β-adrenergic system.

H. W. Strauss, MD

Cardiovascular Imaging: Who Does It and How Important Is It to the Practice of Radiology?

Levin DC, Parker L, Sunshine JH, et al (Thomas Jefferson Univ, Philadelphia; American College of Radiology, Reston, Va; Georgetown Univ, Washington, DC)
AJR 178:303-306, 2002

10–37

Background.—The Committee for Cardiovascular Imaging was formed by 4 leading national radiology organizations to advance clinical practice, research, and education regarding cardiovascular disease imaging and thus improve patient care. To form a basis for their activities, research was carried out to determine the significance of the role of noninvasive cardiovascular imaging in radiology and the percentage of noninvasive cardiovascular imaging that is performed by various specialists.

Methods.—Data were drawn from the national 1998 Medicare Part B database, from which 460 procedure codes were reviewed. Of the 65 thought to be specifically related to the cardiovascular system, 5 categories were formed: cardiac MR imaging, MR angiography, cardiovascular nuclear medicine, echocardiography, and vascular sonography. Nationwide examination volume, utilization rate per 1000 Medicare fee-for-service enrollees, Part B physician reimbursements, and percentages of evaluations done by radiologists, cardiologists, surgeons, and other physicians were determined for each of the code categories.

Results.—In the 5 categories, 19,244,001 noninvasive cardiovascular imaging examinations were performed (utilization rate of 603 per 1000), and Medicare Part B reimbursements were $1,709,687,577. Two thirds of all examinations were echocardiography, 19.9% were vascular sonography, and 15.8% were nuclear medicine; MR angiography and cardiac MR imaging together amounted to less than 1% of the procedures. Radiologists performed only 1.6% of the echocardiography studies, but 44.8% of the vascular sonography and 37.8% of the cardiovascular nuclear medicine studies; they strongly predominated in the performance of MR angiography and cardiac MR imaging (Table 2). Most of the cardiovascular nuclear medicine and echocardiographic examinations were performed by cardiologists. Nearly 24% of the vascular sonography examinations were done by surgeons, who were overall responsible for only a fraction of the cardiovascular imaging. Other physicians did 18.4% of the echocardiography and 20.0% of the sonography (10.3% internists, 5.3% neurologists, and 3.5% thoracic surgeons). For echocardiography, 15.2% of the total 18.4% of studies done by other physicians were conducted by internists. Of all the cardiovascular imaging examinations noted, radiologists did 16.7%, cardiologists did 61.5%, surgeons did 4.8%, and other physicians did 16.9%. In terms of payment, radiologists received 13.8% of the Medicare Part B reimbursements, cardiologists 63.4%, surgeons 4.4%, and other physicians 18.4%. In

TABLE 2.—Noninvasive Cardiovascular Imaging Performed by Radiologists, Cardiologists, Surgeons, and Other Physicians in 1998

Category*	Performed by Radiologists (%)	Performed by Cardiologists (%)	Performed by Surgeons (%)	Performed by Other Physicians (%)
Cardiac MR imaging (n = 1,017)	85.7	13.6	0.0	0.7
MR angiography (n = 154,764)	95.3	0.0	0.1	4.5
Cardiovascular nuclear medicine (n = 3,045,452)	37.8	53.8	0.1	8.2
Echocardiography (n = 12,207,754)	1.6	79.8	0.2	18.4
Vascular sonography (n = 3,835,014)	44.8	11.3	23.8	20.0

Note: Data are based on the national 1998 Health Care Financing Administration Physician/Supplier Procedure Summary Master Files of claims made for physician services to the 31.9 million fee-for-service enrollees in the Medicare Part B program that year.

*Of 460 procedure codes for noninvasive diagnostic imaging in the database, 65 that were specifically related to the cardiovascular system were grouped in categories for analysis.

(Courtesy of Levin DC, Parker L, Sunshine JH, et al: Cardiovascular imaging: Who does it and how important is it to the practice of radiology? *AJR* 178:303-306, 2002. Reprinted with permission from the *American Journal of Roentgenology.*)

evaluating diagnostic cardiac catheterization procedures, radiologists did only 0.3% of the cardiac catheterization and coronary and ventricular angiography examinations.

Conclusions.—The practice of radiology is well represented in the performance of noninvasive cardiovascular imaging, except for echocardiography. Thus, noninvasive cardiovascular imaging is an important part of the radiologist's practice.

▶ Noninvasive cardiovascular imaging plays a major role in management of the cardiac patient. The fact that most nuclear cardiology studies are performed by cardiologists may be the result of issues of patient referral and the overall training and qualifications of the individuals performing the test. Nuclear physicians generally know much more about the technology, but less about the patient management issues than cardiologists. For nuclear physicians to continue participating in this important area, training programs should emphasize the clinical role these procedures play in patient care.

H. W. Strauss, MD

Ga-67 SPECT to Detect Endocarditis After Replacement of an Aortic Valve

Pena FJ, Banzo I, Quirce R, et al (Hosp Universitario Marqués de Valdecilla, Santander, Spain)
Clin Nucl Med 27:401-404, 2002   10–38

Background.—Among the complications that can develop in patients who have undergone cardiac valve replacement, one of the most serious is prosthetic valve endocarditis, which affects 2% to 4% of patients. Ga-67 scintigraphy has documented ability to detect the presence of infection in the heart, leading to accurate diagnosis. Ga-67 scintigraphy plus SPECT were used to correctly diagnose infectious endocarditis in a patient who had an aortic valve replacement.

Case Report.—Man, 28, underwent replacement of the ascending aorta and aortic valve, then was hospitalized 5 months later with suppuration from the surgical sternal wound and fever of greater than 1 weeks' duration. *Staphylococcus epidermidis* was cultured, and surgical cleansing was performed 5 days after admission. The patient was discharged on antibiotics, but returned to the hospital 10 days later for persistent fever; a Ga-67 scan was ordered. Planar images were normal 48 and 72 hours after injecting 296 MBq (8 mCi) Ga-67 citrate; only a faint area of increased activity was noted in the area of the heart. SPECT images suggested the presence of an infection, revealing a well-defined doughnut-like pathologic uptake of moderate intensity in the mediastinum and the cardiac origin of the graft (Fig 3). A high-resolution CT scan was negative, so antibiotic treatment was continued and the patient was discharged. He returned 3 weeks later with sepsis and positive culture of *S epidermidis*,

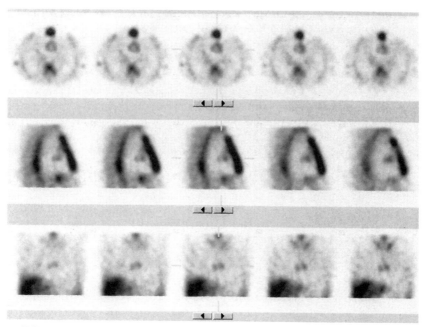

FIGURE 3.—Ga-67 SPECT images show retrosternal doughnut-shaped uptake at the site of the aortic valve prosthesis. (Courtesy of Pena FJ, Banzo I, Quirce R, et al: Ga-67 SPECT to detect endocarditis after replacement of an aortic valve. *Clin Nucl Med* 27(6):401-404, 2002.)

for which antibiotic treatment was begun. A spiral CT scan revealed minor inflammatory changes at the origin of the ascending aorta, and another Ga-67 SPECT study confirmed mediastinal pathologic uptake. A transesophageal US study suggested vegetation in the aortic prosthesis, and the prosthesis was subsequently replaced. During surgery, 2 small foci of purulent fluid were noted in the anastomotic junction of the prosthesis with the native aortic valve annulus, and graft and valve cultures showed *Staphylococcus haemolyticus* and *Staphylococcus hominis*. The surgery and antibiotic treatment cleared the infection.

Conclusions.—The use of Ga-67 plus SPECT was crucial in detecting the valve endocarditis in this patient. The CT scan did not show significant abnormalities, but both transesophageal US and surgery, performed based on the SPECT findings, confirmed the presence of infection. The diagnosis of infectious endocarditis may require the use of Ga-67 scanning along with SPECT views to obtain information that cannot be obtained otherwise.

▶ Gallium can provide the information. It is interesting to wonder whether FDG PET could do it as well or better.

H. W. Strauss, MD

The Safety of Dipyridamole in Patients Undergoing Myocardial Perfusion Scintigraphy Prior to Lung Volume Reduction Surgery

Roman MR, Angelides S, Freeman AP, et al (Prince of Wales and Sydney Children's Hosp, Australia)
Eur J Nucl Med 28:1405-1408, 2001   10–39

Background.—Patients with end-stage chronic obstructive pulmonary disease (COPD) who are undergoing lung volume reduction surgery (LVRS) have a greatly increased risk of perioperative cardiac complications. Their preoperative assessment can be accomplished noninvasively by using myocardial perfusion scintigraphy (MPS), generally with vasodilators such as dipyridamole or adenosine. Although these agents are contraindicated in persons with asthma, their safety in COPD is as yet undetermined, with some studies recommending dipyridamole use and others not recommending its use. The safety of dipyridamole for patients with end-stage nonreversible COPD was evaluated, and the incidence of side effects was compared with that in control patients.

Methods.—The 50 patients enrolled included 25 in the LVRS group (mean age, 65 years) and 25 in the control group (mean age, 66 years), which consisted of patients undergoing dipyridamole MPS before elective noncardiothoracic surgery. The mean forced expiratory volume at 1 minute (FEV$_1$) for the LVRS group was 0.79 L.

Results.—None of the patients demonstrated allergic reactions to dipyridamole, nor did they exhibit hypotension or wheezing. Side effects were found in 14 of the LVRS patients, with 5 cases of dyspnea, 1 of severe hypotension, and 8 cases of headache and flushing; all of these were alleviated by aminophylline. Of the 7 LVRS patients with an abnormal MPS, 3 developed dyspnea. The MPS results led to major management changes in 2 patients of the LVRS group. Perioperative cardiac complications developed in 2 LVRS patients. In the control group, 14 patients developed side effects, with 2 cases of dyspnea, 1 of severe hypotension and bradycardia, 1 of chest pain, and 10 cases with minor complaints; all were alleviated with aminophylline. Of the 6 control patients who had an abnormal MPS study, 1 developed dyspnea. Equivocal MPS abnormalities were found in 6 control patients.

Conclusions.—Although few patients were included and significant comorbidity was present, it appears that dipyridamole MPS can be used safely in patients with severe nonreversible COPD.

▶ This is an important paper because these patients have severe obstructive lung disease. Medication with inhaled bronchodilators appears very efficacious in this group, since only 5 patients developed dyspnea, which responded well to aminophylline.

H. W. Strauss, MD

Recent Rapid Increase in Utilization of Radionuclide Myocardial Perfusion Imaging and Related Procedures: 1996-1998 Practice Patterns

Levin DC, Parker L, Intenzo CM, et al (Thomas Jefferson Univ, Philadelphia; American College of Radiology, Reston, Va)

Radiology 222:144-148, 2002

10–40

Background.—Currently the leading method of noninvasively detecting coronary artery disease uses radionuclide myocardial perfusion imaging (MPI), and its sensitivity and specificity exceed those of exercise electrocardiographic stress testing by itself. Further advances include the use of electrocardiographic gating and technetium 99m–labeled radioisotopes. These developments have led to the addition of 2 new codes in the nuclear medicine section of the *Current Procedural Terminology*, fourth edition, coding manual (Table 1). Overuse of these new techniques has become a concern, so cardiac nuclear medicine practice patterns were investigated among several physician specialty groups to reveal why these examinations have come to be used so frequently so quickly.

Methods.—The 1996 and 1998 databases from National Medicare Part B supplied the data needed to assess the use of 4 primary procedure codes for radionuclide MPI and left ventricular wall motion or left ventricular ejection fraction procedures. The physician groups studied were cardiologists, radi-

TABLE 1.—Cardiac Radionuclide Imaging Codes in 1998

CPT-4 Code	Descriptor	Global Relative Value Units*	No. of Examinations Performed†
78460	MPI; (planar) single study, at rest or stress	3.75	11,740
78461	MPI; (planar) multiple studies, at rest and/or stress, and redistribution and/or rest injection	6.80	55,955
78464	MPI; tomographic (SPECT), single study at rest or stress	9.09	139,644
78465	MPI; tomographic (SPECT), multiple studies, at rest and/or stress and redistribution and/or rest injection	14.67	1,329,884
78478	WM (in addition to primary procedure)	2.57	673,050
78480	EF (in addition to primary procedure)	2.57	493,064
78472	CBPI, gated equilibrium; single study at rest or stress, WM plus EF	7.30	100,957
78473	CBPI, gated equilibrium; multiple studies at rest and stress, WM plus EF	10.89	16,403
78481	CBPI, first pass; single study at rest or stress, WM plus EF	6.99	43,126
78483	CBPI, first pass; multiple studies at rest and stress, WM plus EF	10.53	18,252

*Refers to Medicare relative value units in 1998.
†1998 values.
Abbreviation: CBPI, Cardiac blood-pool imaging.
(Courtesy of Levin DC, Parker L, Intenzo CM, et al: Recent rapid increase in utilization of radionuclide myocardial perfusion imaging and related procedures: 1996-1998 practice patterns. *Radiology* 222:144-148, 2002. Radiological Society of North America)

ologists, and other physicians. Also included was an analysis of the use patterns for cardiac imaging methods that could have been replaced by radionuclide imaging.

Results.—From 1996 to 1998, the total usage per 100,000 Medicare beneficiaries for the 4 codes rose 19.1% (4046 to 4820). For radiologists the increase was 3.7%, for cardiologists it was 36.3%, and for other physicians it was 18.6%. Total use of the 2 add-on procedures increased 264% over the 2 years, with an increase of 277% for cardiologists, 227% for radiologists, and 314% for other physicians. Radiologists initially performed 48.4% of the MPI examinations and cardiologists 43.8%; over the 2-year period, cardiologists increased their performance statistics to 50.1% and radiologists fell to 42.1%. Because the use by radiologists increased over the same period, the increased performance by cardiologists reflects a much more rapid increase in their utilization rather than a shift in procedure volume between the 2 specialties. The ratio of the add-on examinations to the primary MPI for cardiologists was 0.94, and for radiologists it was 0.53. The performance of stress echocardiography testing by cardiologists increased by 24.2% and that of cardiac catheterization and coronary angiography increased 8.7%.

Conclusions.—The usage rate of MPI grew significantly between 1996 and 1998, with the growth nearly all reflecting increased use by cardiologists. The use of add-on procedures grew even more sharply, so that by 1998, the probability that a patient would undergo one of these procedures was greater when a cardiologist performed MPI than when a radiologist did. Other imaging studies that might have been replaced by MPI also showed increases, so the new procedures are not replacing the old.

▶ The clinical use of MPI, with the added analysis of global and regional ventricular function, is continuing to grow in the Medicare population. A surprising observation is that MPI is not replacing other cardiac imaging procedures but is performed in addition to the other procedures.

H. W. Strauss, MD

Relationship Between Altered Sympathetic Innervation, Oxidative Metabolism and Contractile Function in the Cardiomyopathic Human Heart: A Non-Invasive Study Using Positron Emission Tomography
Bengel FM, Permanetter B, Ungerer M, et al (Technischen Universität München, Germany; Kreiskrankenhaus Fürstenfeldbruck, Germany)
Eur Heart J 22:1594-1600, 2001   10–41

Background.—In patients with progressive heart failure, radiolabeled norepinephrine analogues and nuclear imaging techniques have identified changes in the presynaptic sympathetic innervation, the severity of which is linked closely to clinical outcome. Various noninvasive techniques were used to understand the global and regional relationship among sympathetic innervation, contractile function, and oxidative metabolism in human hearts with cardiomyopathy.

Methods.—The 8 men and 2 women (mean age, 53 years) had chronic idiopathic dilated cardiomyopathy and symptomatic heart failure of at least 6 months' duration. PET with C-11 hydroxyephedrine quantified presynaptic catecholamine uptake sites; C-11 acetate measured oxidative metabolism; and tomographic radionuclide angiography assessed global and regional function. Results were compared with those from control groups of healthy individuals.

Results.—Left ventricular performance was moderately to severely limited. Regional variations marked wall motion, with the highest levels found in the basal anterior and lateral segments and the lowest ones in the region approaching the septum, inferior wall, and apex. Three patients had left-bundle branch block possibly responsible for this reduced septal shortening. The myocardial perfusion measure revealed a regionally homogeneous appearance. The cardiomyopathic patients had a significantly lower global clearance constant k(mono), and there was a significant correlation between the k(mono) value and the rate pressure product. The correlation between afterload and k(mono) reached borderline statistical significance. On multivariate stepwise regression analysis, the rate pressure product and the systemic vascular resistance were identified as independent determinants of oxidative metabolism. In the patients with cardiomyopathy, the global myocardial hydroxyephedrine retention was significantly lower and there was mild regional heterogeneity with the lowest retention in the apex. Abnormally low hydroxyephedrine retention occurred in the patients' left ventricles in 58% of cases. A significant correlation was shown between global hydroxyephedrine retention and left ventricular ejection fraction, and a weak—but significant—correlation also existed between regional hydroxyephedrine retention in myocardial segments and regional endocardial shortening. The nearest independent predictor of global hydroxyephedrine retention in patients with cardiomyopathy was ejection fraction.

Conclusions.—Hearts with cardiomyopathy exhibit altered presynaptic sympathetic innervation, shown by the retention of C-11 hydroxyephedrine, and these changes correlate with reduced contractile performance, but not ventricular loading. Rates of oxidative metabolism also showed no correlation with sympathetic innervation state. The major determinants of myocardial oxygen consumption were cardiac work and ventricular afterload.

▶ This article elegantly correlates the interaction among innervation, oxidative metabolism, and contractile function in patients with idiopathic dilated cardiomyopathy. While perfusion was not markedly decreased, oxidative metabolism was reduced by about 33% and presynaptic innervation reduced by about 37% compared with normal subjects. More studies are necessary to determine whether the reductions in innervation and metabolism are the cause or the effect.

H. W. Strauss, MD

Synthesis and Evaluation of ^{18}F-Labeled Choline Analogs as Oncologic PET Tracers

DeGrado TR, Baldwin SW, Wang S, et al (Duke Univ, Durham, NC)

J Nucl Med 42:1805-1814, 2001   10–42

Background.—The unique capacity of PET to evaluate metabolic activity in human neoplasms has proved useful in the evaluation of many forms of cancer. The glucose analogue [^{18}F]FDG has proven useful as an oncologic PET probe for many types of cancer. However, FDG PET has limited sensitivity for the detection of certain cancer types, such as androgen-dependent prostate cancer. These limitations have prompted efforts to develop new oncologic PET tracers. Studies have identified elevated levels of choline (trimethyl-2-hydroxyethylammonium) and choline kinase (CK) activity in neoplasms and have motivated the development of positron-labeled choline analogues for noninvasive detection of cancer with PET. The use of fluoromethyl-dimethyl-2-hydroxymethylammonium [FCH]) as an oncologic probe was evaluated in comparison with several other closely related molecules.

Methods.—The uptakes of FCH, [^{18}F]fluoromethyl-methylethyl-2-hydroxyethylammonium (FMEC), [^{18}F]fluoroethyl-dimethyl-2-hydroxyethylammonium (FEC), and [^{18}F]fluoropropyl-dimethyl-2-hydroxyethylammonium (FPC) were each evaluated for their biologic acceptance for phosphorylation by CK and uptake by cultured PC-3 human prostate cancer cells. FCH PET was also performed on a patient with prostate cancer, a patient with a brain tumor, and a patient with metastatic breast cancer.

Results.—FCH and FMEC revealed in vitro phosphorylation by CK similar to that of choline, whereas rates of phosphorylation of FEC and FPC were 30% and 60% lower, respectively. The accumulations of FCH, [*methyl*-^{14}C] choline (CH), and FPC in cultured PC-3 cancer cells were comparable, whereas the uptake of FEC was about one fifth the uptake of FCH. Dosimetry estimates indicated that the kidneys are radiation-dose-critical organs for FCH. PET images from the patient with recurrent prostate cancer showed uptake of FCH in the prostatic bed and in metastases to lymph nodes. In the patient with metastatic breast cancer, FCH PET showed uptake in the malignancies (Fig 7). In the patient with recurrent brain tumor proved by biopsy, PET revealed FCH uptake with little confounding uptake in normal brain tissues.

Conclusions.—FCH, a fluoromethyl choline analogue, may serve as a probe of choline uptake and phosphorylation in cancer cells. In contrast, fluoroethyl (FEC) and fluoropropyl (FPC) analogues showed relatively poorer biologic compatibility. Preliminary PET studies in patients with prostate cancer, breast cancer, and brain tumor are supportive of the need for further studies to determine the usefulness of FCH as an oncologic probe.

▶ ^{18}F-Fluoromethyl choline is a biologically useful analogue of choline. It is concentrated in patients with gliomas, prostate and breast cancer. Fluorocholine imaging appears to provide data that are complementary to that of FDG.

H. W. Strauss, MD

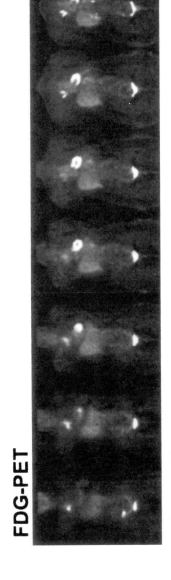

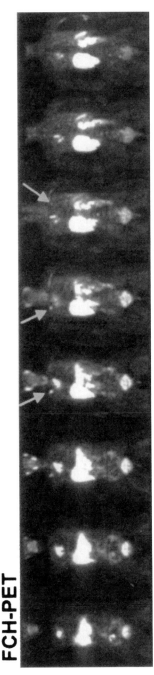

FIGURE 7.—Patient with metastatic breast cancer underwent FCH PET and FDG PET. Myocardial uptake is observed only with FDG, whereas more prominent uptake in salivary glands, liver, and kidneys is seen with FCH, which is consistent with normal uptake of choline by these tissues. Uptake of FDG and FCH is indicated in large metastases associated with sternum, right hilar and paratracheal lymph nodes, and right anterior pelvis. Volume of submanubrial metastasis was significantly larger on FCH PET scan. Smaller regions of focal uptake are observed on FCH PET scan in right chest wall and left lung (*arrows*) that are not seen on FDG PET scan. Uptake pattern of FDG was homogeneous across anterior pelvic metastasis, whereas FCH was taken up preferentially by periphery of this tumor. (Reprinted by permission of the Society of Nuclear Medicine, from DeGrado TR, Baldwin SW, Wang S, et al: Synthesis and evaluation of ^{18}F-labeled choline analogs as oncologic PET tracers. *J Nucl Med* 42:1805-1814, 2001.)

Relationship Between Evaluation by Quantitative Fatty Acid Myocardial Scintigraphy and Response to β-Blockade Therapy in Patients With Dilated Cardiomyopathy

Ito T, Hoshida S, Nishino M, et al (Osaka Rosai Hosp, Japan)
Eur J Nucl Med 28:1811-1816, 2001   10–43

Background.—Patients who have dilated cardiomyopathy (DCM) may also have an impaired myocardial fatty acid metabolism, which has implications for the effectiveness of therapy. Iodine 123 15-(*p*-iodophenyl)-3-*R*,*S*-methylpentadecanoic acid (BMIPP) myocardial scintigraphy can visualize the extent of myocardial injury. The images thus obtained were evaluated to see if the extent of injury is related to the ability of patients with DCM to respond to therapy with β-blockers.

Methods.—BMIPP myocardial scintigraphy was performed before and 6 months after 37 patients with DCM received metoprolol therapy. A quantitative estimate of myocardial BMIPP uptake (%BM uptake) was calculated as a percentage of the total injected count ratio. Other values that were measured included left ventricular end-diastolic and end-systolic dimensions (LVDd, LVDs) and ejection fraction (LVEF).

Results.—On the basis of the functional results at 6 months, patients fell into 2 groups: those improving more than 10% in LVEF (28 patients) and those improving less than 10% (9 patients). For 2 patients, metoprolol was discontinued because their conditions deteriorated with its increased administration; these patients were among the nonresponders. Significant improvements in LVDd, LVDs, and LVEF were achieved with 6 months of metoprolol therapy among the responders, whereas these values remained unchanged from baseline in the nonresponders. Responders had significantly higher %BM uptake values than nonresponders (2.1% compared with 1.0%). By multiple regression analysis, %BM uptake independently predicted the outcome of β-blocker therapy. When %BM was reduced, globally impaired uptake was present. The sensitivity of %BM uptake in detecting responders versus nonresponders was 0.93, and the specificity was 1.00 at a threshold value of 1.4.

Conclusions.—The quantitative method chosen allowed a greater differential evaluation between responders and nonresponders than earlier studies indicated. BMIPP scintigraphy was able to predict the response of patients with DCM to β-blocker therapy, with a threshold value of 1.4%GM uptake of value in differentiating those who will respond from those who will not. The slightly higher BMIPP uptake in the myocardial tissues of responders before therapy is begun may indicate a greater capacity to reverse the damage to the injured myocardium.

▶ This is an impressive study. There have been several articles suggesting that patients with DCM have an altered myocardial metabolic preference—changing from fatty acid to glucose. Although it is unclear whether this is a cause or an effect, this investigation suggests persistent fatty acid uptake is a good predictor of response to β-blocker therapy. Because carvedolol may be even more effective than metoprolol, it would be interesting to see if BMIPP uptake is also predictive with carvedolol.

H. W. Strauss, MD

Comparison of Sestamibi, Tetrofosmin, and Q12 Retention in Porcine Myocardium

Matsunari I, Haas F, Nguyen NTB, et al (Technische Universität München, Munich; Deutches Hezzentrum München, Munich)
J Nucl Med 42:818-823, 2001

10–44

Background.—Stress ^{201}Tl myocardial perfusion imaging has been widely used for 20 years in the evaluation of coronary artery disease (CAD). The low photon energy and the relatively long physical half-life, however, impose limitations on this technique despite its excellent physiologic characteristics. Efforts have been made to develop new myocardial perfusion tracers that can be labeled with ^{99m}Tc, and several ^{99m}Tc-labeled perfusion agents have now been introduced as an alternative to conventional [201]Tl. The most widely used of these is ^{99m}Tc-sestamibi, a lipophilic cationic tracer. Recently 2 other ^{99m}Tc-labeled tracers, ^{99m}Tc-tetrofosmin and ^{99m}Tc-Q12, have been proposed for clinical use. The myocardial retention of these 3 ^{99m}Tc-labeled tracers in a porcine model was assessed.

Methods.—The model included 6 pigs with coronary occlusion and 3 pigs without coronary occlusion. A simultaneous injection was administered of sestamibi and either tetrofosmin (5 pigs) or Q12 (4 pigs) labeled with either ^{99m}Tc or [95m]Tc during pharmacologic vasodilation. The absolute myocardial retention of each tracer was then calculated from the myocardial tracer activity and arterial input function.

Results.—For all 3 tracers, the plot of the tracer versus flow achieved a plateau at a higher flow range. Sestamibi, however, demonstrated a higher mean retention than either tetrofosmin or Q12. In addition, a linear regression analysis of the relationship between retention and microsphere-determined flow showed a greater increment in retention for sestamibi than for tetrofosmin or Q12.

Conclusions.—All 3 ^{99m}Tc-labeled tracers in this study—sestamibi, tetrofosmin, and Q12—showed a nonlinear increase in retention with increasing flow. Sestamibi, however, may show more favorable characteristics as a flow tracer in a porcine myocardium model.

▶ Although retention is important, it is the contrast between lesion and nonlesion that is critical for diagnosis. Although sestamibi had greater retention, it is not clear from this study whether lesion contrast would be better with sestamibi than tetrofosmin or Q12.

H. W. Strauss, MD

Measurement of Ventricular Volumes and Function: A Comparison of Gated PET and Cardiovascular Magnetic Resonance

Rajappan K, Livieratos L, Camici PG, et al (Natl Heart and Lung Inst, London; Imperial College, London)

J Nucl Med 43:806-810, 2002   10–45

Background.—Cardiovascular MR (CMR) is the standard method whereby the parameters indicating left ventricular (LV) and right ventricular (RV) function are determined. Cardiac PET may also be used to obtain information on ventricular function along with myocardial metabolism, perfusion, and receptor density data. Cardiac volumes and function assessment with PET blood-pool imaging were compared with those obtained by ECG gating with CMR.

Methods.—For the 9 patients, measurements were taken with CMR and PET techniques. Parameters included LV and RV end-diastolic volume (EDV), end-systolic volume (ESV), stroke volume (SV), and ejection fractions (EF).

Results.—For LV EF, a slight, but significant, difference was noted between CMR and PET values. For LV SV and LV EDV, the differences between the 2 methods were borderline. All the parameters had correlations between 0.63 and 0.99 (Fig 1). The best agreement was noted for ESV, with underestimations on PET for LV EF and LV EDV and for RV EDV and RV SV. The worst agreement was for LV SV.

Conclusions.—The ventricular function and volume measurements obtained with gated cardiac PET and CMR showed good agreement. Thus, function and volume information can be obtained during a standard PET protocol.

▶ Great correlations!

H. W. Strauss, MD

FIGURE 1.—Scatterplots and Bland-Altman plots for left ventricular parameters measured with cardiovascular MR (*CMR*) and PET. Line of unity (*dashed line*) and linear regression line (*solid line*) with equation, *r*, and probability values are shown on each scatterplot. *Abbreviations: EDV*, End-diastolic volume; *ESV*, end-systolic volume; *SV*, stroke volume; *EF*, ejection fraction. (Reprinted by permission of the Society of Nuclear Medicine, from Rajappan K, Livieratos L, Camici PG, et al: Measurement of ventricular volumes and function: A comparison of gated PET and cardiovascular magnetic resonance. *J Nucl Med* 43:806-810, 2002.)

FIGURE 1

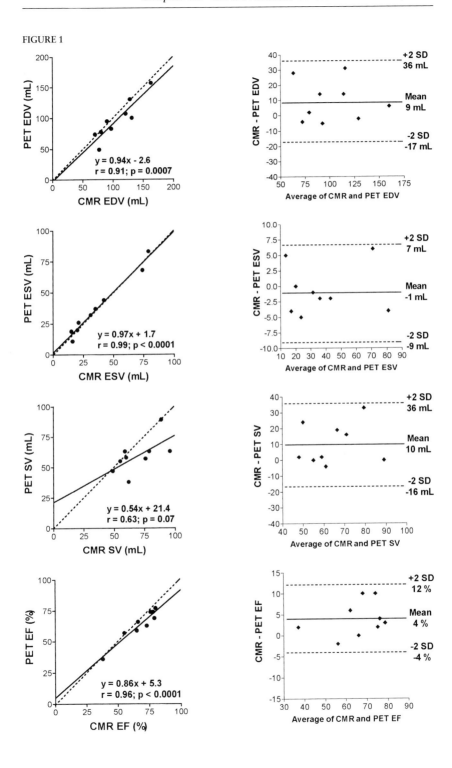

Assessment of Coronary Flow Reserve: Comparison Between Contrast-Enhanced Magnetic Resonance Imaging and Positron Emission Tomography

Ibrahim T, Nekolla SG, Schreiber K, et al (Technischen Universität München, Munich; Kardiologische Abteilung Krankenhaus München-Bogenhausen, Munich)

J Am Coll Cardiol 39:864-870, 2002   10–46

Background.—The noninvasive evaluation of myocardial flow with the use of nuclear imaging techniques has high diagnostic and prognostic value. PET allows regional quantification of absolute coronary flow reserve (CFR), which shows sensitivity for detecting early abnormalities of coronary vascular reactivity that indicate coronary artery disease (CAD). Contrast-enhanced MRI may also be used to evaluate regional blood flow and can detect regional flow abnormalities in patients with CAD. Quantitative flow measurement with PET and MRI estimates of regional myocardial blood flow were compared.

Methods.—Two groups of healthy volunteers believed to have a low likelihood of CAD (based on history and clinical examination) and 25 patients who had angiographically documented CAD were studied. MRI and PET analyses were done at rest and during adenosine stress. The dynamic MRI evaluation included a multislice ultrafast hybrid sequence and a rapid Gd-DTPA bolus injection. N-13 ammonia PET flow reserve measurements were compared with upslope and peak-intensity indices, which had been regionally determined from first-pass signal intensity curves.

Results.—In 20 healthy volunteers, MRI was done during adenosine infusion and produced a significantly increased rate-pressure product. Fourteen volunteers also had a 0.005 mmol/L bolus of Gd-DTPA injected. The variability rates, both intraobserver and interobserver, were very low. Fourteen healthy volunteers were analyzed by PET and showed a rate-pressure product that increased significantly under adenosine. The CFR assessed by PET was significantly higher than the MRI flow ratios in normal volunteers. Comparable values for the rate-pressure product during stress were achieved by PET and MRI. The MRI indices of flow reserve demonstrated a progressive reduction with increasing severity of coronary artery stenosis. Patients with CAD had reduced MRI indices, even when there were no angiographically detected lesions, when compared with the healthy volunteers. MRI indices in patients with CAD were significantly lower than the CFR in PET, which is consistent with findings among the healthy volunteers. The peak-intensity index correlated poorly with PET flow measurements. The CFR and upslope index showed significant correlations.

Conclusions.—With contrast-enhanced MRI, the stress/rest flow ratios calculated from first-pass myocardial time-intensity curves were found to be stable and reproducible measures. Whereas the upslope index had the highest values among the MRI parameters evaluated, the CFR was underestimated as compared with PET, which can be attributed to the myocardium's low extraction fraction for Gd-DTPA. The MRI upslope index and PET flow reserve estimates were closely related, yielding acceptable diagnostic performance for CAD localization.

▶ The investigators observed a relatively poor correlation between MR signal changes and PET signal changes as predictors of CFR. This may be an intrinsic problem with MR, since gadolinium concentration and changes in the MR signal are not linearly correlated.

H. W. Strauss, MD

Assessment of Left Ventricular Systolic and Diastolic Function Based on the Edge Detection Method With Myocardial ECG-gated SPET
Higuchi T, Nakajima K, Taki J, et al (Kanazawa Univ, Ishikawa, Japan)
Eur J Nucl Med 28:1512-1516, 2001   10–47

Background.—ECG-gated myocardial single-photon emission tomography (G-SPET) can evaluate left ventricular functional parameters during a myocardial perfusion study. Various cardiac diseases are associated with specific patterns of impaired cardiac function, which can be predicted by left ventricular systolic ejection and diastolic filling rates. Gated equilibrium blood pool scintigraphy (GBP) is generally used to measure these parameters, but G-SPET can also be used, although its reliability is undetermined. The ejection and filling rates obtained by G-SPET were compared with those by GBP.

Methods.—The 52 patients (aged 28 to 90 years; mean age, 66 years) were evaluated with G-SPET and GBP within 2 weeks. Ejection fraction (EF), peak ejection rate (PER), peak filling rate (PFR), and mean filling rate during the first third of diastolic time (1/3FRm) were determined with edge detection software.

Results.—Both methods obtained measurements of all parameters. Severe perfusion defects in the apical wall (5 patients), anteroseptal wall (2 patients), inferior wall (2 patients), or septum (1 patient) were detected. No significant differences were found in heart rate or blood pressure between the 2 methods. The correlation coefficients between the 2 methods for EF were 0.90; for PER, 0.88; for PFR, 0.80; and for 1/3FRm, 0.82. The dV/dt parameters were slightly lower with G-SPET than with GBP because of the limited number of frames per cardiac cycle. With regard to EF, PER, and 1/3FRm, the correlations between the 2 methods were good.

Conclusions.—Using edge detection software, G-SPET was able to obtain values for ejection and filling parameters in the 52 patients evaluated. Significant correlations with the values obtained with GBP were achieved in the PER, PFR, and 1/3FRm measurements, although G-SPET gave slightly underestimated values.

▶ Although gated blood pool imaging (at 24 frames/cardiac cycle) is a gold standard for evaluating ventricular function, G-SPET provides very similar data when acquired at 12 frames/cardiac cycle with a 360-degree acquisition.

H. W. Strauss, MD

Improved Coronary Disease Detection With Quantitative Attenuation-Corrected Tl-201 Images
Shotwell M, Singh BM, Fortman C, et al (Univ of Cincinnati, Ohio)
J Nucl Cardiol 9:52-61, 2002   10–48

Background.—Nonuniform attenuation artifacts reduce the ease of interpreting myocardial perfusion images and correlating them with the angiographic findings. The best way to handle this is to entirely eliminate the effects of the nonuniform attenuation. Ways to correct the attenuation that are currently available differ in their results. The differences may originate in image acquisition or evaluation methods. The results obtained in attenuation correction of Tl-201 images obtained with the use of a triple-headed gamma camera, fan-beam collimators, a cobalt 57 line source, and image quantitation were reported and assessed for their efficacy in eliminating nonuniform artifacts.

Methods.—Tomographic Tl-201 myocardial imaging was performed in 49 patients who had evidence of coronary artery disease on angiograms (single-vessel disease in 28, double-vessel disease in 12, and triple-vessel disease in 9) and in 69 patients who had a less than 5% likelihood of having coronary artery disease. From this latter group, scintigraphic data from the first 20 men and 20 women allowed the generation of normal reference ranges for the three processing methods, specifically, attenuation correction, attenuation with Compton scatter correction, and no correction.

Results.—For visually interpreted images, the detection rate for coronary artery disease in the left anterior descending artery territory was 79% whether the images were made with attenuation correction or with attenuation-scatter correction but was only 46% with uncorrected images. Normalcy rates for the three processing methods were equal. On the right side, the detection rate was similar for all three, but attenuation-corrected images had a much better normalcy rate than uncorrected images. Overall, the detection rates for the three methods were essentially equal, but a significantly improved normalcy rate was linked to attenuation-corrected images than to the uncorrected images. Thus on visual assessment, the severity of defects was increased by attenuation correction in left anterior descending stenoses and decreased in right coronary artery stenoses. With quantitative analysis, detection rates were nonsignificantly higher with attenuation correction and attenuation-scatter correction. Per-patient analysis showed attenuation correction produced a higher coronary disease detection rate than uncorrected images. Attenuation–scatter corrected images produced a nonsignificant trend toward detecting more stenotic arteries in comparison with uncorrected images.

Conclusions.—Attenuation correction improved the detection of left anterior descending coronary artery stenosis without reducing disease detection elsewhere or reducing the normalcy rate. Quantitative analysis improved overall detection rates and did not reduce the normalcy rate. The detection rate and normalcy rate were also higher in the left anterior descending coronary artery territory with the quantitation method. The attenuation-scatter method did not improve detection rate or normalcy rate over those obtained with attenuation only.

▶ This study documents the importance of attenuation correction in the interpretation of perfusion images. Now, instrument manufacturers need to advance the technology of measuring attenuation to make the procedure seamless in clinical practice.

H. W. Strauss, MD

Dobutamine Stress Echocardiography Versus Quantitative Technetium-99m Sestamibi SPECT for Detecting Residual Stenosis and Multivessel Disease After Myocardial Infarction
Lancellotti P, Benoit T, Rigo P, et al (Univ Hosp of Liège, Belgium)
Heart 86:510-515, 2001   10–49

Introduction.—Dobutamine stress echocardiography (DSE) and technetium-99m sestamibi SPECT (mibi) are useful in the diagnosis and functional evaluation of coronary artery disease, but these techniques have not been compared for their ability to predict residual stenosis of the infarct-related artery and the presence of multivessel disease early after acute myocardial infarction. Seventy-five patients who underwent simultaneous DSE and mibi SPECT were studied prospectively.

Methods.—Patients were 61 men and 14 women with a mean age of 56 years. All had experienced a first noncomplicated acute myocardial infarct and underwent the imaging studies at a mean of 5 days later. Quantitative coronary angiography and left ventriculography were performed within 1 week of DSE and mibi SPECT.

Results.—Sixty-nine patients had significant stenosis (>50%) of the infarct-related artery. Stenosis was mild in 11 patients, moderate in 21, and severe ($\geq$70%) in 17. Elective coronary angiography was performed in 35 patients, 15 of whom had multivessel disease. Residual ischemia was identified with DSE in 55 patients and with mibi SPECT in 49 patients. Sensitivity of the tests was 78% and 70%, respectively; specificity was 83% for both tests. Combining the tests increased sensitivity to 94% but did not improve specificity. In the detection of mild stenosis, mibi SPECT was far more sensitive (73%) than DSE (9%). The findings of wall motion abnormalities with DSE and transient perfusion defects with mibi SPECT outside the infarction zone were sensitive (Fig 2) and highly specific for multivessel disease.

Conclusion.—After early acute myocardial infarction, DSE and mibi SPECT are equally accurate in the detection of residual infarct-related artery stenosis of 50% or greater and the presence of multivessel disease. DSE is more accurate in the prediction of moderate or severe infarct-related artery stenosis. Combining the imaging methods improves only the detection of mild stenosis.

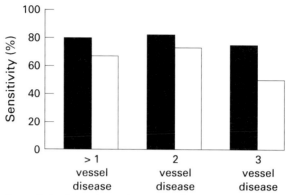

FIGURE 2.—Bar graph showing sensitivity of quantitative ^{99m}Tc sestamibi single-photon emission computed tomography (mibi SPECT) and dobutamine stress echocardiography (DSE) for detecting multivessel disease. *Black bars*, residual ischemia on DSE; *white bars*, residual ischemia on mibi SPECT. (Courtesy of Lancellotti P, Benoit T, Rigo P, et al: Dobutamine stress echocardiography versus quantitative technetium-99m sestamibi SPECT for detecting residual stenosis and multivessel disease after myocardial infarction. *Heart* 86:510-515, 2001. With permission from the BMJ Publishing Group.)

▶ Perfusion imaging was sensitive for detecting lesions with more than 50% stenosis, but much to my surprise, stress echo is better at detecting lesions with 70% narrowing, as well as multivessel disease. These findings are at odds with the generally accepted dictum that radionuclide studies are more sensitive, but echo is more specific.

H. W. Strauss, MD

Evaluation of Left Ventricular Function Using Electrocardiographically Gated Myocardial SPECT With ^{123}I-Labeled Fatty Acid Analog
Nanasato M, Ando A, Isobe S, et al (Nagoya Daini Red Cross Hosp, Japan; Nagoya Univ, Japan)
J Nucl Med 42:1747-1756, 2001   10–50

Background.—The diagnostic and prognostic value of left ventricular (LV) ejection fraction (LVEF) for patients with ischemic heart disease is well documented. LV function is evaluated in many cases by ECG-gated myocardial SPECT with ^{99m}Tc-tetrofosmin, but the accuracy of the variables LVEF, LV end-diastolic volume (LVEDV), and LV end-systolic volume (LVESV) with the use of this method and β-methyl-*p*-^{123}I-iodophenylpentadecanoic acid (BMIPP) is as yet unclear.

Methods.—The 29 men and 7 women (mean age, 61.6 years) had ischemic heart disease and were evaluated with ECG-gated myocardial SPECT with ^{123}I-BMIPP and with ^{99m}Tc-tetrofosmin and left ventriculography (LVG) within 1 week. The variables in question were assessed on gated SPECT and evaluated with commercially available software for automatic data analysis. Visual assessment of the regional wall motion by using these methods was also carried out.

Results.—On ^{123}I-BMIPP, the mean LVEF was 41.1%; on ^{99m}Tc-tetrofosmin it was 44.5%; and on LVG it was 46.0%. Mean values for LVEDV were 113.2, 118.1, and 126.9 mL, respectively; those for LVESV were 69.1, 69.2, and 69.5 mL, respectively. The 2 gated SPECT procedures showed no significant differences in the values of these variables. Excellent correlation was shown between the global LV function and regional wall motion between the 2 gated SPECT methods, but significantly lower correlations were noted between each gated SPECT method and LVG. The interobserver validity was the same for the 2 gated SPECT methods.

Conclusions.—The use of ECG-gated myocardial SPECT with ^{123}I-BMIPP gave accurate LVEF and LV volumes when compared to the use of gated SPECT with ^{99m}Tc-tetrofosmin and LVG. It is possible to assess myocardial fatty acid metabolism and LV function simultaneously with the ^{123}I-BMIPP SPECT method, which increases its desirability in evaluating various cardiac diseases.

▶ It is impressive that administering 111 to 148 MBq of iodine-123 and 550 to 740 MBq of technetium-99m results in gated images of the heart that correlate well in terms of left ventricular wall motion, volumes, and ejection fraction. The data suggest that (1) the quantitative programs are robust, and (2) BMIPP can define both ventricular function and the distribution of fatty acid metabolism.

H. W. Strauss, MD

Usefulness of *Dobutamine* Tc-99m Sestamibi-Gated Single-Photon Emission Computed Tomography for Prediction of Left Ventricular Ejection Fraction Outcome After Coronary Revascularization for Ischemic Cardiomyopathy

Leoncini M, Sciagrà R, Maioli M, et al (Misericordia e Dolce Hosp, Prato, Italy; Univ of Florence, Italy)
Am J Cardiol 89:817-821, 2002   10–51

Background.—Gated SPECT is useful in the assessment of regional and global left ventricular (LV) function. Changes in myocardial perfusion during gated SPECT with low-dose dobutamine infusion allow assessment of myocardial viability. Whether changes in LV ejection fraction (LVEF) between rest and dobutamine nitrate-enhanced technetium (Tc) 99m sestamibi-gated SPECT were predictive of changes in global function after revascularization in patients with ischemic cardiomyopathy were examined.

Methods.—The subjects were 37 patients (33 men and 5 women; mean age, 63) with coronary artery disease and impaired LV function (mean LVEF 32%). Before undergoing complete myocardial revascularization, all patients underwent resting and dobutamine nitrate-enhanced sestamibi-gated SPECT. Within 3 months or more after coronary artery bypass grafting (n = 14) or within 1 month after coronary angioplasty (n = 14), baseline resting sestamibi-gated SPECT was repeated to assess global changes in function. A significant improvement in global function was defined as a change in LVEF of 5% or greater after revascularization.

Results.—The mean LVEF improved significantly from 34% to 39% after revascularization. Nineteen patients (51%) had a significant improvement in global function, whereas 18 patients (49%) had an increase in LVEF of less than 5%. Receiver operating characteristic curve analysis indicated that the optimal cutoff value for predicting a significant improvement in LVEF after revascularization was an increase in LVEF of 5% or greater during dobutamine infusion. The sensitivity, specificity, and accuracy of this cutoff value were 79%, 78%, and 78%, respectively. The increase in LVEF during dobutamine infusion correlated significantly with the increase in LVEF after revascularization ($r = 0.85$).

Conclusion.—An increase in LVEF of 5% or greater during dobutamine-enhanced Tc-99m sestamibi-gated SPECT was a good predictor of a significant improvement in LVEF after revascularization in these patients with ischemic cardiomyopathy.

▶ Low-dose dobutamine imaging with determination of rest and dobutamine ejection fraction is a very effective approach to the identification of viable ischemic tissue.

H. W. Strauss, MD

11 Correlative Imaging

Introduction

This chapter begins with correlative neuro cases, beginning with a discussion of SPECT and MRI for brain perfusion. Tumor grading and a variant of Cushing's disease follow. Finally, two unusual cases, neuro-Behçet's disease and Nipah encephalitis, end the neuro correlative portion. The section ends with correlative bone selections, starting with two unusual examples of neoplasm, and ending with tendonopathy and unusual osteochondral lesions.

Alexander Gottschalk, MD

Quantitative Measurement of Regional Cerebral Blood Flow With Flow-Sensitive Alternating Inversion Recovery Imaging: Comparison With [Iodine 123]-Iodoamphetamin Single Photon Emission CT
Arbab AS, Aoki S, Toyama K, et al (Yamanashi Med Univ, Japan; GE-YMS, Tokyo)
AJNR Am J Neuroradiol 23:381-388, 2002   11–1

Background.—Both SPECT and PET are well-established techniques for the assessment of cerebral perfusion. In addition, regional cerebral blood flow (rCBF) measurements with various brain imaging techniques have a good correlation with the criterion standard rCBF measurements obtained with either radioactive microspheres or xenon 133. Flow-sensitive alternating inversion recovery (FAIR) MR imaging is a technique for the depiction of cerebral perfusion without contrast enhancement. Whether quantification at FAIR imaging can be used to assess rCBF in a manner similar to [iodine 123]-iodoamphetamine (^{123}I-IMP) SPECT was assessed.

Methods.—A group of 9 patients with internal carotid or major cerebral arterial stenosis underwent ^{123}I-IMP SPECT and FAIR imaging at rest and after acetazolamide stress. Values for FAIR and ^{123}I-IMP rCBF were compared and correlated. Receiver operating characteristic analysis was performed to detect hypoperfused segments on FAIR images.

Results.—The rCBF values of normally perfused segments were 41.53 mL/100 g/min for pre-acetazolamide ^{123}I-IMP and 51.91 mL/100 g/min for post-acetazolamide ^{123}I-IMP studies. Corresponding values for pre-acetazolamide and post-acetazolamide FAIR images, respectively, were 46.64 and 59.60 mL/100 g/min with a TI of 1200 milliseconds and 53.23 and 68.17

mL/100 g/min with a TI of 1400 milliseconds. There was significant correlation between ^{123}I-IMP and FAIR results for both the pre-acetazolamide and post-acetazolamide images. Sensitivity in detecting hypoperfused segments was significantly higher with post-acetazolamide images (86%), and specificity (82% to 85%) and accuracy (80% to 82%) were higher with all pre-acetazolamide and post-acetazolamide images (all TIs).

Conclusions.—These findings indicated that FAIR imaging, like nuclear medicine studies, complements routine MR imaging in the assessment of cerebral perfusion.

▶ I have often complained about comparisons of antiquated MRI sequences to modern nuclear medicine techniques. This article gives you an example of why I have made that complaint. If their MRI technique is widely accepted, it could seriously dent *or* replace brain perfusion studies in nuclear medicine. Furthermore, "fusion" would be automatic.

A. Gottschalk, MD

Pre-operative Grading of Intracranial Glioma: Comparison of MR-Determined Cerebral Blood Volume Maps With Thallium-201 SPECT
Lam WW-M, Chan K-W, Wong W-L, et al (Chinese Univ, Hong Kong)
Acta Radiol 42:548-554, 2001   11–2

Background.—Low-grade gliomas often evolve into high-grade gliomas, and the incidence of evolvement can be as high as 50%. In patients with low-grade gliomas that are treated conservatively, monitoring of the lesion allows early detection of transformation and active proliferation and timely management. Several different imaging modalities have been used in previous studies to assess the grading of the glioma. The accuracy of MRI-determined cerebral blood volume (CBV) maps was compared with the accuracy of SPECT imaging with thallium-201 in the preoperative grading of intracranial glioma.

Methods.—Nineteen patients (7 women, 12 men) with a mean age of 46.8 years with intracranial gliomas were examined with MR perfusion imaging before surgery. Sixteen of these patients were also evaluated with SPECT imaging with thallium-201. The main outcome measures were the tumor-to-contralateral-white-matter negative integral and tracer uptake ratios. These ratios were compared in high- and low-grade tumors.

Results.—Grades I and II gliomas had maximum CBV ratios that were significantly lower than the maximum CBV ratio of grades III and IV gliomas. No statistical difference was found when the CBV ratios of grades I and II, graded II and III, and grades III and IV gliomas were compared. No difference in tumor uptake ratio was seen on thallium SPECT imaging between low- and high-grade gliomas.

Conclusions.—Negative integral determination with MRI was found to be useful for preoperative grading of intracranial gliomas; however, SPECT thallium-201 imaging was not useful for this evaluation.

▶ This is discouraging. I worry that these usually "ring enhancing" lesions, that is, a necrotic center with extensive peripheral tumor neovascularity, may be averaged for the lower resolution thallium data and not for MRI. This could compromise the thallium analysis because uptake in the necrotic center should be minimal, and image averaging would blend this into the image data as a whole.

A. Gottschalk, MD

Serendipitous Detection of Cushing's Disease by FDG Positron Emission Tomography and a Review of the Literature
Komori T, Martin WH, Graber AL, et al (Vanderbilt Univ, Nashville, Tenn)
Clin Nucl Med 27:176-178, 2002   11–3

Background.—A patient with progressive dementia had adrenocortico-tropic hormone–producing pituitary adenoma diagnosed as a serendipitous finding on FDG-PET images. The patient had Cushing's disease associated with dementia-like neuropsychiatric symptoms.

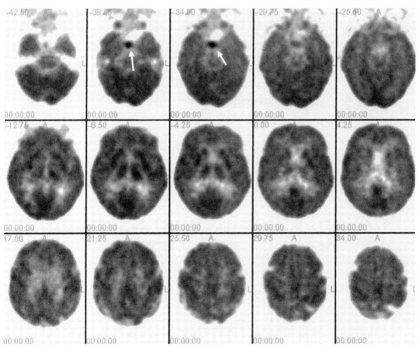

FIGURE 1.—Axial FDG-PET images show hypermetabolism in the pituitary gland (*arrow*) and global decreased uptake in the cortical and subcortical gray matter. The distribution of FDG does not suggest a degenerative dementia. (Courtesy of Komori T, Martin WH, Graber AL, et al: Serendipitous detection of Cushing's disease by FDG positron emission tomography and a review of the literature. *Clin Nucl Med* 27 (3):176-178, 2002.)

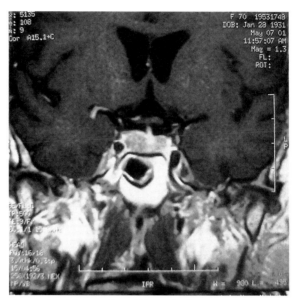

FIGURE 2.—A coronal gadolinium-enhanced T1-weighted MR image shows 2 foci of abnormal enhancement within the pituitary gland. The largest on the right measures 1 × 0.8 cm, and the left focus measures 0.7 × 0.6 cm. These were most consistent with dual adenomas. (Courtesy of Komori T, Martin WH, Graber AL, et al: Serendipitous detection of Cushing's disease by FDG positron emission tomography and a review of the literature. *Clin Nucl Med* 27(3):176-178, 2002.)

Case Report.—Woman, 70, was evaluated for progressive dementia and bizarre behavioral changes and underwent FDG-PET imaging of the brain to assess the presence of degenerative dementia. The patient had a history of hypertension and diabetes mellitus, but she did not manifest the phenotypic features of Cushing's disease. Her serum glucose level was elevated to 179 mg/dL at the time of FDG administration. The FDG-PET images showed marked uptake of FDG in the pituitary gland and global diffusely decreased uptake in the cortical and subcortical gray matter (Fig 1). The distribution of FDG in the cortex was unremarkable otherwise and was not typical of Alzheimer's dementia. An MR image showed 2 enhancing lesions in the pituitary gland, 1 measuring 1 cm on the right and the other measuring 0.7 cm on the left (Fig 2). Endocrinologic evaluation revealed Cushing's disease. The tumors were resected. Pathologic examination revealed a pituitary adenoma with corticotropic cells in the right pituitary gland and enlarged acini of corticotrophs within normal adenohypophysis, consistent with corticotropic hyperplasia, in the left pituitary gland. The patient's dementia and behavioral changes subsided gradually after surgery.

Conclusions.—Normal pituitary glands do not accumulate FDG and are not visualized by FDG PET, but the most common intrasellar tumors, pituitary adenomas and craniopharyngiomas, do accumulate FDG to a high degree despite being benign. It is speculated that abnormal cerebral glucose metabolism might be a contributing factor to the cognitive and psychiatric abnormalities that are frequently observed in patients with Cushing's disease.

▶ A nice case with a happy outcome.

A. Gottschalk, MD

Brain Perfusion SPECT in Juvenile Neuro-Behçet's Disease
Vignola S, Nobili F, Picco P, et al (Univ of Genoa, Italy)
J Nucl Med 42:1151-1157, 2001   11–4

Background.—Behçet's disease is a systemic vasculitis characterized by recurrent oral and genital ulcerations and relapsing uveitis. Virtually any organ or system, including the CNS, may also be affected to some extent. Some of the subtle, at times equivocal, syndromes related to involvement of the CNS in Behçet's disease, such as mild cognitive deterioration and headaches, may result in misinterpretation and may contribute to an underestimation of the actual prevalence of Behçet's disease. In this study, regional cerebral blood flow was evaluated by ^{99m}Tc-hexamethylpropyleneamine oxime SPECT in juvenile patients with Behçet's disease and signs or symptoms of CNS involvement at some time in their clinical history.

Methods.—Of 7 patients enrolled in the study (age range, 7-18 years; mean age, 9.1 years), 3 patients experienced seizures, 3 patients experienced severe, persistent headaches refractory to common analgesic and nonsteroidal anti-inflammatory drugs, and 1 patient had recurrent episodes of acute intracranial hypertension. All patients underwent electroencephalography; 5 patients also underwent MRI, and 1 patient underwent CT. Brain SPECT was performed with a high-resolution, brain-dedicated camera.

Results.—Hypoperfusion was observed in all patients by both visual and asymmetric analyses and was localized primarily in the basal ganglia, the thalami, and the temporal cortex, including the medial portion of the temporal cortex. Temporal perfusion was observed mainly in patients with seizures, whereas hypoperfusion of deep gray nuclei was found primarily in other patients. Impairment of brain function was noted on electroencephalography in 5 of 6 patients, and MRI revealed multiple bilateral white matter lesions in 1 patient with persistent headaches.

Conclusions.—Perfusion SPECT seems to be quite sensitive to brain abnormalities in children and adolescents with Behçet's disease and signs or symptoms of CNS involvement, even when findings on brain MRI are negative.

▶ This series details an interesting facet of an interesting disease. It points out that, although no consistent SPECT perfusion pattern is characteristic, one should watch for hypoperfusion in the basal ganglia, the thalami, and the temporal lobe cortex. It would be interesting to have before and after SPECT scans after steroid therapy and clinical relief to see by how much the perfusion deficit has been corrected.

A. Gottschalk, MD

Relapsed and Late-Onset Nipah Encephalitis
Tan CT, Goh KJ, Wong KT, et al (Univ of Malaya, Malaysia; Seremban Hosp, Malaysia; Kuala Lumpur Hosp, Malaysia)
Ann Neurol 51:703-708, 2002   11–5

Background.—From September 1998 to June 1999 there was an outbreak of a previously undescribed encephalitis in several pig-farming villages in Malaysia and Singapore. A total of 265 patients developed acute encephalitis and were admitted to hospitals throughout Malaysia, and 105 of these patients died. The causative agent was determined to be a new paramyxovirus, subsequently named *Nipah virus*. Genomic sequencing has established the Nipah virus as a new paramyxovirus closely related to the Hendra virus. The primary manifestation of Nipah virus infection was a severe acute encephalitic syndrome. While many patients made a full recovery, it was observed that some patients might develop neurological manifestations for the first time several months after recovery from acute nonencephalitic or asymptomatic infection. A preliminary investigation has indicated that these late complications may result from direct viral attack rather than postinfectious demyelination. The first comprehensive report of relapsed and late-onset encephalitis after acute Nipah virus infection in Malaysia more than 2 years after the initial outbreak was presented.

Methods.—After the initial outbreak of Nipah virus infection, approximately 160 patients who recovered from acute encephalitis and 89 patients who had either nonencephalitic or asymptomatic infection were followed up at various treatment centers.

Results.—A total of 12 survivors (7.5%) of acute encephalitis had recurrent neurological disease (relapsed encephalitis). Of the patients who initially had acute nonencephalitic or asymptomatic infection, 10 patients (3.4%) had late-onset encephalitis. The mean time between the first neurologic episode and the time of initial infection was 8.4 months. Three patients had a second neurologic episode. The onset of the relapsed or late-onset encephalitis was usually acute. Common clinical features in these patients were fever, headache, seizures, and focal neurologic signs. There were 4 (18%) deaths among the 22 relapsed and late-onset encephalitis patients. Magnetic resonance imaging typically revealed patchy areas of confluent cortical lesions, and serial SPECT showed the evolution of focal hyperperfusion to hypoperfusion in the corresponding areas. Necropsy in 2 patients revealed changes in focal encephalitis with positive immunolocalization for Nipah virus antigens, but there was no evidence of perivenous demyelination.

Conclusions.—In Nipah virus infection of the CNS, a unique relapsing and remitting encephalitis or late-onset encephalitis may develop.

► This seems far out. But, I thought West Nile Virus was far out also. So, if in the future we hear more about either the Nipah or Hendra virus, remember that you heard it here first.

A. Gottschalk, MD

A Case of Aseptic Vertebral Necrosis in the Context of Metastatic Lumbar Disease
Panow C, Valavanis A (Radiologie Florissant, Geneva; Universitätsspital Zürich, Switzerland)
Neuroradiology 44:249-252, 2002   11–6

Introduction.—Aseptic necrosis of vertebral bodies usually appears as the main feature of Scheuermann disease in adolescence or as Kümmell disease in elderly patients with osteoporosis. A case was reported in which metastatic Ewing sarcoma involving the vertebral spine was the origin of vertebral body necrosis.

Case Report.—Man, 19, had undergone 5 years of treatment for metastatic Ewing sarcoma of the lower extremity. Three weeks after a regular bone scintigraphy appeared normal, the patient was seen with acute lumbar pain after minor trauma. Repeat bone scintigraphy revealed peripheral captation of the vertebral body of L1, with a photopenic center. Overt local metastatic disease was not apparent on MRI, and no abnormality was seen on conventional radiography. The patient was seen 11 months later with progressive lumbar pain, voiding problems, and L5 radicular symptoms on both sides. Extensive metastatic involvement was shown on MRI and confirmed by vertebral body biopsy.

Conclusion.—Although metastatic disease of Ewing sarcoma was not apparent initially on MRI or Tc-99m bone scintigraphy, it proved to be the origin of vertebral body necrosis. A neoplastic condition should be included in the differential diagnosis of avascular necrosis of the vertebral body.

► I once saw melanoma do this. I always thought that metastatic compression of the vascular network to the vertebral body was the cause. If you look carefully at the early MRI, you can find a small anterior perispinal mass, which is easy to see on the late MRI exam. This could be the culprit because compression would markedly decrease or even abolish tracer delivery.

A. Gottschalk, MD

Metastatic Clear-Cell Sarcoma of the Capitate: A Case Report

Reichert B, Hoch J, Plötz W, et al (Med Univ of Lübeck, Germany)
J Bone Joint Surg Am 83-A:1713-1717, 2001   11–7

Background.—Clear-cell sarcoma is a very rare tumor that occurs in intimate association with tendons or aponeuroses and has phenotypic features in common with malignant melanoma; it is therefore referred to as melanoma of the soft parts. Clear-cell sarcoma occurs more commonly in women than in men. Patients are usually between 20 and 40 years of age. The most common sites for this highly malignant tumor are the limbs, particularly the region of the foot and ankle. Metastases to the bones of the hand are very rare and account for 0.1% of all metastases. The capitate has not previously been reported as the initial metastatic site of soft-tissue sarcoma.

Case Report.—Man, 29, presented with a 4-week history of pain in the right foot. Physical examination showed the plantar surface of the foot to be swollen and tender. MRI showed a well-defined, ellipsoid mass measuring 8 × 4 × 3.8 cm between the metatarsal bones and the plantar aponeurosis. CT showed erosion of the fifth metatarsal. Open biopsy revealed a circumscribed, lobulated nodular mass. Histologic examination of the mass demonstrated a uniform pattern that consisted of compact nests of rounded or fusiform cells with a pale or clear cytoplasm. A network of collagenous tissue was seen between the cells. On immunohistochemical analysis, the tumor cells expressed antigens for S-100 protein and melanoma-associated antigen, reflecting melanin synthesis. Antibodies reactive to epithelial membrane antigen and cytokeratin were negative. The diagnosis of clear-cell sarcoma was made. Staging examinations did not reveal metastatic dissemination. A transtibial amputation was performed 18 days after the biopsy. At the amputation site, both soft tissue and bone marrow from the tibia were free of tumor-cell infiltration. Two months after initial diagnosis, the patient fell onto both hands. One week later he sought medical attention for continued pain, and a fracture of the capitate with osteolysis was found on examination of the left wrist. An open biopsy of the capitate revealed malignant tissue resembling a clear-cell sarcoma. The diagnosis was confirmed histopathologically. Multiple metastases were later found in the left humerus, axilla, and clavicle and within the superior mediastinum. Additional widespread metastases developed, and the patient died 10 months after the initial presentation.

Conclusions.—The average age of patients at the first manifestation of clear-cell sarcoma is approximately 25 years, and the most frequent site for the primary tumor is the foot. The mass is moderately sized and grows slowly. Pain is reported by only half of patients, so there may be several years between the first occurrence of the tumor and treatment. Once a metastatic clear-cell sarcoma in the hand or wrist has been confirmed, further spread of tumor is likely. A limb-preserving procedure rather than amputation through the forearm should be performed whenever possible because the prognosis for clear-cell sarcoma is very poor. The unique feature of the present case is the initial metastasis to the capitate, which has not previously been documented.

▶ A most unusual case. This tumor seems to have grown so fast the doubling time could be measured in microseconds. However, in describing these tumors, the authors note the typical clinical mass "grows slowly." This suggests that widespread latent metastases are hanging around—in this case in the capitate. It makes me wonder what a whole-body PET scan with FDG would have looked like.

A. Gottschalk, MD

Case Report: Positive Bone Scan Findings in Grade I Posterior Tibial Tendon Dysfunction
Ameglio PJ, Philbin T, Pomeroy G (Integrated Orthopaedics, Exeter, NH; Portland Orthopaedic Foot and Ankle Ctr, South Portland, Me; Univ of New England, Portland, Me)
Foot Ankle Int 22:953-955, 2001   11–8

Background.—Two patients with grade I posterior tibial tendon dysfunction after inversion-type ankle injuries had bone scan findings suggestive of a medial malleolus fracture. The patients had not responded to nonoperative treatment. A bone scan and MRI had not delineated the correct diagnosis. The patients were seen at the authors' clinic at 5 and 7 months, respectively, from their injuries, with complaints of persistent medial ankle pain.

 Case 1.—Woman, 44, was referred with a 5-month history of medial ankle pain after an inversion-type ankle injury. Radiographic findings obtained in the emergency department at the time of her injury were negative. Her ankle was placed in a U-stirrup for 4 weeks, after which the patient was told to follow up with her primary care physician. The patient began physical therapy after her initial visit to the primary care physician but failed to improve. A bone scan was requested because of persistent pain in the medial aspect of the ankle, and findings were suggestive of a fracture of the medial malleolus. After 2 months with no improvement, an MRI was performed; the findings suggested an occult osteochondral injury. The patient was placed in a short-leg, non–weight-bearing cast for 6 more weeks, but her symptoms did not improve. A CT scan showed complete disruption of the medial ligament complex, but the adjacent tendons were intact. The patient underwent surgical exploration of the posterior tibial tendon and was found to have a longitudinal tear in the posterior tibial tendon, which was repaired and augmented with a flexor digitorum longus tendon transfer.

Case 2.—Woman, 38, was seen after a 7-month history of medial ankle pain after an inversion-type ankle injury while playing basketball. The findings from the initial radiographic examination were negative for a fracture. The patient's ankle was placed in a U-stirrup for 4 weeks; she was then allowed to resume normal activities. However, she had persistent ankle pain for 9 weeks after the initial injury. A findings of a bone scan suggested an occult fracture or bone bruising. Findings on MRI were consistent with bone bruising and possible trabecular microfractures within the midposterior and medial malleolar portions of the talus and medial malleolus. After 6 more weeks of treatment with a short-leg cast, an ankle lace-up brace, orthotics, and nonsteroidal anti-inflammatory medications, all of which were unsuccessful in relieving her persistent medial ankle pain, the patient was referred to the clinic. She was given a diagnosis of grade I posterior tibial tendon insufficiency, and surgery was advised. A longitudinal tear was discovered in the posterior tibial tendon, along with a thickened periosteum and tendon sheath. It was repaired, and the posterior tibial tendon was augmented with a flexor digitorum longus tendon transfer. The patient healed uneventfully and had complete resolution of her symptoms.

Conclusions.—In both patients, a diagnosis of grade I posterior tibial tendon insufficiency was made and confirmed by findings at surgery. The diagnosis of stage I posterior tibial tendon dysfunction should be considered in a patient who is seen with persistent medial ankle pain after an ankle sprain and a bone scan suggestive of a fracture.

▶ Usually, in articles like this, I complain that one of the techniques is not state-of-the-art and is compared with another that is. In this case, I think both techniques are not up to par. The bone scan could use a pinhole collimator to provide good detail and show precisely where the bone lesion was. The MRI should have either an inversion recovery or a fast spin-echo fat suppression proton density sequence.

I have heard well-known ankle orthopedic surgeons plea for a bone scan to be done before MRI because this allows the MRI sequences to be altered to fit the lesion (eg, the angulation of the foot in relation to the axial slices). In this case, axial slices oriented along the long axis of the calcaneus (instead of oriented perpendicular to the tibia as shown in the article) would display the entire length of the posterior tibial tendon better, and the fat suppressed or inversion recovery images would probably show the tear and the associated contusion, which is usually very difficult to see on the T2-weighted slices shown here.

A. Gottschalk, MD

Bilateral Distal Tibial Osteochondral Lesion: A Case Report

Sopov V, Liberson A, Groshar D (Technion-Israel Inst of Technology, Haifa)

Foot Ankle Int 22:901-904, 2001   11–9

Introduction.—Osteochondral lesion (OCL) is defined as a localized defect in the cartilaginous and subchondral tissue of the bone. The most common location of this condition is the talar dome. The imaging characteristics of OCL are well recognized on MRI; however, no study describing the scintigraphic appearance of this type of lesion has been done. The scintigraphic and MRI findings of bilateral OCL in the distal tibia are discussed.

Case Report.—Woman, 20, was a military recruit with 6 months of persistent pain in both ankle joints. She had been involved in intensive physical training for several months and had no history of acute trauma. Physical examination showed tenderness of the anteromedial aspect of both ankle joints. No anatomical or biomechanical abnormalities were noted in the lower extremities. Findings were normal on anteroposterior and true lateral foot radiographs. Bone-scintigraphy revealed focal increased uptake of technetium-99m methylene diphosphonic acid (^{99m}Tc-MDP) in the blood flow and blood pool, and, in the late phase of the study, at the anteromedial aspect of both distal tibias. An MRI examination showed an OCL in the anteromedial aspect of both tibial plafonds. The patient refused surgery and was treated conservatively with rest and nonsteroidal anti-inflammatory drugs. A month after discontinuing active training, her pain was diminished. At 3 years of follow-up, she continued to experience mild anterior ankle pain during intensive physical training.

Conclusion.—The patient had findings similar to the scintigraphic pattern of OCL in the talar dome. The cause and development of this disease should be further investigated.

▶ I have often seen talar dome osteochondral defects (OCds), but bilateral distal tibial OCds is new to me. The possibility of a genetic predisposition suggested by the authors is intriguing.

A. Gottschalk, MD

12 Physics, Instrumentation, and Dosimetry

Introduction

It is interesting to note that some continuing themes are mixed with new directions in instrumentation, as reflected in the selections for this year's chapter of the YEAR BOOK.

The first three selections deal with established concepts of performance characteristics, quality control, and calibration of camera systems. Two of these three articles deal with PET cameras, which I believe is consistent with the new emphasis on F-18 imaging in our field.

The fourth through seventh articles in this year's chapter represent the renewed interest in registering functional information with anatomy. We remember the initial interest in registering functional and anatomical brain images (appearing approximately 5-7 years ago), and now this has extended to the more difficult problem of registering such pairs of images in the thorax and abdomen. The most direct way of doing this is to build a combined nuclear medicine and x-ray scanner, which by now every major manufacturer has developed. For those clinics not yet fortunate enough to have these combined scanners, some of the software methods for registration described here offer a less expensive alternative.

The next four articles represent some of the more classical contributions that we have seen in years past. Crosstalk corrections for dual isotope SPECT imaging (scatter correction), as well as attenuation correction improvements undergo incremental changes from year to year. In this section of the chapter, the use of statistical parametric mapping (SPM) reminds us that the quantitative improvements gained by scatter and attenuation correction result in more quantitative "clinical interpretations" afforded by statistical analysis of the images.

The 12th through 14th articles represent one of the strongest new directions in our field of nuclear medicine imaging. Firstly, we note the emphasis on "molecular imaging," whereby we delve past the mere macroscopic functional characteristic of organs and look deeper into cellular mechanisms including gene expression. Secondly, the studies are first being carried out in animals; over the past few years we have seen a very strong movement toward the development of imaging instrumentation, specifically with small animals in mind. We have finally moved beyond placing animals into human-sized cameras, and many of our prominent research institutes maintain and operate small animal imagers for developing new radioligands. The resolution in these small animal instruments is truly impressive.

As always, we complete this chapter with an array of articles documenting new methods for calculating dosimetric quantities and evaluations of internal dosimetry of new radiopharmaceuticals. As they do every year, such articles demonstrate the continuing development of new tracers for studying new molecular systems and assure us that the radiation doses delivered to human subjects remain at acceptable risk levels.

I. George Zubal, PhD

Multicenter Comparison of Calibration and Cross Calibration of PET Scanners

Geworski L, Knoop BO, de Wit M, et al (Univ of Berlin; Hannover Med School, Germany; Univ Hosp Eppendorf, Hamburg, Germany; et al)

J Nucl Med 43:635-639, 2002   12–1

Background.—Calibration is the establishment of the relationship between the measured count rate per volume and the true activity concentration. The basic calibration method is similar for all dedicated PET scanners and must be performed for each mode of data acquisition. Procedures differ, however, on the basis of scanner manufacturer and type. Ideally, the calibration involves measurement of a phantom containing a known and homogeneous activity concentration, preferably determined with the on-site dose calibrator. An aliquot of the phantom content has to be withdrawn for cross calibration of the well counter. In practice, however, a manufactured calibration phantom is often used; the manufactured phantom contains a certified activity of the long-lived positron emitter ^{68}Ge in solid matrix, which prevents withdrawal of a sample to check either the dose calibrator or the well counter. The volume of matrix carrying the activity is not certified, resulting in uncertainty regarding the activity concentration. The recommended procedure in this case is to cross calibrate the matrix volume against another cylindrical phantom containing a short-lived positron emitter of known activity and volume, such as ^{18}F. The calibration of PET scanners and their cross calibration to peripheral devices were compared in a multicenter study.

Methods.—Standardized protocols were applied to the evaluation of 23 dedicated PET scanners. Dose calibrators were checked using ^{68}Ge standards to ensure the exact determination of the activity used.

Results.—An error of less than 5% was observed in 9 of 19 3-dimensional acquisition modes and in 11 of 20 two-dimensional acquisition modes. Four scanners displayed an error of 10% in 3-dimensional modes, and 5 scanners displayed an error of 10% in 2-dimensional modes. All other scanners demonstrated errors of 5% to less than 10%. The measurements obtained with one scanner could not be adequately analyzed because of hardware and software problems.

Conclusions.—The calibration of scanners must be carefully checked beforehand for clinical multicenter studies that rely on quantitative analysis of PET data. Thorough application of straightforward, standard procedures can provide an accuracy of at least 5% to 10% error for almost all of the dedicated PET scanners tested. However, permanent monitoring of these scanners is needed to maintain this level of accuracy.

▶ We know, of course, that absolute quantitation of activity is not always essential for clinical diagnosis. Indeed, semiquantitation (or relative uptake determination of radiopharmaceuticals within the body) is typically what clinicians use to make a diagnostic evaluation. However, more clinically important data can be reported by knowing the absolute uptake of the structures we image in nuclear medicine. As we try to attain this better standard of using absolute uptake as a clinical measure, we see that average errors of approximately 10% are somewhat encouraging; however, the occasional error of greater than 20% warns us that as a community, we need to work a little harder to improve our measurement accuracy.

I. G. Zubal, PhD

Decaying Source Method for Scintillation Camera Resolving Times
Woldeselassie T (Addis Ababa Univ, Ethiopia)
Med Phys 28:2336-2343, 2001   12–2

Introduction.—Scintillation camera systems may be effectively described by using the resolving times T and τ_0 of the dominant nonparalyzable and paralyzable components—the detector system and the computer interface, respectively. The decaying source method for scintillation camera resolving times is described.

Methods.—When used with a full spectrum window, the scintillation camera has a lower nonparalyzable and an upper paralyzable operating range with normalized threshold input rate $n_t = N_t \tau_0 = \ln(1 + k_T n_t)$, where $k_T = T/\tau_0$. The correct determination of T and τ_0 necessitates that both r_{12} and r in the normalized 2-source equations $k_T = (2/r_{12} - 1/r)$ and $k_0 = (r_{12}/2r^2)\ln(2r_{12})$ come from the nonparalyzable ($n \leq n_t$) ranges and paralyzable ($n \geq_t$) ranges, respectively. Thus, an important constraint of the 2-source method is that the large ratio $a = n_{12}/n = 2$ can cause an input rate range (n, n_{12}); this includes the threshold point n_t, in which neither T nor τ_0 can be measured accurately. The decaying-source method constitutes a refinement of the 2-source method, which allows smaller ratios $1 < a < 2$ to be used. It also includes the 2-source method as a special case ($a = 2$). This new method needs 2 consecutive readings on a single decaying source, as opposed to 3 measurements on 2 sources of activity, for every determination of T or τ_0; this minimized staff exposure.

Conclusion.—Because only count rates and time intervals need to be recorded, this new method greatly simplifies computerization of the data acquisition and analysis activities. It is obvious that there is potential for real-time applications. The method allows T and τ_0 to be determined accurately and with adequate resolution to show possible variations with input rate. Long measurement times with a decaying source can be bypassed, if needed, by using a set of decaying sources simultaneously to cover various portions of the count rate range.

▶ There are 3 interesting aspects to this publication. First, although the accepted National Electrical Manufacturers Association (NEMA) method requires that 2 sources be used (individually and combined) to measure deadtime, the use of a decaying source while obtaining multiple camera count rate measurements is a more "pleasing" method. It has the added advantage of demonstrating the graphic relationship between measured and actual flux. Second, this article is a fresh review on essential camera performance characteristics, including the mathematical equations. In addition, the follow-up article by the same author published in the same journal[1] continues with this good scientific overview. Finally, I find it encouraging that investigators in lands as far away as Ethiopia support the efforts and science of nuclear medicine and make important contributions to the field.

I. G. Zubal, PhD

Reference

1. Woldeselassie T: Precise real-time correction of anger camera deadtime losses. *Med Phys* 29:1599-1610, 2002.

Performance of a Whole-Body PET Scanner Using Curve-Plate NaI(T1) Detectors

Adam L-E, Karp JS, Daube-Witherspoon ME, et al (Univ of Pennsylvania, Philadelphia)

J Nucl Med 42:1821-1830, 2001   12–3

Background.—The C-PET scanner is one of a new generation of clinically oriented PET scanners (Fig 1, B). This whole-body scanner, without interplane septa, is designed to achieve high performance in clinical applications. It is unique in the use of 6 curved thallium-doped sodium iodide (NaI[T1]) detectors (2.54 cm thick). The scanner has a ring diameter of 90 cm, a patient port diameter of 56 cm, and an axial field of view of 25.6 cm. NaI(T1) has relatively low stopping power compared with other scintillator materials used in PET, but this is partially compensated for by the large axial field of view and the ability to scan without septa. These are possible because of the energy resolution of 11% for NaI(T1); the lower energy threshold can be raised to 435 keV to limit the scattered events without reducing the true events. A ^{137}Cs source is used for transmission scans. The clinical and physical performance of the C-PET scanner was characterized.

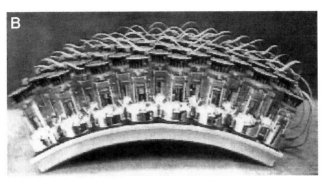

FIGURE 1, B.—CurvePlate crystal (Bicron, Newbury, OH) with 48 photomultiplier tubes. Dimensions of crystal are 47 cm (circumferential) × 30 cm (axial) × 2.54 cm (thick). (Reprinted by permission of the Society of Nuclear Medicine, from Adam L-E, Karp JS, Daube-Witherspoon ME, et al: Performance of a whole-body PET scanner using curve-plate NaI(T1) detectors. *J Nucl Med* 42:1821-1830, 2001.)

Methods.—The relevant protocols of the International Electrotechnical Commission (IEC) (IEC 61675-1) and the National Electrical Manufacturers Association (NEMA) (NU2-1994 and NU2-2001) were used to determine the performance characteristics of the C-PET scanner. An image-quality phantom and patient data were used to evaluate image quality under clinical scanning conditions. The data were rebinned with Fourier rebinning into 2-dimensional (slice-oriented) datasets and reconstructed with an iterative reconstruction algorithm.

Results.—In comparison with previous PENN PET scanners, the C-PET scanner has an improved count-rate capability and spatial resolution. The current NU2-1994 and IEC measurements with the 19-cm-long phantoms characterize the best performance for PET imaging, whereas the new proposed measurements—with longer phantoms for scatter, count rate, and sensitivity measurements—better characterize the performance under clinical conditions and better characterize 3-dimensional whole-body scanning. The clinical count-rate behavior is better predicted by the 70-cm-long phantom than by the IEC whole-body phantoms. The longer phantoms also allow better comparison between scanners with different axial fields of view.

Conclusions.—Single-event transmission scans interleaved between sequential transmission scans allow the completion of a whole-body study in less than 1 hour. Overall, the C-PET scanner is a cost-effective PET scanner that performs well in many clinical applications.

▶ This article points to 2 very interesting developments within our field. Some very interesting dedicated camera designs are being engineered to accommodate the increased need for PET as a routine clinical modality. This curved-plate design is meant to improve efficiency and resolution of this PET instrument. However, as this Year Book goes to print, it is not clear whether such instruments are considered to be an "acceptable instrument." The Center for Medicare and Medicaid Services is in the process of deciding whether only full-ring systems can be used to obtain reimbursement for PET scans. They are also considering whether NaI is an acceptable detector for 511 keV scanning.

It seems odd that such an agency is deciding on the actual types of technologies that may be used in the clinic.

I. G. Zubal, PhD

Registration of Emission and Transmission Whole-Body Scintillation-Camera Images
Sjögreen K, Ljungberg M, Wingårdh K, et al (Lund Univ, Sweden; Middlesex Hosp, London)
J Nucl Med 42:1563-1570, 2001   12–4

Background.—Whole-body (WB) scintillation-camera imaging is frequently used to measure the uptake and retention of activity in organs and tissues. The measurements are required for assessment of absorbed dose, for radiation protection in diagnostic nuclear medicine, and for dose planning in radionuclide therapy. WB activity quantification can be performed by using the conjugate method, which can also be applied directly to the WB images. The quantification method used in this methodology assumes that the patient position is the same for each imaging session. Image registration is required if the anterior and posterior images are acquired sequentially and the patient has moved between the scans, for alignment of images from a series of acquisitions, and for alignment to a transmission scan acquired on a separate occasion. A method for registration of WB images was presented that can be applied to between-emission image registration and to registration of transmission and emission images.

Methods.—Registration in this technique is performed by maximization of the mutual information. The spatial transformation has been tailored for the registration of WB images and comprises global and local transformations, including rigid, projective, and curved transformations. A coarse registration is performed first, using cross-correlation and direct pixel scaling. Optimization is then performed in a sequence, beginning with the 2 legs independently, followed by the upper body and head. Evaluation was performed for clinical images of an ^{131}I-labeled monoclonal antibody and for Monte Carlo–simulated images. The simulations were accomplished with an anthropomorphic WB computer phantom especially modified to match the patient position during WB scanning.

Results.—For the simulated images, the registration errors are within 1 pixel (<3.6 mm) for a sufficient image count level. Separate evaluation of the influence of noise demonstrated that the errors increase below a total image count of about 10^5 (signal-to-noise ratio of about 4). For clinical evaluations, the deviations between point markers are 9 ± 5 mm.

Conclusions.—An automatic registration system for WB images has been developed that is applicable to emission-emission and transmission-emission registration. This method has been found to be reliable in more than 50 clinical studies.

▶ Here is an interesting application for registering emission and transmission scans. Typically, transmission and emission scans are combined for attenuation corrections applied to cardiac SPECT. Here however, the transmission scan is used for optimizing conjugate view quantitation of uptake activities in various organs. This report is additionally interesting, since it looks at some of the problems associated with such registration techniques. By generating simulated images with Monte Carlo algorithms, we can look at different noise realizations of the same distribution, and learn about the effect of noise on registration accuracies.

I. G. Zubal, PhD

An Activity Quantification Method Based on Registration of CT and Whole-Body Scintillation Camera Images, With Application to [131]I
Sjögreen K, Ljungberg M, Strand S-E (Lund Univ, Sweden)
J Nucl Med 43:972-982, 2002   12–5

Introduction.—Recent advances in radionuclide therapy and radioimmunotherapy have underscored the need for in vivo quantification of activity distributions as a basis of individualized patient dosimetry. A new method for conjugate view activity quantification for ^{131}I-labeled monoclonal antibody distribution is presented.

Methods.—The new method was based on the combined use of images from whole-body (WB) scintillation camera scanning, WB transmission scanning with [57]Co, and CT. All images were coaligned by using a recently created program for the registration of WB images. Corrections for attenuation, scatter, and septal penetration were performed by using image space. Compensation for scatter and septal penetration was performed by deconvolution, with point-response functions ascertained from Monte Carlo simulations. Attenuation correction was performed by implementing a patient-specific 364-keV narrow-beam attenuation map obtained through a combination of information from the CT and transmission scans. A relationship for the conversion of the CT numbers to mass density is presented. The attenuation- and scatter-compensated image was converted from counts to activity by using a sensitivity value for 364-keV photons in air, then was analyzed for the activity of volumes of interest by using 2-dimensional regions of interest ascertained from the CT investigation. The CT was initially resliced into coronal slices. A maximum-extension region of interest was outlined that enclosed the volume of interest. Compensation for background activity and overlapping organs was performed on the basis of total patient thickness in the projection line and on precalculated organ-background thickness fractions.

Results.—The method evaluation was performed by using data from both experimental measurements and the Monte Carlo simulations (Fig 2). The use of an attenuation map taken directly from the CT investigation was also assessed. An accuracy of 10% or more was obtained to determine organ activity quantification. For smaller-diameter tumors, deviations were greater

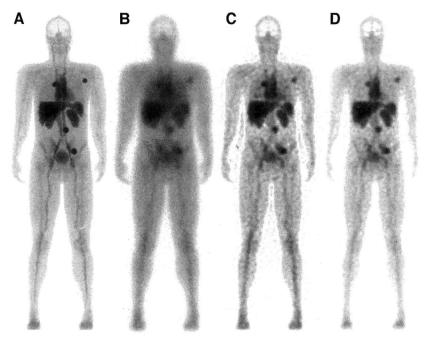

FIGURE 2.—Simulated images of activity distribution that mimic current patient group. Images were obtained as the geometric mean of anterior and posterior projections. **A,** Image representing defined activity distribution, obtained by analytic integration. **B,** Monte Carlo simulated image for the camera system used. **C,** Image corrected for scatter and septal penetration. **D,** Image corrected for attenuation, scatter, and septal penetration. (Reprinted by permission of the Society of Nuclear Medicine, from Sjögreen K, Ljungberg M, Strand S-E: An activity quantification method based on registration of CT and whole-body scintillation camera images, with application to [131]I. *J Nucl Med* 43:972-982, 2002.)

because of a lack of correction for the background-dependent partial-volume effect.

Conclusion.—Registration of CT and WB scintillation camera images was successful in improving activity quantification by the conjugate view method.

▶ This article continues with the function-to-anatomy registration theme discussed in the previous article. It makes an additional interesting point by realizing that the images shown here are *not* of a human subject. This anatomy and radiopharmaceutical distribution exist nowhere else except in the memory of a laboratory computer. I believe we are approaching the capability of being able to evaluate certain technical aspects of imaging radiopharmaceutical distributions in humans by running computer simulations instead of resorting to imaging human volunteers. This becomes more and more possible as our computer-simulated images look more and more humanlike. Had you not stopped to read the title abstract and comments for this article, you probably would have never suspected that these images were just a computer simulation.

I. G. Zubal, PhD

Influence of Implementation Parameters on Registration of MR and SPECT Brain Images by Maximization of Mutual Information

Zhu Y-M, Cochoff SM (Philips Med Systems, Cleveland, Ohio)
J Nucl Med 43:160-166, 2002   12–6

Introduction.—Mutual-information maximization is a popular algorithm for automatic image registration. Several implementation issues have not been assessed in a single, coherent context. The use of various implementation strategies were assessed in MR and SPECT brain image registrations to ascertain the best implementation strategy.

Methods.—Twenty-one registrations between MR and SPECT brain images in 8 patients were accomplished by mutual-information maximization with different implementation strategies. The results of a popular strategy were selected as the standard. All other results were compared with the standard. The statistics of misregistrations were determined. Registration speed, accuracy, precision, and success rate were examined.

Results.—Compared with trilinear interpolation, nearest-neighbor interpolation slightly sped the registration process; however, the success rate was lower. The number of bins used to estimate the probability density function influences the speed and robustness. The use of fewer bins produced a less robust registration. Adaptively altering the number of bins increased the registration speed and robustness. Simplex optimization increased the registration speed markedly, producing a slightly degraded success rate. Simplex optimization with adaptive bin strategy enhanced the success rate and further reduced the registration time. Multiresolution optimization produced a better success rate, with little impact on the accuracy and precision of registration. An increase in the number of resolution levels increased the rate of success. Multisampling optimization also enhanced the success rate. The results were less accurate and precise than those obtained with multiresolution optimization, with an increase in the number of levels, diminishing the performance. Segmentation affected the registration speed and success rate. Because segmentation is problem-specific, the effect was not conclusive.

Conclusion.—The various implementation strategies considerably affect the performance of automatic image registration by mutual-information maximization. The optimal implementation strategy would include trilinear interpolation, adaptive change of the number of bins when estimating probability density function, and exploitation of a simplex optimization algorithm with a multiresolution scheme.

▶ PET and SPECT cameras are now being manufactured with CT scanners mounted on the gantry. The percentage of these dual-modality units will remain small compared with the number of single-modality cameras that are operated in radiology departments. Hence, the need for improved software algorithms for automatically registering functional SPECT and PET with anatomical CT and MRI images continues to play an important role in localizing radionuclide uptakes onto physiologic structures. Indeed, the method of mutual information works so well for neurologic evaluations that I venture to say that, for brain scans, there is really no need to do these on combined dual-modality gan-tries for good registered function to anatomy-fused images.

I. G. Zubal, PhD

An Iterative Transmission Algorithm Incorporating Cross-Talk Correction for SPECT
Narayanan MV, King MA, Byrne CL (Univ of Massachusetts, Worcester and Lowell)
Med Phys 29:694-700, 2002   12–7

Introduction.—Simultaneous emission/transmission acquisitions in car-diac SPECT with a ^{99m}Tc/^{153}Gd source combination allow nonuniform at-tenuation correction. Cross-talk of ^{99m}Tc photons downscattered into the ^{153}Gd energy window contaminates the reconstructed transmission map used for attenuation correction. The estimated cross-talk contribution can be subtracted before transmission reconstruction or incorporated into the reconstruction algorithm itself. An iterative transmission (MLTG-S) algo-rithm based on the maximum-likelihood transmission gradient (MLTG) al-gorithm specifically accounts for this cross-talk estimate.

Methods.—A simultaneous emission/transmission protocol was used to acquire clinical images on a 3-headed PRISM 3000 system in which 2 cam-era heads with parallel-hole collimators acquired ^{99m}Tc emission images while the third head, with a 65-cm fan-beam collimator opposed to a ^{153}Gd line source, acquired transmission projections. Two patient studies were evaluated to demonstrate the ability of the MLTG-S algorithm to recon-struct patient-specific attenuation maps.

Results.—Subtracting the cross-talk estimate before transmission recon-struction can produce negative and zero values if the estimate is larger than or equal to the count in the transmission projection bin, particularly with increased attenuator size or amount of cross-talk. This produces inaccurate attenuation coefficients for MLTG reconstructions with cross-talk subtrac-tion. Conversely, the MLTG-S reconstruction generated better estimates of attenuation maps by avoiding the subtraction of the cross-talk estimate.

Conclusion.—A comparison of emission slices corrected for nonuniform attenuation shows that inaccuracies in the reconstructed attenuation map resulting from cross-talk can artificially enhance the extracardiac activity, confounding the ability to see the left ventricular walls.

▶ When imaging ^{99m}Tc, it is desirable to select transmission isotopes with en-ergies below 140 keV. This allows for simultaneous emission and transmission imaging, whereby the transmission scan does not introduce unwanted counts into the emission scan. However, the opposite does in fact occur, and the "somewhat corrupted" transmission scan can lead to errors in the attenuation correction. This article represents new developments in the iterative recon-struction algorithms that minimize the effect of scattered photons. Such scatter correction methods can, of course, also be applied to dual-isotope emission SPECT studies.

I. G. Zubal, PhD

The Value and Practice of Attenuation Correction for Myocardial Perfusion SPECT Imaging: A Joint Position Statement From the American Society of Nuclear Cardiology and the Society of Nuclear Medicine
Hendel RC, Corbett JR, Cullom SJ, et al (Society of Nuclear Medicine, Reston, Va)
J Nucl Med 43:273-280, 2002   12–8

Background.—Tissue attenuation significantly affects the accuracy of SPECT myocardial perfusion imaging. The effects of photon attenuation require correction techniques that so far have been indirect and have included breast binding, prone imaging, and ECG-gated SPECT methods. The most recent developments in attenuation correction were reviewed, its clinical usefulness was assessed, and recommendations were offered.

Techniques and Trials.—Because all available techniques involve limitations, the presence of attenuation has made interpretation difficult. The clinical trials focusing on coronary artery disease have demonstrated the effectiveness of a 3-detector system (2 parallel-hole collimators to collect emission data and a third that has a fan-beam collimator to acquire transmission data from an Am-241 line source) in improving diagnostic accuracy (Table 1). One trial noted that specificity improved from 48% to 82% with Tc-99m sestamibi SPECT imaging. Similar gains were made in sensitivity and accuracy in various other trials. An important limitation in the first multicenter trial was a reduced ability to detect multivessel disease when attenuation-scatter correction was used; this may affect prognostication. Significant gains in overall specificity, increased normalcy, and improved test sensitivity were noted when the imaging algorithm included a motion correction algorithm with attenuation correction and depth-dependent resolution compen-

---

TABLE 1.—Diagnostic Value of Attenuation Correction Systems

			Sensitivity (%)		Specificity (%)		Normalcy (%)	
Author	System	*n*	NC	AC	NC	AC*	NC	AC
Ficaro	U Mich	119	78	84	48	82	88	98
Hendel	ADAC	200	76	78	44	50	86	96
Links*	SMV	112	84	88	69	92	69	92
Gerson†	Picker	113	85	90	NA	NA	72	70
Gallowitsch	Eiscint	49	89	94	69	84	NA	NA
Lenzo†	Siemens	171	93	93	84	88	78	85
Composite		764	81	85	64	81	80	89

*Includes motion correction and depth-dependent blur correction.
†Includes scatter correction.
Abbreviations: NC, Non-n-attenuation-corrected SPECT; AC, attenuation-corrected SPECT; NA, not available.
(Reprinted by permission of the Society of Nuclear Medicine, from Hendel RC, Corbett JR, Cullom SJ, et al: The value and practice of attenuation correction for myocardial perfusion SPECT imaging: A joint position statement from the American Society of Nuclear Cardiology and the Society of Nuclear Medicine. *J Nucl Med* 43:273-280, 2002.)

sation. Clinically, enhanced sensitivity with attenuation correction remains unclear, although some evidence indicates that the detection of defects as well as multivessel and left main disease may be improved with second-generation systems. Other applications that have shown improvement with attenuation correction techniques include triage for patients with chest pain, detection of areas of viable myocardium, better correlation with PET results, and improved ability to predict functional recovery after revascularization. Because accurate attenuation correction depends on high-quality transmission images, quality control measures have been developed. In particular, count densities need to be sufficient to overcome the intrinsic inconsistencies of scans that have poor signal-to-noise ratios. Other important quality control issues that are related to transmission maps include body truncation, patient motion, scaling of attenuation coefficients to correct tissue densities, accurate registration of attenuation maps and emission data, and gating artifacts. Also, correct windowing of relevant photopeaks for attenuation-corrected SPECT imaging is essential. Reference transmission scans should be done every day to ensure optimal equipment performance and should include quantitative analysis. Education of interpreting physicians, physicists, and technologists is an important part of the quality assurance process. Scatter correction and depth-dependent resolution issues were also addressed.

Conclusions.—Substantial progress has been made in the area of attenuation correction SPECT techniques, and areas contributing to increased sensitivity, specificity, and accuracy have been identified, such as effective quality control, scatter correction, and resolution compensation. Not all commercially available systems have been clinically validated, and the impact of these methods on diagnostic accuracy compared with other techniques is not yet determined. Providers are advised to add hardware and software that have been clinically validated and include appropriate quality control tools. Both corrected and noncorrected images should be included in all reviews and incorporated into final reports.

▶ I find it somewhat surprising to learn that attenuation correction for cardiac nuclear medicine studies is often not applied. I believe the reasons for not using this correction include the wide variety of transmission geometries developed over the years (which is "better"?), and the nuisance of truncation artifacts. This article is very important in that it demonstrates that these attenuation corrections (using whichever geometry) do in fact increase the sensitivity and, particularly, the specificity of the diagnostic value. Table 1 strongly supports how very substantial these percent improvements are.

I. G. Zubal, PhD

The Effect of Scatter Correction on ^{123}I-IMP Brain Perfusion SPET With the Triple Energy Window Method in Normal Subjects Using SPM Analysis

Shiga T, Kubo N, Takano A, et al (Hokkaido Univ, Sapporo, Japan)

Eur J Nucl Med 29:342-345, 2002   12–9

Introduction.—Scatter correction (SC) with the triple-energy window method has recently been used for brain perfusion SPET. The effect of SC with triple-energy window method on *N*-isopropyl-*p*-[^{123}I]iodoamphetamine (^{123}I-IMP) SPET was examined in 15 normal right-handed research subjects.

Methods.—The SPET data were acquired from 20 to 40 minutes after injection of 167 MBq of IMP; a triple-head gamma camera was used. The images were reconstructed with SC and without SC. A 1.5-Tesla scanner was used to obtain 3-dimensional T1-weighted MR images. The IMP images with and without SC were coregistered to the 3-D MR images. The 2 coregistered IMP images were normalized by means of SPM96, and a *t* statistic image for the contrast condition effect was constructed. The areas were analyzed by using a voxel-level threshold of 0.001; the corrected threshold was 0.05. Compared with findings obtained without SC, the IMP distribution with SC was significantly reduced in the peripheral areas of the cerebellum, cortex, and ventricle and also in the lateral occipital cortex and the base of the temporal lobe. The IMP distribution with SC was significantly increased in the anterior and posterior cingulate cortex, the insular cortex, and the medial part of the thalamus.

Conclusion.—The differences in the IMP distribution with and without SC exist in the peripheral areas of the cerebellum, cortex, and ventricle, in addition to the occipital lobe, the base of the temporal lobe, the insular cortex, the medial part of the thalamus, and the anterior and posterior cingulate cortex. These differences are important to consider and must be recognized for adequate interpretation of IMP brain perfusion SPET after scatter correction.

▶ The importance of SC is dramatically illustrated in Fig 1 in the original journal article. Note the enhanced contrast between the gray and white matter in the transverse slices in the top half of Fig 1 in the original journal article. By removing scattered events in this group of subjects, the enhanced contrast directly leads to a better appreciation of smaller internal structures like the striatum and thalamus. This serves as a strong argument for applying scatter correction methods to our routine clinical images, and indeed we see that scatter correction is evolving toward more routine use in many manufacturers' reconstruction and image-processing software packages.

I. G. Zubal, PhD

Molecular Imaging of Small Animals With Dedicated PET Tomographs

Chatziioannou AF (Univ of California, Los Angeles)
Eur J Nucl Med 29:98-114, 2002   12–10

Background.—In recent years, many of the traditional clinical medical imaging technologies such as x-ray CT, MRI, US, SPET, and PET have been adapted for imaging small laboratory animals. The development of dedicated small animal PET scanners, and the opportunity for bringing together technology for high-resolution PET tomographs with the methods and techniques of modern molecular biology research and drug development were discussed.

Overview.—The most important features in the design of dedicated small animal PET scanners were considered, along with the basic performance characteristics of several first-generation systems. Among the advantages of PET imaging is that imaging can be performed repeatedly before and after interventions, which allows each animal to be used as its own control. Positron-labeled compounds that target a range of molecular targets are being synthesized, with examples of biologic processes ranging from receptors and synthesis of transmitters involved in cell communication, to metabolic processes and gene expression. PET imaging has been used extensively in studies of nonhuman primates and other large animals, but new detector technology has improved spatial resolution, which has made it possible to perform PET imaging of the laboratory mouse, the most important model in modern biology. The challenges involved in PET imaging of small animals such as the mouse were described, including reduction of the number of channels needed to read out the matrix of scintillator elements and the need for continued improvement in sensitivity. One important area for additional research is the application of iterative statistical reconstruction algorithms that accurately model the physics and geometry of the scanner and minimize the statistical errors in the reconstruction process. Another area for further improvement is the development of software for accurate quantification and robust, objective analysis of data obtained from small animal investigations.

Conclusions.—The role of small animal PET in modern biology and pharmaceutical discovery and evaluation is still being determined, and valuable in vivo information will likely be obtained from future studies.

▶ Of course, PET geometries lead the development of new radiopharmaceuticals that can be investigated in small animals. In addition to the excellent overview of small animal PET scanners developed over the last several years, this article also highlights the very substantial improvement that advanced, iterative methods bring to reconstructed resolutions (Fig 7 in the original journal article). This article predicts that reconstructed resolutions for such small animal scanners also lie below 1.0 mm.

I. G. Zubal, PhD

Evaluation of High-Resolution Pinhole SPECT Using a Small Rotating Animal

Habraken JBA, de Bruin K, Shehata M, et al (Univ of Amsterdam)
J Nucl Med 42:1863-1869, 2001   12–11

Background.—Ex vivo animals are used frequently to study the biologic behavior and dosimetry of new radiopharmaceuticals under development. However, there are many benefits to the use of an in vivo technique such as SPECT. SPECT imaging offers the opportunity to obtain measurements at more than 1 point in time after administration of a radiopharmaceutical, which is a significant benefit in determining temporal behavior. In addition, SPECT imaging simplifies the assessment of drug therapy effects, because it can be repeated over a long period on the same animal by using serial injections of the radiopharmaceutical. If it were possible to adequately image small organs, in vivo SPECT would replace these ex vivo measurements in a relatively large number of cases. The pinhole collimator has been used extensively in planar imaging to obtain greater detail, but the pinhole collimator is difficult to use in SPECT because it requires a heavy collimated detector to rotate around a small object with a constant radius of rotation. A newly developed animal pinhole SPECT system that minimizes the mechanical misalignment was tested.

Methods.—In this technique, the gantry and collimator are fixed, and the animal rotates. Hollow cylinders of different sizes were made to enable imaging of a variety of small animals, including mice, hamsters, and rats. Calibration experiments were performed to ensure that the axis of rotation was exactly in the middle of the cylinder. Phantom experiments were performed to assess sensitivity, spatial resolution, and uniformity of the system and to test the system for distortion artifacts. A brain dopamine transporter rat study and a hamster myocardial study were performed to test the clinical feasibility of the system.

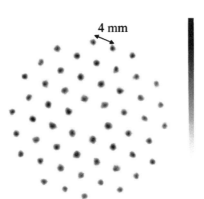

FIGURE 2.—Transverse slice of multiple line source phantom. (Reproduced by permission of the Society for Nuclear Medicine, from Habraken JBA, de Bruin K, Shehata M, et al: Evaluation of high-resolution pinhole SPECT using a small rotating animal. *J Nucl Med* 42:1863-1869, 2001.)

Results.—In the line source experiment, the spatial resolution in air was 1.3 mm full width at half maximum, with a radius of rotation of 33 mm. The system also has good uniformity and is capable of detecting cold spots of 2-mm diameter. The animal studies demonstrated the feasibility of imaging receptors or transporters and organs with adequate detail in a practical setup (Fig 2).

Conclusions.—The feasibility of a rotating cylinder mechanism for pinhole SPECT was demonstrated. This technique provides the same characteristics as conventional pinhole SPECT with a rotating camera head and without distortion artifacts. This technique allows pinhole SPECT to replace many ex vivo animal experiments.

▶ Several new systems are being developed for small animal imaging. As can be inferred from the transverse slice of a hot spot phantom shown here, a resolution of approximately 1.5 mm is routinely achievable with these newly developed pinhole geometries. Since sensitivity can be increased by simply adding more pinholes, I believe that a reconstructed resolution of under 1.0 mm will be soon documented in our Year Book within the next few years.

I. G. Zubal, PhD

Towards In Vivo Nuclear Microscopy: Iodine-125 Imaging in Mice Using Micro-Pinholes
Beekman FJ, McElroy DP, Berger F, et al (Univ Hosp Utrecht, The Netherlands; Univ of California, Los Angeles; Univ of California, Davis)
Eur J Nucl Med 29:933-938, 2002   12–12

Introduction.—Positron-sensitive gamma-radiation detectors equipped with collimators have been used for the in vivo imaging of the distribution of radiolabelled molecules in both animals and human beings. The best image resolution that has been realized to date in a rodent is on the order of 1 mm. A method for constructing a basic and compact gamma camera for in vivo radionuclide imaging in small animals at much higher spatial resolution is reported.

Camera Construction.—Resolution improvements were obtained by combining dense, shaped, micropinhole apertures with iodine-125 (^{125}I), an isotope with low energy emissions, ease of incorporation into a vast range of molecules, and straightforward translation into the clinic by other isotopes of iodine that are appropriate for nuclear medicine imaging. The ^{125}I images of test distributions and a mouse thyroid were obtained at a resolution of up to 200 μm by using this new, simple bench-top camera.

Discussion/Conclusion.—Combining tiny high-density pinholes with ^{125}I permits details of a few hundred micrometers to be resolved in the thyroid of a living mouse, even with the use of a basic positron-sensitive gamma detector. The future development of ultra–high-resolution SPET systems will permit the 3-dimensional evaluation of the distribution of several radiolabelled tracers. The labor-intensive in vitro or ex vivo methods may be replaced in several instances by the imaging of intact living animals at the submillimeter level. This will also permit accurate longitudinal trial designs and may facilitate the development of new diagnostic or therapeutic agents. In vivo imaging with iodine may mean many translational opportunities.

▶ Whereby coincidence imaging's spatial resolution is limited to a few millimeters because of the physical properties of the isotope's emissions, single photon imaging's spatial resolution is ultimately limited only by the hole-size of the collimator placed between the source distribution and detector. The substantially better than 1-mm spatial resolution demonstrated in Fig 4 in the original article points toward imaging studies that could approach the cellular level. Admittedly, sensitivity is a challenge here, but duplication of many such collimators and detectors is a straightforward way of increasing the count efficiency.

I. G. Zubal, PhD

Breast Milk Activity During Early Lactation Following Maternal ^{99}Tc^m Macroaggregated Albumin Lung Perfusion Scan
McCauley E, Mackie A (Univ Hosp of North Durham, England)
Br J Radiol 75:464-466, 2002   12–13

Introduction.—A breast-feeding infant may receive a radiation dose from ingesting breast milk after the administration of a radiopharmaceutical to the mother. The Administration of Radioactive Substances Advisory Committee recommends interruption times for breast-feeding to decrease the radiation dose to the infant of less than 1 mSv from ingested activity. The Administration of Radioactive Substances Advisory Committee recommends not using these interruption times in the period of early lactation when colostrum is being produced. Information regarding radioactivity in colostrum is minimal. Measurements of radioactivity are needed on serial samples of early breast milk to estimate any need for breast-feeding interruption.

Methods.—Woman, 26, underwent a lung scan for the assessment of pulmonary embolism approximately 15 hours post partum. The patient received ^{133}Xenon and 86 MBq of ^{99m}Tc macroaggregated albumin (MAA) for the ventilation and perfusion investigations, respectively. The absence of significant quantities of free ^{99m}Tc pertechnetate in the ^{99m}Tc MAA was verified (labelling efficiency, 98.8%). An electric pump was used to express milk as completely as possible every 4 hours during the day only. The radioactivity concentration of every sample was ascertained by means of a gamma counter of known counting efficiency, applying a decay correction to consider the time since expression. The spectrum of several samples was evaluated to verify the absence of contaminating radionuclides.

Results.—The radioactive concentration rose initially, reached a peak at about 15 hours, and decayed monoexponentially. The half-life was approximately 4.8 hours. The estimated dose to the infant from the ingestion alone, had breast-feeding not been interrupted, was approximately 0.02 mSv.

Conclusion.—An interruption in breast-feeding may not be needed after the administration of up to the diagnostic reference level of ^{99m}Tc MAA during early lactation.

▶ The table in the original article gives interesting data regarding ^{99m}Tc activity in breast milk. Despite the 6-hour half-life of ^{99m}Tc, the activity in breast milk does not reach a peak until approximately 15 hours after administering MAA. The levels of activity in this table are such that the United Kingdom's recommendation of 1 mSv ingested by infants would not have been exceeded and suggests that the interruption of breast-feeding would be unnecessary. The authors make the added point that the "cuddle dose" received by the infant from the mother's holding and hugging should not be neglected when estimating the total dose received by the infant.

I. G. Zubal, PhD

Preliminary Data on Biodistribution and Dosimetry for Therapy Planning of Somatostatin Receptor Positive Tumours: Comparison of ^{86}Y-DOTATOC and ^{111}In-DTPA-Octreotide
Förster GJ, Engelbach M, Brockmann J, et al (Univ Hosp Mainz, Germany; Univ of Basel, Switzerland; Research Centre Jülich, Germany)
Eur J Nucl Med 28:1743-1750, 2001   12–14

Background.—^{90}Y-DOTATOC, a somatostatin analogue, is used to treat patients with neuroendocrine tumors. Individual planning of the optimal therapeutic strategy could be performed if accurate pretherapeutic dosimetry could be accomplished. The biodistribution and resulting dosimetric calculation for therapeutic exposure of critical organs and tumor masses based on the PET tracer ^{86}Y-DOTATOC, which is chemically identical to the therapeutic agent, were compared with results based on the use of ^{111}In-DTPA-octreotide, the tracer commonly used for somatostatin receptor scintigraphy.

Methods.—Scintigraphy with ^{111}In-DTPA-octreotide and a PET investigation with ^{86}Y-DOTATOC were performed within an interval of 1 week in 3 men aged 46 to 67 years. Medication with somatostatin analogues was discontinued for at least 4 weeks. All 3 patients had serum creatinine levels within the normal range, and all had a histologically confirmed carcinoid tumor of the gastrointestinal tract and liver metastases and were candidates for ^{90}Y-DOTATOC therapy. Recent morphologic imaging with US and CT had confirmed metastatic disease in all 3 patients. Tumor masses were calculated on the basis of CT images.

Results.—The patients showed no clinical adverse reaction and no side effects after the IV injection of ^{86}Y-DOTATOC or ^{111}In-DTPA-octreotide. In all the patients, the activity in blood decreased to less than 10% within the first 3 hours and to less than 1% within 13 to 15 hours. Residence times were calculated and doses for potential therapy with ^{90}Y-DOTATOC were estimated on the basis of the regional tissue uptake kinetics. There were no relevant differences in the serum kinetics and urinary excretion of both tracers, and estimated liver doses were similar for both tracers. Dose estimation for organs with the highest level of radiation exposure—the kidneys and the spleen—showed differences of 10.5% to 20.1%, depending on the tracer. The largest discrepancies in dose estimation (23.1%-85.9%) were found in tumor masses. There was also a wide intersubject variability in the organ kinetics.

Conclusions.—These findings suggest that dosimetry based on [86]Y-DOTATOC and ^{111}In-DTPA-octreotide yields similar organ doses, while there are relevant differences in estimated tumor doses. It would appear that individual pretherapeutic dosimetry for ^{90}Y-DOTATOC therapy is necessary because of the large differences in organ doses between individual patients. When possible, this dosimetry should be accomplished by using the chemically identical tracer [86]Y-DOTATOC.

▶ Nuclear medicine continues to make strides in tumor diagnostic and associated therapies. Dosimetry data on these agents continue to be updated, and the list of possible agents increases from year to year.

I. G. Zubal, PhD

MIRD Dose Estimate Report No. 19: Radiation Absorbed Dose Estimates From ^{18}F-FDG
Hays MT, for the MIRD Committee (VA Palo Alto Health Care System, Calif; et al)
J Nucl Med 43:210-214, 2002   12–15

Background.—[18]F-FDG is used intravenously as a bolus to enhance scans of various organs as well as whole-body scans. Although widely used, few studies have alone provided the human kinetic data required to perform dosimetry calculations and offer a dose estimate report. The radiation doses to the different organs were estimated based on a review of current literature.

Methods.—The half-life of ^{18}F is 109.77 minutes, then ^{18}F decays to stable [18]O by positron emission. Among the biologic data evaluated were various residence times, which were determined from 4 sources, all well-documented human studies. Absorbed doses were estimated by using the residence times.

Results.—Residence times were obtained for the heart, liver, lungs, plasma, erythrocytes, and urine in healthy human beings by using model-generated time–activity curves that incorporated physical decay. Urine data provided biologic parameters for input into the MIRD dynamic bladder model to allow calculation of the dose experienced by the urinary bladder wall surface under various circumstances. Healthy Japanese subjects were evaluated with the use of quantitative organ time–activity curves for 1 hour after intravenous injection of ^{18}F-FDG, focusing specifically on brain and bladder activity in these smaller subjects. Adjustments for the size differences between the MIRD and Japanese standard man models produced compa-

TABLE 1.—Estimated Absorbed Doses From Intravenous Administration
of ^{18}F-FDG (Mean ± SD)

Target Organ	Absorbed Dose Per Unit of Administered Activity	
	mGy/MBq	rad/mCi
Brain	0.046 ± 0.012	0.17 ± 0.044
Heart wall	0.068 ± 0.036	0.25 ± 0.13
Kidneys	0.021 ± 0.0059	0.078 ± 0.022
Liver	0.024 ± 0.0085	0.088 ± 0.031
Lungs	0.015 ± 0.0084	0.056 ± 0.031
Pancreas	0.014 ± 0.0016	0.052 ± 0.0060
Red marrow	0.011 ± 0.0017	0.040 ± 0.0062
Spleen	0.015 ± 0.0021	0.056 ± 0.0078
Urinary bladder wall*	0.073 ± 0.042	0.27 ± 0.16
Ovaries†	0.011 ± 0.0015	0.041 ± 0.0055
Testes†	0.011 ± 0.0016	0.041 ± 0.0057
Whole body	0.012 ± 0.00077	0.043 ± 0.0023

*Dose to urinary bladder wall is based on 120-minute void intervals, starting 120 minutes after dosing, using traditional static MIRD model.
†Doses to ovaries and testes include doses from residence times in urinary bladder and remainder of body as calculated from data in Hays and Segall. *Editor's note:* Hays and Segall is reference 2 in the original journal article.
(Reprinted by the Society of Nuclear Medicine, from Hays MT, for the MIRD Committee: MIRD dose estimate report no. 19: Radiation absorbed dose estimates from ^{18}F-FDG. *J Nucl Med* 43:210-214, 2002.)

rable residence times. Continuous external counting of bladder ^{18}F activity was used to obtain bladder residence times, and brain residence times were derived from 1-hour brain ^{18}F-FDG dynamic studies wherein data were obtained at 5-minute intervals and integrated numerically with the trapezoidal rule. Minor differences in residence times were apparent between men and women. Residence times from individual patient data were combined with S values to estimate the radiation absorbed dose estimates on a personal basis. Absorbed doses were derived for the brain, heart wall, liver, kidneys, pancreas, spleen, urinary bladder, red marrow, lungs, whole body, and gonads (Table 1).

Conclusions.—The published literature was reviewed to yield the data required for a dose estimate report of radiation doses received by human organs after a bolus of ^{18}F-FDG is injected intravenously. Data used and assumptions made were outlined.

▶ Without a doubt, the number of FDG scans conducted each year is on the rise. An update to the dosimetry of FDG is most timely and of great utility. The reproduction of the estimated absorbed doses to the most important organs of the human body shown here serves as a handy reference.

I. G. Zubal, PhD

Calculating the Absorbed Dose From Radioactive Patients: The Line-Source Versus Point-Source Model

Siegel JA, Marcus CS, Sparks RB (Nuclear Physics Enterprises, Cherry Hill, NJ; Univ of California, Los Angeles; CDE Dosimetry Services, Inc, Knoxville, Tenn)
J Nucl Med 43:1241-1244, 2002   12–16

Background.—Patients who are undergoing treatment with radiopharmaceutical agents are radioactive, making exposure to them a possible source of apprehension. They are counseled to stay a reasonable distance from others, and the potential doses to others have been calculated. However, these calculations have generally assumed an unattenuated point source and used the inverse square law. In nuclear medicine patients, the wide dispersal of activity distribution is more accurately depicted in a line-source model, which should be easy to use routinely.

Methods.—The dose rate per unit activity was calculated for a point source and for line sources measuring 20, 50, 70, 100, and 174 cm. The ratios of the point-source calculations to the line-source values were determined. Conversion factors were developed to allow conversion of the exposure rate constants to dose rates per activity for the line-source lengths at varying distances.

Results.—The ratios calculated indicate that the inverse square law approximation is not accurate for a line source until a specific distance is reached, which depends on the line-source length (Table 1). The dose rate

TABLE 1.—Ratios of Line-Source Values to Point-Source Values as Function of Line-Source Length and Distance

Distance (cm)	$l = 20$ cm	$l = 50$ cm	$l = 70$ cm	$l = 100$ cm	$l = 174$ cm
1	0.147	0.061	0.044	0.031	0.018
5	0.554	0.275	0.204	0.147	0.087
10	0.785	0.476	0.369	0.275	0.167
15	0.882	0.618	0.500	0.384	0.241
20	0.927	0.717	0.601	0.476	0.309
25	0.951	0.785	0.679	0.554	0.371
30	0.965	0.834	0.739	0.618	0.427
35	0.974	0.868	0.785	0.672	0.478
40	0.980	0.894	0.822	0.717	0.524
45	0.984	0.913	0.850	0.754	0.566
50	0.987	0.927	0.872	0.785	0.603
55	0.989	0.939	0.891	0.812	0.637
60	0.991	0.947	0.905	0.834	0.667
65	0.992	0.955	0.917	0.852	0.694
70	0.993	0.960	0.927	0.868	0.719
75	0.994	0.965	0.936	0.882	0.741
80	0.995	0.969	0.943	0.894	0.761
85	0.995	0.973	0.949	0.904	0.779
90	0.996	0.975	0.954	0.913	0.795
95	0.996	0.978	0.958	0.921	0.810
100	0.997	0.980	0.962	0.927	0.823

values estimated for the line-source lengths evaluated with the inverse square law approximation are within about 10% of the values that are obtained with the line-source approach at distances of 20, 45, 60, 85, and 145 cm. When the distance is less than these, using the point-source model overestimates both the dose rate and the radiation absorbed dose to exposed persons; this overestimation may be significant. Corrections are required for individual patient attenuation and scatter.

Conclusions.—Calculations of radiation doses to persons who are exposed to patients containing radiopharmaceuticals have assumed a point-source model, yet a line-source model is more accurate, more realistic, and more practical.

▶ It is interesting to note the error associated with calculating the exposure dose from patients when assuming the patient source distribution is a simple point. It is probably more accurate to assume that the radioisotope is somewhat evenly distributed throughout the length of the patient (from head to toe). Hence, the exposure to personnel, friends, and family members of the patient under the assumption that the patient is a line source will give improved exposure dose estimates. The errors associated with point source–based calculations are highest when close to the patient. For distances larger than 1 m from the patient, the point-source estimates are in error by less than 20%. It is consoling to realize that when in closer proximity to the patient, we have in the past erred to the conservative. Realizing that exposure doses (particularly to relatives of the patient) have in the past been higher than the better estimates presented here, we have good evidence that we need not be so strict in some of our release policies for patients.

I. G. Zubal, PhD

Subject Index

A

Acetazolamide
  effect, delayed appearance in chronic cerebrovascular ischemic disease, 220
Adenoma
  hepatic, multiple, Tc-99m RBC SPECT of, 177
  parathyroid, preoperative localization with delayed Tc-99m sestamibi SPECT, 105
    with Doppler ultrasound *vs.* nuclear medicine scintigraphy, 108
Adolescents
  neuro-Behçet's disease in, brain perfusion SPECT in, 309
Adrenal
  lesions detected on CT or MRI, characterization by FDG PET, 111
β-Adrenoceptor
  myocardial, density measurement by PET, 282
    with *(S)*-CGP 12388 tracer, 283
Age
  differences in brain perfusion SPECT, 232
Air
  leak, diagnosis by radionuclide scan, 16
Albumin
  human serum, technetium-99m, protein-losing enteropathy detected on scintigraphy with, 171
  macroaggregated, technetium-99m, maternal lung perfusion scan with, breast milk activity during early lactation after, 333
Algorithm
  iterative transmission, incorporating cross-talk correction for SPECT, 326
Alzheimer's disease
  cerebral metabolic decline in, FDG PET of, 206
  memory impairment in, episodic, neural substrates of, FDG PET of, 207
  morphologic and functional changes in same patients with, longitudinal evaluation of, 208
  predictor of, novel, 210
Ammonia
  N-13, PET with, *vs.* contrast-enhanced MRI for assessment of coronary flow reserve, 298

Anatomic
  standardization and reference to normal data, analysis of clinical brain SPECT data based on, 228
Angiogenesis
  fluorodeoxyglucose uptake and, in lung metastases, 20
Angioplasty
  coronary, percutaneous transluminal left ventricular function and myocardial perfusion after, Tc-99m scintigraphy for, 251
  primary, early prediction of regional functional recovery with single-injection resting ECG-gated SPET after, 236
Angiotensin
  -converting enzyme inhibition *vs.* angiotensin receptor blockade for renography in renal artery stenosis, 143
Animals
  small
    molecular imaging with dedicated PET tomographs of, 330
    rotating, evaluation of high-resolution pinhole SPECT using, 331
Antibody
  monoclonal
    anti-CD 15, technetium-99m, imaging in appendicitis with, 159
    81C6, murine I-131 antitenascin, in newly diagnosed malignant gliomas, 80
Anti-CD
  15 monoclonal antibody, technetium-99m, imaging in appendicitis with, 159
Antigen
  prostate-specific, initial levels, effect on need for bone scans in newly diagnosed prostate cancer, 89
Antitenascin
  monoclonal antibody 81C6, murine I-131, in newly diagnosed malignant gliomas, 80
Antithyroid
  drugs, effect on outcome of radioiodine therapy in Graves' disease and toxic nodular goiter, 117
Aortic
  reconstruction, prosthetic, preoperative Tc-99m HMPAO-leukocyte total-body scans in, 185

Q

Author Index

A

Aboagye EO, 58
Acampa W, 237
Adachi Y, 240
Adam L-E, 320
Agarwal DM, 12
Aizawa T, 89
Akabani G, 80
Akhurst T, 26, 55
Alavi A, 1
Alcocer E, 164
Alexander EK, 122
Alexander GE, 206
Alnafisi N, 111
Alpert NM, 141
Altehoefer C, 113
Alzahrani AS, 75
Ameglio PJ, 313
Ammannati F, 201
Ando A, 302
Angelides S, 288
Anjos AC, 176
Antonescu C, 148
Aoki S, 305
Aquino SL, 7
Arai H, 210
Arbab AS, 305
Arena S, 135
Aronchick JM, 1
Arslan N, 134
Arveschoug AK, 106
Asano E, 227
Asmuth JC, 7
Aung W, 121
Avery RA, 191
Aygit AC, 188

B

Baeza R, 251
Bajc M, 12
Baker CSR, 275
Bakheet S, 75
Baldwin SW, 292
Banzo I, 286
Baron J-C, 207
Barreras JR, 12
Barrington SF, 280
Baum JK, 63
Bax JJ, 273
Becherer A, 143
Beekman FJ, 332
Beggs AD, 5
Beller GA, 263
Belzberg AC, 281

Bengel FM, 290
Bennink RJ, 65
Benoit T, 301
Beppu T, 226
Berger F, 332
Bergert ER, 127
Bergkvist L, 68
Berman DS, 244
Bertelsen H, 106
Biggi A, 10
Bitzén U, 12
Blanksma PK, 282
Blomquist L, 162
Bommer M, 52
Boon P, 195
Börner AR, 140
Bos R, 28
Both M, 40
Boubaker A, 148
Brady F, 58
Brem RF, 64
Britton KE, 73
Brockmann J, 334
Bromhead SE, 85
Buccheri G, 10
Buck AK, 6, 52
Burger C, 62
Burnand KG, 187
Buscema M, 135
Byrne CL, 326

C

Calnon DA, 266
Camici PG, 296
Candell-Riera J, 245, 254
Capezzone M, 71
Carrasquillo JA, 112
Casara D, 107
Castro MR, 127
Castro PF, 251
Catafau AM, 219
Catalano MF, 164
Cavalieri RR, 118
Chaly T, 204
Chan K-W, 306
Chang CY, 209
Chantarujikapong SI, 192
Chareonthaitawee P, 275
Chatham JR, 146
Chatziioannou AF, 330
Chen K, 206
Cheon GJ, 249
Cheze-LeRest C, 60
Chiou Y-Y, 151
Chiu N-T, 92

Choe G, 193
Christensen R, 67
Christian TF, 242
Ciccoli CDF, 225
Civelek AC, 102, 104
Claessens RAMJ, 145
Coates T, 157
Cochoff SM, 325
Cohen MS, 134
Colbert M, 67
Coleman RE, 80
Conti A, 246
Cooke CD, 268
Corbalan R, 251
Corbett JR, 327
Correia DJA, 141
Cosson E, 184
Costa DC, 60
Costanzo E, 246
Cuchiara A, 2
Cullom SJ, 327
Cuocolo A, 237
Curran KM, 5
Curti T, 154
Cybulla M, 147

D

Da Silva AJ, 253
Daube-Witherspoon ME,
    320
de Bruin K, 331
de Geus-Oei L-F, 72
DeGrado TR, 292
Dehdashti F, 134
de Jong RM, 282
deKemp RA, 271
Demus D, 243
Dence C, 276
De Potter T, 42, 78
DePuey EG, 281
Desgranges B, 207
de Wit M, 318
Dhawan V, 204
Dierckx RA, 232
di Luzio AS, 201
Dimitrakopoulou-Strauss
    A, 84
Domingo E, 245
Donnemiller E, 200
Donovan P, 104
Dörner J, 98
Doss AL, 266
Downey RJ, 26
Doze P, 283
Drenth JPH, 37